D1572883

DATE DUE

Neuro-Gastroenterology

Neuro-Gastroenterology

Eamonn M. M. Quigley, M.D., F.R.C.P., F.A.C.P., F.A.C.G., F.R.C.P.I.

Professor of Medicine and Human Physiology, Head of the Medical School,
National University of Ireland, Cork; Consultant Physician and Gastroenterologist,
Cork University Hospital, Cork, Ireland

Ronald F. Pfeiffer, M.D.

Professor and Vice Chair, Department of Neurology, University of Tennessee Health
Science Center, Memphis, Tennessee

With 26 Contributing Authors

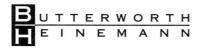

An Imprint of Elsevier Inc.

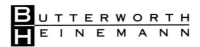

FIRST EDITION

Butterworth-Heinemann is an imprint of Elsevier Inc.

Copyright 2004, Elsevier Inc. (USA).

Medicine is an ever-changing field. Standard safety precautions must be followed but as new research and clinical experience broaden our knowledge, changes in treatment and drug therapy may become necessary or appropriate. Readers are advised to check the most current product information provided by the manufacturer of each drug to be administered to verify the recommended dose, the method and duration of administration, and contraindications. It is the responsibility of the treating physician, relying on experience and knowledge of the patient, to determine dosages and the best treatment for each individual patient. Neither the Publisher nor the author assumes any liability for any injury and/or damage to persons or property arising from this publication.

Every effort has been made to ensure that the drug dosage schedules within this text are accurate and conform to standards accepted at time of publication. However, as treatment recommendations vary in the light of continuing research and clinical experience, the reader is advised to verify drug dosage schedules herein with information found on product information sheets. This is especially true in cases of new or infrequently used drugs.

Recognizing the importance of preserving what has been written, Elsevier Inc. prints its books on acid-free paper whenever possible.

Library of Congress Cataloging-in-Publication Data

Neurogastroenterology: gastrointestinal dysfunction in neurological disease / [edited by]
    Eamonn M.M. Quigley, Ronald F. Pfeiffer.—1st ed.
      p. ; cm.
    ISBN 0–7506–7356–7
      1. Gastrointestinal system—Diseases. 2. Nervous system—Diseases—Complications.
3. Gastrointestinal system—Innervation. I. Quigley, Eamonn M. M. II. Pfeiffer, Ronald.
    [DNLM: 1. Gastrointestinal Diseases—etiology. 2. Nervous System
Diseases—complications. WI 140 N494 2004]
    RC817.N487 2004
    616.3′3—dc21
                                                        2003052356

British Library Cataloguing-in-Publication Data

A catalogue record for this book is available from the British Library.

The publisher offers special discounts on bulk orders of this book.
For information, please contact:

Manager of Special Sales
Elsevier Inc.
625 Walnut Street
Philadelphia, PA 19106
Tel: 215-238-7800
Fax: 215-238-8483

Editor: Susan F. Pioli
Assistant Editor: Laurie Anello

For information on all Elsevier publications available, contact our World Wide Web home page at: http://www.elsevierhealth.com

10 9 8 7 6 5 4 3 2 1

Printed in the United States of America

Contents

Contributing Authors

Waseem Ashraf, M.D., F.R.C.P.
Consultant Gastroenterologist, Department of Gastroenterology, King George Hospital, London, United Kingdom

Adil E. Bharucha, M.D.
Associate Professor of Medicine, Division of Gastroenterology and Hepatology, Department of Internal Medicine, Mayo Clinic, Rochester, Minnesota

Felix Bokstein, M.D.
Instructor, Department of Neurology, Tel-Aviv University; Physician in Charge of Neuro-Oncology Service, Department of Oncology, Tel-Aviv Medical Center, Tel-Aviv, Israel

Kirsteen N. Browning, Ph.D.
Assistant Research Scientist, Department of Internal Medicine – Gastroenterology, University of Michigan, Ann Arbor, Michigan

Michael Camilleri, M.D.
Professor of Medicine, Mayo Medical School; Consultant in Gastroenterology, Mayo Clinic, Rochester, Minnesota

Jeffrey L. Conklin, M.D.
Professor, Department of Internal Medicine, University of California, Los Angeles, School of Medicine; Director, Esophageal Center, Department of Internal Medicine, Cedars-Sinai Medical Center, Los Angeles, California

Francis Creed, F.R.C.Psych., M.D.
Professor of Psychological Medicine, School of Psychiatry and Behavioural Sciences, Manchester Royal Infirmary, and Victoria University of Manchester, Manchester, United Kingdom

Lorraine L. Edwards, M.D.
Staff Neurologist, Mary Lanning Hospital, Hastings, Nebraska

Richard A. Gillis, Ph.D.
Professor, Department of Pharmacology, Georgetown University School of Medicine, Washington, D.C.

Elspeth Guthrie, M.B., Ch.B., M.R.C.Psych., M.Sc., M.D.
Professor of Psychological Medicine and Medical Psychotherapy, School of Psychiatry and Behavioural Sciences, Manchester Royal Infirmary, and Victoria University of Manchester, Manchester, United Kingdom

Peter J. Kahrilas, M.D.
Gilbert H. Marquardt Professor of Medicine, Division of Gastroenterology, Department of Medicine, The Feinberg School of Medicine, Northwestern University; Chief, Division of Gastroenterology, Department of Medicine, Northwestern Memorial Hospital, Chicago, Illinois

Kenneth L. Koch, M.D.
Professor of Internal Medicine-Gastroenterology; Head, Section of Gastroenterology, Wake Forest School of Medicine, The Bowman Gray Center, Winston-Salem, North Carolina

Amos D. Korczyn, M.D., M.Sc.
Chair of Neurology, Sackler Faculty of Medicine, Tel-Aviv University, Ramat-Aviv, Tel-Aviv, Israel

Phillip A. Low, M.D.
Professor of Neurology, Department of Neurology, Mayo Foundation, Rochester, Minnesota

Joseph A. Murray, M.D.
Professor of Medicine, Department of Internal Medicine, Mayo Medical School; Consultant, Division of Gastroenterology and Hepatology, Department of Internal Medicine, Mayo Clinic, Rochester, Minnesota

Thomas V. Nowak, M.D.
Consultant in Gastroenterology, St. Vincent Hospital, Indianapolis, and St. John's Medical Center, Anderson, Indiana

Ronald F. Pfeiffer, M.D.
Professor and Vice Chair, Department of Neurology, University of Tennessee Health Science Center, Memphis, Tennessee

Eamonn M. M. Quigley, M.D., F.R.C.P., F.A.C.P., F.A.C.G., F.R.C.P.I.
Professor of Medicine and Human Physiology, and Head of the Medical School, National University of Ireland, Cork; Consultant Physician and Gastroenterologist, Cork University Hospital, Cork, Ireland

Mark A. Ross, M.D.
Assistant Professor, Mayo Medical School, Rochester, Minnesota; Consultant, Mayo Clinic Scottsdale, Scottsdale, Arizona

Kia Saeian, M.D., M.Sc.Epi.
Assistant Professor of Medicine, Division of Gastroenterology and Hepatology, Medical College of Wisconsin, Milwaukee, Wisconsin

Reza Shaker, M.D.
Professor of Medicine, Radiology and Otolaryngology, and Chief, Division of Gastroenterology and Hepatology, Department of Medicine, Medical College of Wisconsin; Chief, Division of Gastroenterology and Hepatology, Department of Medicine, Froedtert Memorial Lutheran Hospital, Zablocki VA Medical Center, Milwaukee, Wisconsin

Charles A. Sninsky, M.D.
Digestive Disease Associates, Gainesville, Florida

David Thompson, M.D., F.R.C.P., F.Med.SCI.
Professor of Gastroenterology, The University of Manchester Medical School, Hope Hospital, Manchester, United Kingdom

R. Alberto Travagli, Ph.D.
Associate Professor, Department of Internal Medicine – Gastroenterology, University of Michigan, Ann Arbor, Michigan

G. Nicholas Verne, M.D.
Assistant Professor of Medicine, University of Florida College of Medicine; Staff Physician, Malcom Randall VAMC, Gainesville, Florida

Arnold Wald, M.D.
Professor of Medicine, and Associate Chief for Education and Training, Division of Gastroenterology, Hepatology, and Nutrition, University of Pittsburgh Medical Center, Pittsburgh, Pennsylvania

Preface

The impetus to develop this monograph came from our involvement in the evaluation and management of patients with neurological disease who had gastrointestinal symptoms. It soon became apparent to us that these problems had not received the attention they deserved, and available information tended to be dissipated among a variety of journals and monographs. In contrast to this relative paucity of information on gut-central nervous (CNS) interactions at the clinical level, there has been a tremendous explosion in our understanding of their interrelationships at the biochemical, physiological, and pharmacological levels. The complexity of the enteric nervous system has been revealed and its similarities, in terms of neuronal structure and function, to the CNS continue to become more evident. It has also become clear that the gut can no longer be looked upon as a mere passive responder to directions that emanate from the high centers! At the same time, there have been considerable advances in techniques for the assessment of the gastrointestinal motor function and dramatic progress in the area of imaging the central nervous system.

It appeared to us, therefore, that we are on the threshold of being able to translate scientific advances in the area of gut-brain interactions into an understanding of the pathophysiology of gastrointestinal problems among patients with neurological diseases. With this in mind, we brought together a group of gastroenterologists, neurologists, and basic scientists to review this area in this book that attempts to provide an up-to-date overview of the new field of *Neuro-gastroenterology*.

The goals of this monograph are twofold. First, to review the current status of our understanding of the neural function of the gut and its interaction with the central nervous system. And secondly, to survey, with these neurophysiological concepts in mind, the spectrum of gastrointestinal problems that may arise in the patient with neurological disease. Through this monograph we hope to bring this exciting new area of basic and clinical research to a wider audience and to, thereby, promote a better understanding of gastrointestinal symptoms and dysfunction in the patient with neurological disease.

We hope to serve two audiences; the neurologist and the gastroenterologist, and promote a closer interaction between these specialties in the management of the patient with symptoms that reflect the involvement of the gastrointestinal and nervous systems. Therein lies a challenge: how to present material that will be well known to one and relatively new to the other without boring one and failing to satisfy the curiosity of the other. A further difficulty lies in the fact that for many neurological disorders relatively little literature exists on related gastrointestinal dysfunction despite a recognized prevalence of clinically significant gastrointestinal symptomatology.

To address these challenges we have arranged the book into four sections. The first provides an overview, accessible to gastroenterologists and neurologists alike, of our current understanding of the anatomy and physiology of the myoneural apparatus of the gut and of its interactions with the CNS. The second section provides the neurological perspective and reviews the prevalence, evaluation, and implications of gastrointestinal dysfunction in various CNS disorders. The third section describes the major clinical gastrointestinal disorders that may occur in the neurological patient. These discussions, consequent on a paucity of specific information on neurological diseases, frequently draw upon information derived from primary gastrointestinal disorders to guide evaluation and investigation. The final section provides guidance on the management of the major clinical issues that present in these patients.

Eamonn M. M. Quigley
Ronald F. Pfeiffer

Neuro-Gastroenterology

Color Plates

Color Plate I

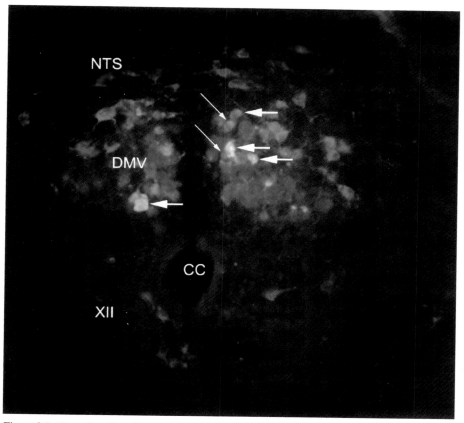

Figure 2.5. Coronal section of caudal DMV. Note that the gastric-projecting TH positive DMV neurons *(thick arrows)* do not contain NOS-IR *(thin arrows).* For clarity, only a few selected gastric-projecting neurons have been highlighted. Computer generated colors indicate: Blue–Fluorogold; Green–TH-IR; Red–NOS-IR.

Color Plate II

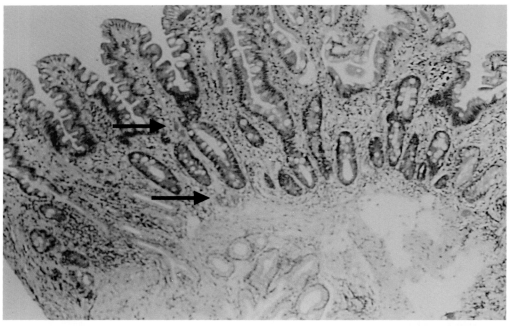

Figure 12.3. A, Small intestinal amyloid deposition *(arrow)* in the small bowel of a patient whose underlying condition was multiple myeloma with monoclonal gammopathy.

Chapter 1

The "Big" Brain and the "Little" Brain: Interactions Between the Enteric and Central Nervous Systems in the Regulation of Gut Function

Eamonn M. M. Quigley and Jeffrey L. Conklin

This book explores the common, but underappreciated, clinical problem of gastrointestinal dysfunction in the patient with neurological disease. That gastrointestinal symptoms should be such a frequent occurrence in the neurological patient will come as no surprise to the neuro-anatomist or neuro-physiologist knowledgeable of the existence of a complex nervous system within the gut, of the many similarities between this enteric, neural apparatus and the central nervous system (CNS), and of the complex interactions between the "big" brain in the cranium and the "little" brain in the gut. Before going on to detail the many gastrointestinal problems that may afflict these nervous systems, let us pause a while to explore the basic science that underpins these clinical phenomena.

THE REGULATION OF GUT FUNCTION

Through its role in digestion, absorption, secretion, and excretion, the gastrointestinal tract and its associated organs play a central role in homeostasis. The various physiological functions of the gastrointestinal tract sub-serve these roles. Thus, motility propels food, chyme, and stool along the gut, promotes mixing of chyme with intestinal enzymes to promote digestion, and increases contact time between luminal contents and the mucosa, promoting absorption. In a similar fashion, the enterocyte adjusts, as appropriate, the balance between net absorption of fluid and electrolytes from the lumen and net secretion; the latter, usually in the ascendancy, lubricating the food bolus and facilitating transit and propulsion. The intestinal smooth muscle cell and the enterocyte have thus become, from a physiological perspective, the two primary targets of regulatory input, be it neural or hormonal. Given that disorders of muscle and nerve are the basis for this monograph, let us explore briefly the physiology of the enteric neuromuscular apparatus and how it relates to "big brother," in the CNS. This is not to deny a role for hormonal or other factors in gut homeostasis; a consideration of all of the factors involved in the regulation of all gut functions is simply beyond the bounds of this overview. For the same reason, our focus will be on the regulation of motor activity rather than of the mucosal enterocyte.

Gut motor function is regulated by an elaborate neuro-humoral system. Levels of control include (Figure 1.1):

- gut muscle, through its intrinsic properties and the close connections (nexi) that exist between individual smooth muscle cells,
- the enteric nervous system,
- the extrinsic (autonomic) nervous input to the gut, and
- the central nervous system.

GUT MUSCLE: THE MOTOR OF MOTILITY

Gut muscle and nerve are integrated to sub-serve intestinal homeostasis.[1-3] Throughout most of the gastrointestinal tract, gut muscle is arranged in two layers—an outer longitudinal and an inner circular layer. The stomach contains an

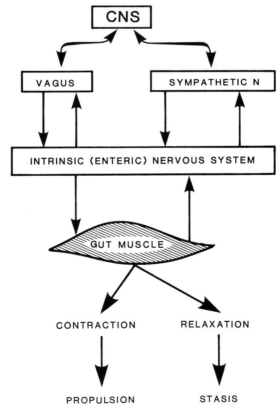

Figure 1.1. The levels of control of gastrointestinal motor activity. Note that the vagi and the sympathetic innervation contain both motor and sensory fibers.

additional oblique layer. The oropharynx and the proximal part of the esophagus contain striated muscle. In the middle third of the esophagus, smooth muscle and striated (skeletal) muscle interdigitate while the distal one third of the esophagus and the lower esophageal sphincter are composed entirely of smooth muscle.[4] A similar interaction between smooth and striated muscle occurs at the other end of the gastrointestinal tract where smooth muscle fibers of the internal anal sphincter function in concert with striated muscle of the external anal sphincter and pelvic floor musculature.[5] These areas also represent an interface between autonomic and somatic nervous systems, and are especially prone to involvement in neurological disease. Sphincters represent another specialized area of gut muscle; these are found at the upper and lower ends of the esophagus, at the pylorus, at the choledocho-duodenal and ileo-colonic junctions, and in the distal anal canal.

Intracellular recordings from gut muscle have revealed its distinctive properties. In the stomach, small intestine, and colon, these cells generate an omnipresent slow wave, a depolarization of the resting membrane potential which does not reach the critical level for firing of the action potential (Figure 1.2). While, in general, slow waves do not generate contractions, they do determine the frequency of contractions, given that action potentials (or spikes), which do cause contractions, occur on the summit of slow waves (Figure 1.2). In this manner, the frequency of phasic contractions, in a given part of the gut, is "phase-locked" to its slow wave frequency. Tone, a state of more sustained contraction, is an important function in some parts of the gut, such as the gastric fundus, colon,[6] and several sphincters.

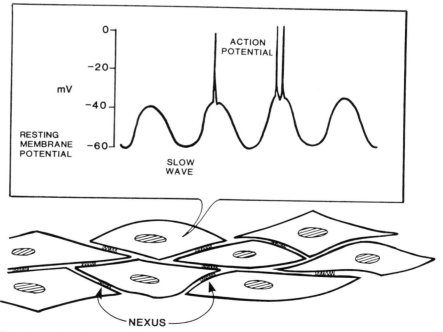

Figure 1.2. Basic electrophysiology of enteric smooth muscle. Individual smooth muscle cells are linked by low-resistance pathways (nexi) which facilitate transmission of electrical events. Note the omnipresent slow wave with superimposed action potential.

Areas of close contact (nexi) between smooth muscle cells facilitate the transmission of electrical events between smooth muscle cells, allowing smooth muscle to function as a syncytium (Figure 1.2). Action potentials may result from neurogenic or neurochemical stimuli; the response of the smooth muscle cell to an incoming stimulus may also be influenced by modulatory events at the neuromuscular junction.

In this manner, the intrinsic electrophysiological properties of the intestinal smooth muscle cell, together with the facility provided by nexi to allow the propagation of signals to adjacent cells, provide the first level of regulation of gut motor function.

THE ENTERIC NERVOUS SYSTEM: THE "LITTLE BRAIN"

The most important level of control of gut function resides within the gut itself, in the neurons and plexi of the enteric nervous system (ENS). It is now abundantly evident that the ENS is capable of generating and modulating many functions within the gastrointestinal tract without input from the autonomic or central nervous systems. Through variations in morphology in the interconnections between neurons and plexi, as well as through the presence of a wide variety of neurotransmitters and neuromodultors, the ENS is capable of exhibiting striking plasticity in generating responses to stimuli, be their origin in the lumen, in the gut wall, or external to the gut.[1–3,7–9] This plasticity is illustrated by the regulation and modulation of transmission of an electrical signal within the ENS. Such transmission may be influenced at either the pre-synaptic or post-synaptic level. For example, inhibitory or excitatory post-synaptic potentials may either "down-regulate" or "upregulate"/prime the post-synaptic neuron and, thereby, either diminish or accentuate, respectively, the likelihood of an action potential traveling down the pre-synaptic neuron and generating a response in the post-synaptic neuron. By virtue of variations in the longitudinal, circumferential, or cross-sectional extent of neuronal interactions, the ENS can generate highly varied, complex and, where appropriate, extensive responses to local stimuli. Such responses can involve one or both muscle layers in concert with, or in isolation from, the mucosa, as appropriate. Support for the concept of the ENS as a "mini-brain" comes from the recognition that the neurally-isolated gut can generate and propagate such sophisticated motor events as the peristaltic reflex and the migrating motor complex.[1] Indeed, it has become increasingly clear that input to the gut from the traditional branches of the autonomic nervous system, influences gut function, not through direct synapses with the effector organs, gut muscle, and mucosa, but through the modulation of enteric neurons.[1,7–9]

The Basic Morphology of the ENS

Ganglionated Plexus

The characteristic structural feature of the enteric nervous system is the ganglionated plexus. There are two major ganglionated plexi within the walls of the hollow viscera of the gut, the submucosal (Meissner's) plexus, and the myenteric (Auerbach's) plexus. The submucosal plexus is located in the submucosa, and the more prominent myenteric plexus is found in the plane between the longitudinal and circular layers of the muscularis propria. The submucoal plexus actually comprises two plexi that are linked by nerve fibers passing from one to the other. One component of the submucosal plexus, the plexus submucosus externus (Shabadasch's plexus), is located in the submucosa near the circular muscle layer. The other component of the submucosal plexus, the plexus submucosus internus (or true Meissner's plexus), is located in proximity to the muscularis mucosa. The submucosal and myenteric plexi consist of numerous ganglia, localized collections of nerve cell bodies extensively interconnected by nerve bundles or strands. This gives the plexi the appearance of a flat meshwork with nodes (ganglia) at junctions in the mesh. The myenteric plexus is architecturally more than a network of ganglia and interconnecting nerve bundles; it also has a secondary structure that consists of nerve bundles that do not connect ganglia, and a tertiary structure consisting of fine nerve fibers that ramify over the smooth muscle within the plane of the myenteric plexus. The plexi are continuous around the circumference of the gut wall and along the length of the gastrointestinal tract. The ganglia of the myenteric plexus are larger and contain more nerve cell bodies than do those of the submucosal plexus. The number and size of ganglia within each plexus, as well as its geometric conformation, varies from organ to organ; the functional significance of these architectural variations is poorly understood. The neural elements constituting ganglionated plexi include:

- the intrinsic innervation, neurons arising from cell bodies in the ganglia of the plexus and projecting to other ganglia (interneurons), or outside the plexus to structures in the gut wall, and
- the extrinsic innervation, axons arising outside the gastrointestinal tract that innervate neurons intrinsic to the ganglionated plexi or travel through the plexus to innervate structures outside the plexus.

The vast majority of neural elements in the ganglionated plexi are intrinsic in origin. Nerve bundles do run between the myenteric and submucosal plexi, thereby providing communication between them. The ganglia also contain glial cells. The neurons and the glial cells of enteric ganglia are tightly packed together so that only a basal lamina is present between them. Not even connective tissue elements or blood vessels penetrate the ganglion. Ganglia are partially enclosed by interstitial cells and connective tissue elements found between the muscle layers or in the submucosa. The lack of a continuous connective tissue sheath means that neuronal cell bodies, dendrites, and glial cells, covered only by a basal lamina, are exposed to the extracellular milieu. Therefore, neurohumoral agents in the interstitial fluid have ready access to cells of the ganglia. Small blood vessels, in close proximity to ganglia of the myenteric plexus, create periganglionic networks in some species.

Enteric Neurons

Enteric neurons, like other nerve cells, consist of a cell body, dendrites (arborisations of the plasma membrane that receive signals from other neurons), and an axon that conducts the action potentials that signal neurotransmitter release. Enteric nerve cells are structurally and functionally heterogenous. Nerve cell processes that course through the intramural plexi and muscle layers are varicose in appearance; they have bulbous expansions, varicosities, that occur every few microns along the length of the axon. An abundance of membrane bound vesicles, analogous to

the synaptic vesicles found in somatic nerve endings, are concentrated in these varicosities. These vesicles serve as storage sites for neurotransmitters. As each enteric
neuron may have up to thousands of varicosities along its length, it becomes possible for an individual neuron to innervate a much larger area than would be possible
were neurotransmission to occur at the nerve ending alone. However, such an
arrangement does not allow for precise spatial control of target tissues. Given their
aforementioned diversity, it should come as no surprise that the classification of
enteric neurons presents somewhat of a challenge. Enteric neurons are, by conven-
tion, classified in three ways:

1. On the basis of electrophysiological properties. Although four electrophysiologically distinguishable types of neurons are known, the bulk of enteric neurons fall into one of two categories: type 1 or S (S/type 1) and type 2 or AH
   (AH/type 2). Type 2 neurons are so named because they produce a prolonged
   after-hyperpolarization following an action potential. S/type 1 neurons are
   tetrodotoxin-sensitive; AH/type 2 are not, as the action potential in these
   neurons may result from either sodium or calcium currents, whereas action
   potentials in S/type 1 neurons are associated with sodium alone. While S/type
   1 neurons typically feature a brief response whose duration is proportional to
   that of the stimulus, AH/type 2 neurons are capable of producing a prolonged
   response to a single brief stimulus.
2. On the basis of their neurotransmitters. At least 30 potential neurotransmitters have been identified in enteric neurons.[7,10] In many instances, more than
   one neurotransmitter may be identified in the same neuron, a phenomenon
   referred to as co-localization. Inhibitory neurotransmitters include nitric
   oxide, vasoactive intestinal polypeptide (VIP), and pituitary adenylyl cyclase-
   activating peptide. Acetylcholine is a primary neurotransmitter of excitatory
   motor neurons that innervate gastrointestinal muscle. Most cholinergic motor
   neurons also contain and release one or more tachykinins (substance P, neurokinin A, neuropeptide K and neuropeptide γ), which also contract gastrointestinal muscle. A small percentage of neurons in the myenteric plexus
   contains serotonin (5-hydroxytryptamine, 5-HT) and acetylcholine. These are
   thought to be interneurons that participate in enteric reflex activity. In the
   submucosal plexus, neurons containing substance P, calcitonin gene-related
   peptide (CGRP), and acetylcholine are likely to act as sensory, and VIP as
   secretomotor neurons.
3. On the basis of morphological characteristics. Dogiel, in his classification of
   enteric neurons, identified six different types of neurons on the basis of morphology (Figure 1.3). Type I neurons featured flat, oval-shaped bodies from
   which projected one slender axonal process and varying numbers of broad flat
   dendrites. Type II neurons had a smoother and more spherical body, and both
   axons and dendritic processes were long and slender. In type III neurons, the
   cell body was spherical or oval in shape and featured a single smooth axon
   and several dendrites of intermediate length that ramified extensively. Types
   IV, V and VI featured various combinations of the above. Most Dogiel type I
   neurons behave electrophysiologically as S/type 1 cells and can be further
   sub-classified according to their constituent neurotransmitter(s); sub-types
   include VIP/nitric oxide-, acetylcholine/substance P-, 5-HT-, and enkephalin-
   containing neurons. Dogiel type II neurons, in contrast, tend to behave as
   AH/type 2 neurons.

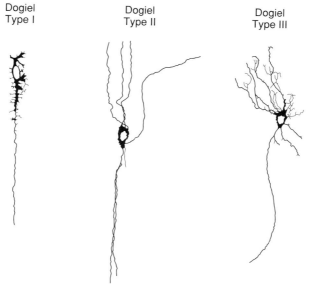

Figure 1.3. The most common varieties of enteric neurons according to the morphological classification of Dogiel. For details see text.

The Neuromuscular Unit

Unlike the somatic neuromuscular unit that consists of a single striated muscle fiber and a motor neuron, one intestinal motor neuron influences whole groups of intestinal smooth muscle cells. This occurs for two reasons. First, each intestinal motor neuron forms many branching processes. Each process runs for several millimeters within the muscle tissue and has many varicosities along its length. Neurotransmitters are released from varicosities by the passage of an action potential along the axon. Since the length of a muscle cell is only 100 to 300 microns, this arrangement ensures that each neuron may directly and simultaneously influence many muscle cells. Secondly, muscle cells are arranged in bundles that are partially separated from one another by connective tissue sheaths. A cross-section of an individual bundle may reveal several hundred cell profiles. Smooth muscle cells within each bundle are closely packed and often coupled electrically to one another by gap junctions, allowing neurally-mediated changes in membrane potential of a muscle cell to spread to contiguous cells and bundles which do not receive any independent innervation. Since branching processes of a motor neuron run parallel to the long axes of muscle cells in the muscle layer, each neuron tends to influence a narrow band of muscle tissue either a part of the way around (in the case of the circular muscle layer) or a part of the way along (in the case of the longitudinal muscle layer) the intestine. This pattern of innervation produces a diffuse neuromodulation of ongoing motor function in a band of muscle tissue, rather than the pinpoint control required in the somatic motor system.[3]

Interstitial Cells of Cajal

These cells are found at various locations in the gut wall, including within the myenteric plexus and at the interface between the circular muscle and the submucosa.[11]

While their morphology varies according to location and may, in some instances, bear some resemblance to smooth muscle cells, it is now evident that these cells are neither neurons nor smooth muscle cells, and are more likely to be derived from fibroblasts.[12] The recognition of the distinctive morphological, electrophysiological, and biochemical properties of the interstitial cells of Cajal (ICCs) has prompted a re-evaluation of the primacy of smooth muscle cells as the originators of gastrointestinal slow wave activity.[13] In the stomach, ICCs located in the myenteric plexus (IC-MY) are responsible for the generation of slow wave activity; these cells are electrically coupled to smooth muscle cells via gap junctions. There is now, indeed, convincing evidence to propose that the slow wave mechanism is an exclusive feature of the interstitial cells, and that the active propagation of slow waves occurs through the interstitial cell network.[13] Slow waves are then electrotonically conducted into and depolarize smooth muscle cells. Another group of ICCs lie in close proximity to enteric nerves. These ICCs receive more neural input than the adjacent muscle; through these neural synapses and by virtue of gap junctions with smooth muscle cells, IC-IM play a central role in neuro-muscular interactions. Throughout the gut, ICC density closely parallels that of inhibitory innervation; in the gastric fundus, for example, ICCs are heavily innervated by inhibitory neurons, and may serve as the conduit for the transmission of those inhibitory signals that regulate tone in this part of the organ. It should come as no surprise that absence of, or abnormalities in, ICCs have been demonstrated in a variety of clinical disorders of intestinal motility.[14–17]

GUT SENSATIONS: RELATING TO THE "LITTLE" BRAIN AND THE "BIG" BRAIN

Unlike the skin, specialized sensory receptors are not a feature of the intestinal mucosa; here, free nerve endings act as polymodal receptors responding to touch, acid, and other chemical stimuli.[18] Sensory information is conveyed from receptors in one of three types of primary afferent neuron:

- intrinsic primary afferent neurons (IPANs) whose cell bodies lie in the submucous or myenteric plexus,
- vagal afferents whose cell bodies lie in the nodose ganglion and input primarily to the nucleus of the tractus solitarius, and
- splanchnic or spinal primary afferents whose cell bodies lie in the dorsal horn of the spinal cord and who synapse with second order neurons that ascend in the spinothalamic and spinoreticular tracts and the dorsal columns.

IPANs provide the sensory arm of intrinsic enteric reflexes, while vagal and splanchnic afferents facilitate vago-vagal and spinal reflexes, and also the transmission of visceral sensory input to the higher centers. IPANs are present in both myenteric and submucosal ganglia, and respond to luminal chemical stimuli, mechanical deformation of the mucosa, and muscle stretch and tension. IPANs may also be activated by serotonin, released locally in a paracrine fashion by enterochromaffin cells. Visceral sensory axons are almost exclusively thin myelinated Aδ or unmyelinated C fibers. Spinal afferents include a population of capsaicin-sensitive unmyelinated C fibers, which contain neuropeptides such as CGRP, VIP, somatostatin, and dynorphin, and the tachykinins substance P and neurokinin A, and are the primary route for the transmission of a variety of nocicepitve stimuli from the gut.[18,19] These fibers respond to a variety of inflammatory mediators, stimuli which also awaken silent nociceptor fibers. Vagal afferent axons ramify extensively in the enteric plexi, and infiltrate muscle sheets where they course with interstitial cells of Cajal. Vagal afferents include mucosal chemosensitive and mechanosensitive neurons, as well as neurons conveying input from tension receptors in the muscle layers. Mucosal receptors on vagal afferents are primarily activated by "physiological" mechanical and chemical stimuli; their proximity to entero-endocrine and mast cells suggests that they may also be activated by serotonin (e.g., in the induction of nausea and vomiting) and other neuropeptides. In the stomach, these afferents mediate the sensory response to intraluminal acid; several mediators are involved, including CCK, secretin, and a direct action of acid on sensory nerve endings. CCK is also thought to be involved in triggering the sensory response to a variety of other intraluminal stimuli. While vagal afferents are viewed as predominantly involved in the transmission of non-noxious stimuli, they should not be viewed as irrelevant to nociception. Indeed, vagal fibers may not only transmit nociceptive input, but may also play an important role in the modulation of nociceptive information traversing other pathways, through the activation of antinociceptive descending spinal pathways.

THE AUTONOMIC NERVOUS SYSTEM: THE CONDUIT BETWEEN THE GUT AND THE CNS

As reviewed in Chapter 5 in this volume, gastrointestinal dysfunction features prominently in disorders of the autonomic nervous system. This should come as no surprise given the role of autonomic nerves as the extrinsic nerves to the gut and, thus, the lines of communication between the gut and the central nervous system.

Most of the constituent nerve fibers of the vagus nerve are afferent neurons, that is, neurons carrying sensory information away from the gut and toward more central nervous structures. Studies using tracer substances to label afferent neurons indicate that afferent vagal fibers supply the mucosa and myenteric ganglia of the esophagus. Vagal afferents also originate in the mucosa, submucosa, myenteric ganglia, and muscularis propria of the stomach. The role of vagal afferents in the transmission of sensory information from the gut has already been detailed above.

Vagal efferent fibers, that is, neurons carrying information from the CNS to the gastrointestinal tract, arise from cell bodies in the dorsal motor nucleus of the vagus and the nucleus ambiguous. Efferent vagal fibers that arise in the nucleus ambiguous are the somatic motor neurons that innervate the striated muscle of the proximal esophagus. Those originating in the dorsal motor nucleus are preganglionic parasympathetic fibers that project to the smooth muscle esophagus, stomach, and the small intestine. Tracer studies indicate that these efferent fibers terminate in the myenteric ganglia, but that most of the neuronal elements in the ganglia are not contacted by the vagal efferent fibers. The density of the vagal efferent innervation decreases steadily from the stomach to the ileocecal junction. Such is the importance of the vagal nuclei in the regulation of gut function and in relaying signals from the "big" brain to the "little" brain that this issue is dealt with in detail in Chapter 2.

The mesenteric nerves arise in the prevertebral (celiac, superior mesenteric, and inferior mesenteric) ganglia, and travel through the mesentery to the stomach and intestine. Most of the axons in the mesenteric nerves are efferent adrenergic fibers arising from cell bodies in the prevertebral ganglia. These are the postganglionic sympathetic fibers that make up the adrenergic neural supply to the gut. Neurons of the prevertebral ganglia receive synaptic inputs from the preganglionic sympathetic fibers which, in turn, arise from cell bodies in the inferomediolateral columns from levels T4 to L4 of the spinal cord. They also receive inputs from afferent neurons located in the wall of the gut.

The pelvic plexus is a ganglionated plexus that is located on either side of the rectum. Nerves from this plexus project to the aboral part of the gastrointestinal tract and to the urogenital organs.

The autonomic nerves act not only as the conduit for information between the gut and the CNS, but also function as the afferent and efferent arcs of so-called "long" reflexes in the gut, such as the gastro-colic and intestino-intestinal reflexes.[20] In this manner, the autonomic nerves permit the rapid transmission of information between distant parts of the gut and, thereby, the generation of rapid responses in one organ, to a stimulus in another. Were these signals to be transmitted through gut muscle and the enteric nervous system, the response would be much delayed or non-existent.

THE "BIG" BRAIN AND GUT FUNCTION

The role of the vagal nuclei in the regulation of gut function is detailed in Chapter 2. Another area of well-documented interaction between the CNS and the gut relates to the effects of stress on gut function. While the precise neuro-anatomy and neuro-physiology of the responsible pathways have not been completely delineated in man, we have learned much about the interactions between the brain and the gut in the stress response from animal models, as well as from well-validated paradigms of both acute and chronic stress in man. Suffice it to stay that a variety of stressors have been clearly and consistently demonstrated to profoundly affect gut motor and absorptive function through both neural and hormonal mechanisms. The hypothalamic-pituitary-adrenal (HPA) axis plays a key role in the latter.[21,22] The development of relatively non-invasive and accurate techniques for dynamic cerebral imaging has, recently, permitted an exploration of the afferent side of the interaction, the responses of the brain to gut events.[23,24] Such studies have also revealed the role of the cortex in the regulation of gut motor function by demonstrating the cortical topography of the swallowing mechanism and, thereby, providing an explanation for the recovery of swallowing function following stroke.[25,26]

CONCLUSIONS

The enteric nervous system provides the gut with a neural apparatus capable of accomplishing many intestinal functions. Input to and from the central nervous system, provided by the autonomic nerves,[27] can modulate this activity and also maintain central awareness of what is going on in the gut.[28] There are many opportunities for dysfunction of this axis in neurological disease. Whether because shared morphological characteristics render both prey to the same afflictions, or because diseases of the central or autonomic systems disrupt the balance between center and periphery, it is commonplace for patients with neurological disease to exhibit gastrointestinal symptoms and dysfunction.

REFERENCES

1. Goyal RK, Hirano I. The enteric nervous system. N Engl J Med 1996;334:1106–1115.
2. Gabella G. Structure of muscles and nerves in the gastrointestinal tract. In LR Johnson (ed), Physiology of the Gastrointestinal Tract, 2nd Ed. New York: Raven Press, 1987; 335–381.
3. Conklin JL. Anatomy of the neuromuscular apparatus of the gastrointestinal tract. In S Anuras (ed), Motility Disorders of the Gastrointestinal Tract. New York: Raven Press, 1992;1–25.
4. Morrell RM. The neurology of swallowing. In ME Groher (ed), Dysphagia and its Management. Woburn, MA: Butterworth–Heinemann, 1984;12–18.
5. Fernandez-Fraga X, Azpiroz F, Malagelada J-R. Significance of the pelvic floor muscles in anal incontinence. Gastroenterology 2002;123:1441–1450.
6. Camilleri M, Ford MJ. Colonic sensorimotor physiology in health and its alteration in constipation and diarrheal disorders. Aliment Pharmacol Ther 1998;12:287–302.
7. Furness JB, Costa M. The Enteric Nervous System. Edinburgh: Churchill Livingstone, 1986.
8. Gabella G. Innervation of the gastrointestinal tract. Int Rev Cytol 1979;59:129–193.
9. Gershon MD, Kirchgessner AL, Wade P. Functional anatomy of the enteric nervous system. In LR Johnson (ed), Physiology of the Gastrointestinal Tract, 3rd Ed. New York: Raven Press, 1994;381–422.
10. Costa MJ, Furness J, Llewellyn-Smith IJ. Histochemistry of the enteric nervous system. In LR Johnson (ed), Physiology of the Gastrointestinal Tract, 2nd Ed. New York: Raven Press, 1987;1–40.
11. Thuneberg L. Interstitial cells of cajal. In S Schultz, JD Wood, BB Rauner (eds), Handbook of Physiology, Vol 1, Motility and Circulation. Bethesda: Am Physiological Soc, 1989;349–386.
12. Gershon MD. Genes, lineages and tissue interactions in the development of the enteric nervous system. Am J Physiol 1998;275:G869–G873.
13. Sanders KM. A case for interstitial cells of Cajal as pacemakers and mediators of neurotransmission in the gastrointestinal tract. Gastroenterology 1996;111:492–515.
14. He CL, Burgart L, Wang L, et al. Decreased interstitial cells of Cajal volume in patients with slow-transit constipation. Gastroenterology 2000;118:14–21.
15. Pardi DS, Miler SM, Miller DL, et al. Paraneoplastic dysmotility: loss of interstitial cells of Cajal. Am J Gastroenterol 2002;97:1828–1833.
16. Boeckxstaens GE, Rumessen JJ, de Wit L, et al. Abnormal distribution of the interstitial cells of Cajal in an adult patient with pseudo-obstruction and megaduodenum. Am J Gastroenterol 2002;97:2120–2126.
17. Wedel T, Speigler J, Soellner S, et al. Enteric nerves and interstitial cells of Cajal are altered in patients with slow-transit constipation. Gastroenterology 2002;123:1459–1467.
18. Grundy D. Neuroanatomy of visceral nociception: vagal and splanchnic afferent. Gut 2002;51:i2–i5.
19. Mayer EA, Gebhart GF. Basic and clinical aspects of visceral hyperalgesia. Gastroenterology 1994;107:271–293.
20. Miolan JP, Niel JP. The mammalian sympathetic prevertebral ganglia: integrative properties and role in the nervous control of digestive tract motility. J Auton Nerv Syst 1996;58:125–138.
21. Williams CL, Peterson JM, Villar RG. Corticotrophin-releasing factor directly mediates colonic responses to stress. Am J Physiol 1987;16:G582–G586.
22. Tache Y, Martinez V, Million M, et al. Stress and the gastrointestinal tract III. Stress-related alterations of gut motor function: role of brain corticotrophin-releasing factor receptors. Am J Physiol 2001;280:G173–G177.
23. Mertz H. Role of the brain and sensory pathways in gastrointestinal sensory disorders in humans. Gut 2002;51:i29–i33.

24. Silverman DH, Munakata J, Ennes H, et al. Regional cerebral activity in normal and patho-logical perception of visceral pain. Gastroenterology 1997;112:64–72.

25. Hamdy S, Jilani S, Price V, et al. Modulation of human swallowing behaviour by thermal and chemical stimulation in health and after brain injury. Neurogastroenterol Motil 2003;15:69–78.

26. Hamdy S, Rothwell JC. Gut feelings about recovery after stroke: the organization and reor-ganization of human swallowing motor cortex. Trends Neurosci 1998;21:278–282.

27. Cachetto DF, Saper CB. Role of the cerebral cortex in autonomic function. In AD Loewy, KM Spyer (eds), Central Regulation of Autonomic Function. New York: Oxford University Press, 1990;208–223.

28. Smith DS, Mertz H. The enteric nervous system in health and disease. Clin Perspect Gastroenterol 2001;4:225–234.

Chapter 2

The Dorsal Motor Nucleus of the Vagus (DMV): A Major CNS Center for Controlling Vagal Outflow to the Upper Gastrointestinal Tract

R. Alberto Travagli, Kirsteen N. Browning, and Richard A. Gillis

The origins of the bulk of the parasympathetic innervation of the gastrointestinal tract (GI) are the bilaterally paired dorsal motor nuclei of the vagus nerve (DMV) located in the dorsomedial medulla oblongata. Preganglionic motor neurons in each DMV provide axons to ipsilateral vagus nerves which, in turn, synapse onto post-ganglionic parasympathetic neurons at all levels of the upper GI tract as well as associated organs such as the liver and pancreas. The DMV also receives extensive inputs from other areas of the brain and the periphery, and thus has to be considered as a major CNS center influencing upper GI function.

Because of the enormous influence that the DMV has on GI function, we have been interested in the cellular organization of this nucleus as well as in the factors that alter the activity of these neurons. We have focused our attention on the organization of the DMV, on the membrane properties of these neurons, and on the synaptic inputs to these neurons, as well as on the neurotransmitters released by the inputs to the DMV.

Data from the published scientific literature suggests that the DMV is organized in an organotopic manner such that each target organ is innervated by neurons with discrete membrane properties and neurochemical phenotypes, different synaptic inputs, and diverse responses to pharmacological agents. The main tools that have been used to confirm and extend these data are anatomical tracing techniques, morphological techniques combined with electrophysiological studies performed in vivo, patch clamp electrophysiological recording technique applied to single DMV neurons in an in vitro brain slice preparation, immunocytochemical techniques, and pharmacological tools. The primary animal species that has been used for these studies is the rat.

The DMV has a Columnar Organization in which the Origins of Subdiaphragmatic Vagal Branches are Arranged Mediolaterally

Retrograde tracing experiments have determined that there is a mediolateral organization within the rat DMV, such that the medial portion of the nucleus contains the somata of neurons that contribute axons to the vagal gastric branches (anterior and posterior), the lateral portion of the DMV contains the somata that send axons to the vagal celiac branches (celiac and accessory celiac), and the hepatic branch originates from scattered somata of the medial portion of the left DMV.[1–6]

The scheme in Figure 2.1 illustrates the location of the neurons that contribute axons to the five branches of the subdiaphragmatic vagus. The mediolateral organization of the DMV columns is not maintained, however, when the target organs of the various vagal branches are analyzed. In fact, gastric branches innervate the entire stomach and the proximal part of the duodenum, the hepatic branch innervates the liver, pylorus and proximal duodenum with minor projections to distal antrum and proximal intestine, and the celiac branches innervate the duodenum, jejunum, ileum, caecum, and colon.[6] This lack of target organ specificity suggests that coordinated gastrointestinal activity is controlled by patches of neurons that have their terminals within the same vagal branch.

Morphological Differences in DMV Neuronal Subgroups

Morphological diversity (soma size and shape, number of dendritic branches, and extent of the dendritic arborization) has been reported in both the rat and the human DMV.[7–10] Both Fogel et al.[9] and Jarvinen and Powley[10] reported four morphologically distinct groups of neurons in the DMV of the rat, although it is difficult to compare quantitative data between studies due to different planes of section, fixation techniques, and measurement strategies. It has also been observed previously that the size of rat DMV neurons is non-uniform, with the largest neurons being located in the lateral DMV and the smallest in the medial DMV.[7]

In a recent study, the morphological properties of DMV neurons were analyzed with respect to their gastrointestinal projections.[11] Differences in morphology were apparent with regard to two cellular features, namely soma size and the number of dendritic branch segments. In detail, DMV neurons that projected to the fundus had a smaller soma area than neurons that projected to the corpus, duodenum, or caecum.

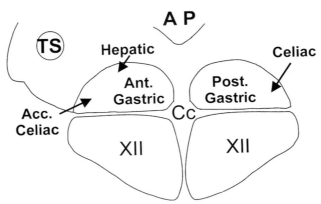

Figure 2.1. Schematic representation of the DMV in a coronal section rostral to obex. Note the mediolateral distribution of origin of the subdiaphragmatic vagus where the anterior gastric, the accessory celiac and the hepatic branches are in the left DMV while the posterior gastric and the celiac branches are in the right DMV.

Conversely, the neurons that project to the caecum had the largest somata compared to the fundus and antrum/pylorus. The second major morphologic feature that was distinctive within the DMV neurons sampled was the number of dendritic branch segments; neurons that projected to the fundus had a smaller soma size and fewer dendritic branches than the neurons that projected to the duodenum or caecum (Figure 2.2).

Such data obtained in the rat DMV seem to support the hypothesis formulated by Huang et al. that neuronal DMV subgroups may form functional units innervating specific organs.[8] Fogel and colleagues have recently provided strong evidence for the existence of a relationship between structure and function in the DMV.[9] These investigators used simple in vivo techniques to demonstrate that DMV neurons responsive to gastric or intestinal distension can be classified into four separate morphological groups. A feature of these subgroups is that the extracellular recorded action potentials in *all* the groups have a *different* shape, which would suggest the possibility of an underlying different arrangement of electrical membrane properties within DMV neurons.

Electrophysiological Differences in DMV Neuronal Subgroups

Diversity in electrophysiological properties is supported by data from previous studies in which a large array of unevenly distributed membrane currents in DMV neurons were observed.[11–18] In a more recent electrophysiological study, our group

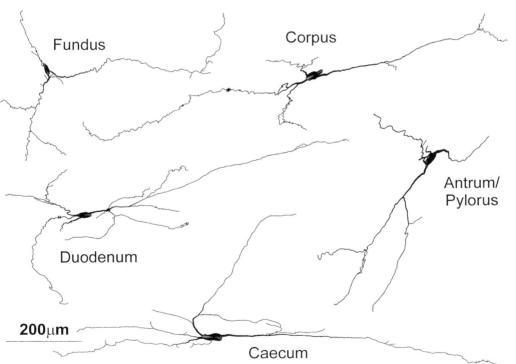

Figure 2.2. Computer-aided reconstruction of five representative neurons projecting to the various targets. Note that the DMV neuron projecting to the fundus has a smaller soma diameter and fewer dendritic branches when compared to the other neurons depicted.

has demonstrated that DMV neurons are heterogeneous. Subpopulations of DMV neurons can be distinguished based on their electrophysiological and morphological properties, and can be correlated to the target organs they innervate.[11] While using the current clamp configuration, Browning et al. showed that DMV neurons can be easily identified as projecting to either the stomach (fundus, corpus, or antrum/pylorus) or to the intestine (duodenum or caecum) by the characteristic shape and duration of the afterhyperpolarization (AHP), i.e., intestinal projecting neurons have a much larger and slower AHP compared to the smaller and faster AHP of gastric-projecting neurons (Figure 2.3). In more detail, neurons projecting to the caecum are the only ones that show the presence of a potassium-mediated inwardly rectifying current, have the largest and slowest AHP (Figure 2.4A), and are more likely to have a slow A-type current. It is not surprising then that they have the slowest frequency response (Figure 2.4B). On the other hand, neurons projecting to the corpus have a relatively fast A-type current and a very high incidence of the non-selective cationic current, I_H, while neurons projecting to the antrum/pylorus have a very short action potential and high occurrence of I_H, making these neurons more likely to respond to depolarization with a higher frequency response. Neurons projecting to the duodenum, instead, combine two opposite characteristics, a large and slow AHP (which would reduce their excitability) and a very large I_H (which would increase their excitability and reduce the inhibition by the AHP). The final result is a frequency response intermediate between the fast gastric- and the slow caecal-projecting neurons (Figure 2.4B). The distinctive characteristic of neurons projecting to the fundus is their elevated input resistance. Though no evident current can be associated with this high input resistance, it is interesting that these neurons show the lowest probability of having the I_M.[11]

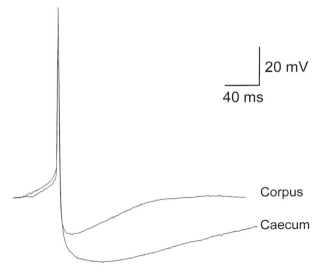

Figure 2.3. Single action potentials were evoked in neurons projecting to the corpus and caecum, respectively. Neurons were current clamped at a holding potential of −55mV before injection of a short (30ms) depolarising current pulse of intensity sufficient to evoke a single action potential at the offset of the current pulse. Note that while the amplitude and duration of the action potentials were similar in the neurons, the caecum-projecting neuron had a much larger and longer-lasting afterhyperpolarization.

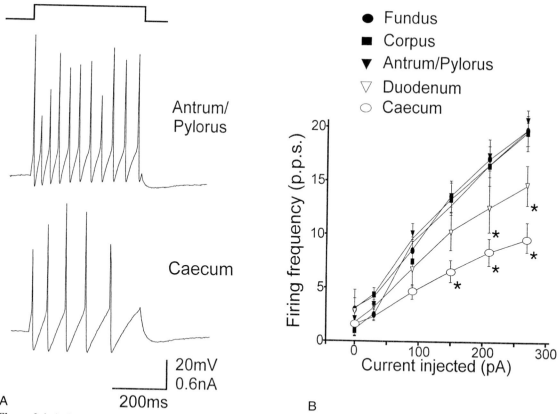

Figure 2.4. A. Representative traces showing repetitive action potentials evoked following injection of a 400 ms-long current pulse (270 pA). Note the faster frequency of firing in the neuron projecting to the antrum/pylorus *(upper panel)* compared to the caecum-projecting neuron *(lower panel)*. The full extent of the action potential is not represented due to software-sampling limitations. **B.** Frequency-response curves for DMV neurons projecting to various regions of the gastrointestinal tract. Note that neurons projecting to the duodenum and caecum fire fewer action potentials at higher frequencies of stimulation than neurons projecting to the gastric fundus, corpus or antrum/pylorus. Holding potential = −55 mV. Asterisks indicate statistically significant differences vs. gastric-projecting neurons.

Morphological and Electrophysiological Correlations

By correlating morphological and electrophysiological properties, Browning et al. demonstrated that differences in neuronal membrane properties between DMV groups were independent of neuronal size, but rather reflected intrinsic differences in membrane properties.[11] While such an observation of morphological differences in GI-projecting DMV neurons may not provide information with respect to function, this observation may have a counterpart in the diverse electrophysiological properties of the neuronal subgroups. Hence, such results suggest that morphological and electrophysiological differences in neuronal groups may reflect underlying functional differences in the GI-projecting DMV neurons as well as reflect an extension of the "size principle."[19]

The size principle, which is widely accepted for motor neuron activation and recruitment, states that neurons with the smallest cell bodies have the lowest threshold for synaptic activation and therefore can be activated by weaker synaptic inputs. As described above, gastric-projecting DMV neurons, particularly fundic neurons, are generally smaller and have a higher input resistance than intestinal-projecting neurons. Thus, these neurons should respond to a greater range of synaptic inputs than the larger intestinal-projecting neurons. Additionally, the larger frequency-responses of gastric neurons should permit the encoding and transmission of synaptic information over a much wider input range. The resting membrane potential of gastric smooth muscle is non-uniform with a gradient from approximately −48mV in the proximal stomach to −70mV in the distal stomach.[20] Since the threshold for contraction is around −50mV,[21] the proximal stomach is in a constant state of partial tone or contraction, and thus relatively small changes in membrane potential can have dramatic effects on muscle tone. In fact, as seen by the effects of vagotomy on GI motor function, extrinsic innervation exerts a greater degree of influence over tonic gastric (particularly fundic) function.[22]

Immunocytochemical Differences in DMV Neuronal Subgroups

Several investigators have reported the differential distribution of putative neurotransmitters or neuromodulators in the DMV.[23-27] The differential distribution of neurotransmitters in the DMV could potentially serve as a template for specific vago-vagal reflexes to convey selective activation of viscera.

Such immunohistochemical findings may have a counterpart in physiological responses. It is well established that the DMV in general, and its caudal portion in particular, comprise neurons that show tyrosine hydroxylase immunoreactivity (TH-IR).[24,28-32] The caudal DMV neurons immunoreactive for TH have been reported as also displaying choline acetyltransferase (ChAT) immunoreactivity, making them likely candidates as vagal motor neurons that project to peripheral targets.[24,30] Immunocytochemical detection of the immediate-early genes encoding for the c-Fos protein reveals the activation of neurons following a wide variety of stimuli. Increased c-Fos expression in response to administration of the gastric relaxant cholecystokinin (CCK) or following gastric distention has been reported in neurons located in the same area of the caudal DMV as TH-IR positive neurons.[32,33]

Recent studies have also focused on the presence and role of nitric oxide (NO) in the brainstem vagal nuclei. We have shown that a subpopulation of DMV neurons containing nitric oxide synthase immunoreactivity (NOS-IR) projects selectively to the gastric fundus.[34] Anatomical and physiological evidence points to a possible role of the NOS-IR positive DMV neurons in vagally-mediated gastric relaxation.[27,34,35] In a recent study which combined selective retrograde tracing and immunohistochemical techniques with physiological stimuli (i.e., in vivo esophageal distention), we have shown: 1) TH-IR positive neurons in the caudal DMV project selectively to the gastric corpus; 2) the TH-IR positive DMV neurons comprise a neuronal subpopulation distinct from the NOS-IR positive DMV neurons; and, 3) TH-IR positive neurons in the DMV are not activated upon esophageal distention. Such evidence led us to conclude that: 1) The TH-IR positive neurons in the caudal DMV constitute a subpopulation of preganglionic neurons distinct from the NOS-IR neurons. These TH-IR neurons do not seem to be implicated in the activation of NANC inhibitory pathways of the gastric receptive relaxation reflex activated by esophageal distention.[34,36] 2) The discrete population of TH-IR positive neurons in the caudal DMV projecting to the corpus may then comprise the preganglionic motor neurons involved in gastric relaxation obtained *via* withdrawal of cholinergic tone[36,37] or (though less probable), TH-IR neurons in DMV are not involved in gastric distention reflexes but rather in the mucosa protection exerted by dopamine.[38] The latter scenario is unlikely since evidence[32,33,39] provides a rather strong case in favor of involvement of DMV catecholaminergic neurons in gastric relaxation. In addition to the proposed "TH-IR neuronal pathway" present in the caudal DMV, there is even stronger evidence for a parallel efferent pathway comprised of NOS-IR neurons. That is, caudal DMV neurons involved in the inhibitory NANC pathways to the fundus region of the stomach at the onset of the receptive relaxation reflex appear to consist of a pool of DMV neurons that exhibit positive staining for NOS.[27,34] Both sets of neurons, i.e., TH-IR and NOS-IR are shown in Figure 2.5.

Synaptic Inputs from Nucleus Tractus Soliturius (NTS)

Preliminary evidence of discrete synaptic inputs from NTS onto DMV neurons has been provided by several investigators.[36,40–42] Fukuda and colleagues have shown

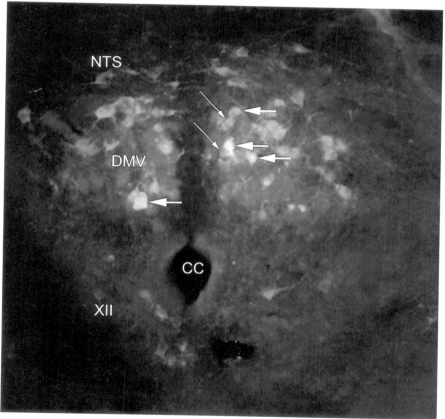

Figure 2.5. Coronal section of caudal DMV. Note that the gastric-projecting TH positive DMV neurons *(thick arrows)* do not contain NOS-IR *(thin arrows)*. For clarity, only a few selected gastric-projecting neurons have been highlighted. Computer generated colors indicate: Blue–Fluorogold; Green–TH-IR; Red–NOS-IR.

that stimulation of the NTS subnucleus commissuralis induced noradrenergic α2-mediated inhibitory potentials in approximately 10% of the DMV neurons.[40] Travagli and colleagues[41] have shown that inhibitory GABA-mediated and/or excitatory glutamate-mediated currents can be evoked by electrical stimulation of the NTS (Figure 2.6). Although the NTS subnuclei responsible for such discrete effects were not identified, such responses (i.e., GABA-only, glutamate only, or both) were determined by the position of the stimulating electrode within the NTS. Willis et al.[42] have shown the existence of a monosynaptic excitatory pathway from NTS to DMV with excitation of DMV neurons being mediated by activation of at least three different glutamatergic receptors: NMDA, AMPA and kainate. Recently, Rogers and colleagues have shown in an in vivo preparation that esophageal stimulation of the NTS subnucleus centralis evoked two types of responses in the DMV: an inhibition in the medial portion, likely mediated by GABA and/or norepinephrine, and an excitation of the more caudal and rostral portions of the nucleus, likely mediated by glutamate[36] (Figure 2.7).

These data would then confirm that DMV neurons receive inputs from NTS that can be differentiated both in terms of origin, i.e., different areas of the NTS (and presumably different areas of the GI tract via specific vagal afferent inputs to their respective NTS subnuclei), as well as in terms of neurotransmitters utilized.

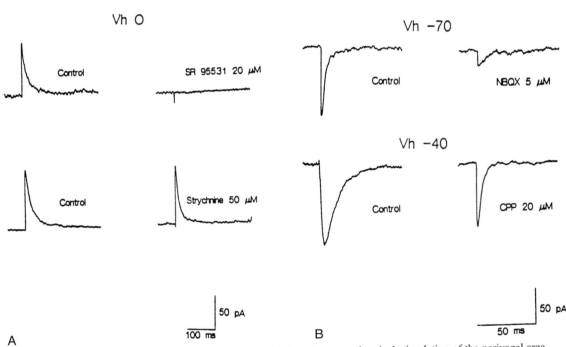

Figure 2.6. A. Inhibitory synaptic current averages in a DMV neuron upon electrical stimulation of the perivagal area. Only GABA currents were present at an holding potential of 0mV and using cesium gluconate, in fact bath perfusion with the GABA_A antagonist SR95531 completely abolished the synaptic current while the glycine antagonist strychnine failed to affect the synaptic current. **B.** Excitatory synaptic current average in a DMV neuron upon electrical stimulation of the perivagal area. GABA currents were abolished by bath perfusion with the GABA_A antagonist picrotoxin. The excitatory currents were identified as mediated by activation of NMDA and non-NMDA receptors because they were attenuated by NBQX and CPP, respectively.

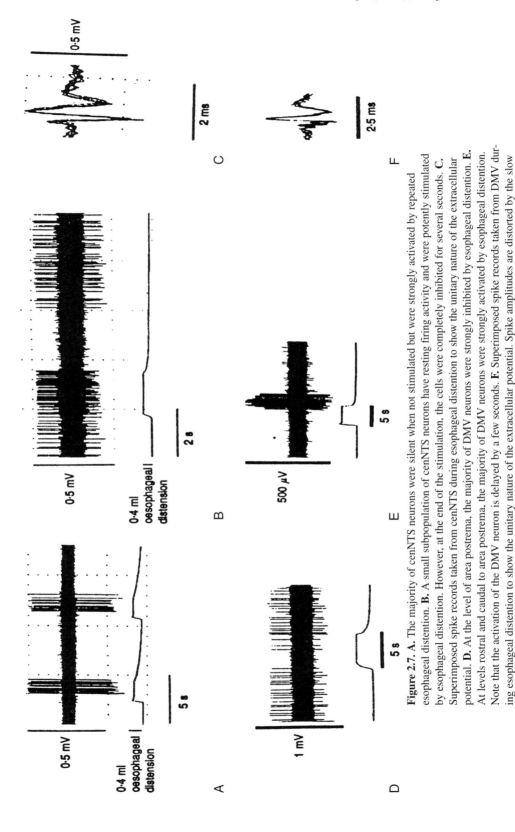

Figure 2.7. A. The majority of cenNTS neurons were silent when not stimulated but were strongly activated by repeated esophageal distention. **B.** A small subpopulation of cenNTS neurons have resting firing activity and were potently stimulated by esophageal distention. However, at the end of the stimulation, the cells were completely inhibited for several seconds. **C.** Superimposed spike records taken from cenNTS during esophageal distention to show the unitary nature of the extracellular potential. **D.** At the level of area postrema, the majority of DMV neurons were strongly inhibited by esophageal distention. **E.** At levels rostral and caudal to area postrema, the majority of DMV neurons were strongly activated by esophageal distention. **F.** Superimposed spike records taken from DMV during esophageal distention to show the unitary nature of the extracellular potential. Note that the activation of the DMV neuron is delayed by a few seconds. Spike amplitudes are distorted by the slow sampling rate.

In conclusion, there is evidence that the synaptic connections between the NTS subnuclei and the DMV neurons are composed of several pathways utilizing different neurotransmitters or different receptor subtypes. The specificity of these pathways, i.e., which neurotransmitters the various NTS subnuclei utilize to project to discrete DMV neurons, though, has not been elucidated.

Synaptic Inputs from the Medullary Raphe Nuclei

The medullary raphe nuclei influence GI reflex activity by providing a selective modulation of NTS-DMV pathways.

It has long been known that serotonin (5-HT)-, thyrotropin releasing hormone (TRH)- and substance P (SP)-containing fibers originating from the medullary raphe nuclei (particularly the raphe obscurus) provide robust input to the dorsal vagal complex (DVC).[43–48] Exogenous application of those substances, both alone and in combination, has been studied in vivo and in vitro.[25,49] Briefly, the function of SP seems to be related mainly to changes in intragastric pressure,[50,51] while the function of both TRH and 5-HT are related primarily to both vagally-mediated acid secretion and tone of the GI tract.[25,52]

Pharmacological Data

Recently, attention has been focused on the role of 5-HT and TRH. The reasons for this focus are that these neurotransmitters are involved in the modulation of the NTS-DMV pathways, and extensive in vitro studies of the mechanism(s) of action of 5-HT and TRH have been carried out.

5-HT.   The importance of 5-HT in the neurophysiology of the dorsal vagal complex (DVC; i.e., NTS and DMV) resides in the powerful modulation of vagal activity exerted by 5-HT rather than the effects of 5-HT *per se*. In fact, even though microinjection of 5-HT in rat DVC has limited effects on gastric function, its coadministration with TRH induces a powerful increase of gastric activity.[44,53,54] The receptor subtype(s) through which 5-HT affects vagal activity has not been unequivocally determined. Autoradiographic localization of 5-HT receptors in the DVC has revealed a rather distinct distribution, with 5-HT1A receptors localized predominantly in the cenNTS, though low quantities were also found in the DMV.[55,56] 5-HT1B receptors are distributed mainly in gelNTS and DMV,[55,57] while 5-HT2 receptors are scattered on DMV somata,[58] and 5-HT3 receptors are present throughout the DVC.[59] These data suggest that a vast array of 5-HT receptor subtypes is present in the DVC, providing the substrate for a finely tuned 5-HT-mediated modulation of vagal activity. Extracellular recordings *in vivo* have provided evidence of diverse responses of DVC neurons to exogenous application of 5-HT. In detail, 5-HT excited ~40% of the NTS neurons studied, but also inhibited ~30% and had no effect on ~20%, the excitatory effect being mediated by 5-HT1A and 5-HT2 agonists.[60] These data would suggest that the 5-HT1A-mediated excitation was obtained as a consequence of presynaptic inhibition of an excitatory input while the 5-HT2-mediated excitation was a consequence of a direct interaction with the recorded units. When the DMV was considered, *in vivo* and *in vitro* recordings have shown that 5-HT2, 5-HT3 and 5-HT4 agonists excited between 60 and 80% of DMV neurons,[16,61–63] while a 5-HT1A agonist excited ~20% but inhibited ~66% of DMV neurons.[64] By studying the effects of 5-HT on gastrointestinal projecting DMV neurons, Browning and Travagli showed that the postsynaptic excitatory effects of 5-HT on the DMV membrane were similarly distributed between gastric and intestinal projecting neurons, though gastric-projecting neurons were more sensitive to the excitatory effects of 5-HT; in any case, the excitation was mediated only by 5-HT2 receptor activation[63] (Figure 2.8). This result is in contrast with an excitatory effect of 5-HT1A agonists on DMV neurons reported by Wang et al.[64] However, in approximately 60% of the DMV neurons, 5-HT decreased the amplitude of inhibitory GABA-mediated

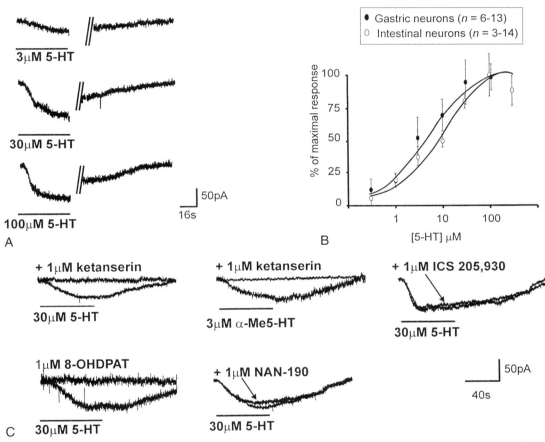

Figure 2.8. A. Representative traces from an intestinal-projecting neuron showing that 5-HT produced a concentration-dependent inward current. Note that the inward current showed little desensitization to 5-HT. The solid lines indicate a break in the recording of approximately 2 minutes. The cell was voltage-clamped at −50mV. **B.** Concentration-response curves for the 5-HT-induced inward current in both gastric- *(solid circles)* and intestinal- *(open circles)* projecting DMV neurons, expressed as a percentage of the maximal response. The EC_{50} for gastric neurons (4μM) was lower than that of intestinal neurons (10μM) although the maximal response was elicited at the same concentration (100μM). **C.** Representative traces showing that the 5-HT-induced inward current was abolished by pretreatment with the 5-HT$_{1C/2}$ receptor antagonist ketanserin (1μM) *(upper left panel)*. Similarly, the inward current induced by the 5-HT$_2$ selective agonist, α-Me5-HT (30μM) was also abolished by pretreatment with ketanserin *(upper middle panel)*. Conversely, the 5-HT$_{1A}$ selective agonist, 8-OH-DPAT (1μM) did not mimic the 5-HT induced inward current *(lower left panel)* and neither the 5-HT$_{1A}$ antagonist, NAN-190 (1μM) *(lower middle panel)* nor the 5-HT$_{3/4}$ antagonist ICS 205,930 (3μM) *(upper left panel)* altered the 5-HT induced inward current. The traces represent recording from different neurons. All the cells were voltage clamped at −50mV.

currents evoked by electrical stimulation of the NTS subnuclei centralis or commissuralis, an inhibition mediated by activation of 5-HT1A receptors, located on the NTS terminals apposing the DMV.[63] This may provide an explanation for the puzzling excitatory effects observed in vivo upon 5-HT1A activation as well as supplying evidence for an in vivo tonic GABA-mediated inhibition of DMV neurons (Figure 2.9).

Overall, these data suggest that the effects of 5-HT are dependent on the receptor subtypes present on the particular DVC cell somata or presynaptic terminals.

TRH. There is a great deal of physiological evidence indicating that TRH is a neurotransmitter/neuromodulator in the central vagal regulation of GI function,[25,52] and such physiological evidence is supported by a comparably large amount of anatomical information. The dense network of TRH-IR terminals present in the DVC has a close relationship to gastric projecting neurons. TRH-IR terminals form symmetrical (inhibitory) synapses onto NTS neurons while asymmetric (excitatory) synapses are observed on DMV neurons.[45,65,66] In vivo electrophysiological studies have shown that a possible effect of TRH to influence GI function is via excitation of DMV neurons,[47] while in vitro electrophysiological studies have shown that TRH does indeed excite DMV neurons via the inhibition of a calcium-dependent potassium current.[13,67] At the level of the NTS, TRH has been proposed to inhibit the neuronal activity of gastric inflation-sensitive cells.[47,68] If, for example, the TRH-mediated inhibition of NTS neuronal activity was targeted to GABA-containing cells projecting to DMV, the end result of TRH release in the DVC would be an extremely powerful increase in vagal output. This may explain the

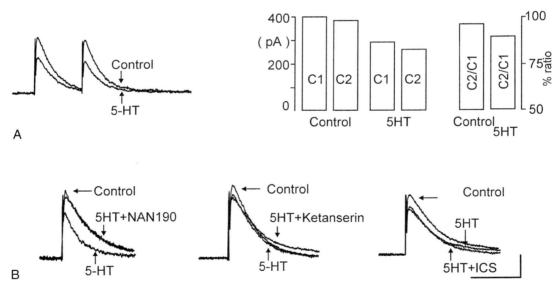

Figure 2.9. A. Decrease in paired pulse ratio. Left, Current traces representing the response to paired pulse stimuli under control conditions and in the presence of 5-HT. Each trace is the average of 3 IPSCs. Middle, Average IPSC amplitude in control and 5-HT (N=20). Right, Average ratio C2/C1 in control and in 5-HT. The ratio is calculated by averaging each C2/C1 ratio in control and in 5-HT. P<0.05; C1= first pulse; C2= second pulse. **B.** Representative traces showing that the 5-HT-induced reduction in IPSC was abolished by pretreatment with the 5-HT$_{1A}$ receptor antagonist NAN 190 (1µM) *(left panel)*. Conversely, neither the 5-HT$_{2A/C}$ selective antagonist, ketanserin (1µM) *(middle panel)* nor the 5-HT$_{3/4}$ antagonist ICS 205,930 (3µM) *(right panel)* attenuated the 5-HT mediated reduction of the IPSC. The traces represent recordings from different neurons. In all traces the stimulus artifact was digitally reduced. Scale bar 400ms, 200pA.

synergistic effect on gastric function observed with the combination of 5-HT and TRH in vivo.[44,53,54] Such effects are not observed at the level of the DMV in in vitro studies, however, and a possible inhibitory effect of TRH on NTS neurons has been postulated.[16]

Using pharmacological and electrophysiological techniques, Browning and Travagli[69] have elucidated at the cellular level this long-standing issue of synergistic interaction of TRH and 5-HT in the DVC. The principal findings were that: 1) exposure to low concentrations of TRH uncover otherwise silent presynaptic 5-HT$_{1A}$ receptors on nerve terminals within the DVC; and, 2) TRH exerts its unmasking capabilities via activation of the cAMP-protein kinase A (PKA) pathway. Indeed, the same 5-HT$_{1A}$ receptors are similarly unmasked by treatments that activate the cAMP-PKA pathway. The net result is that, as a consequence of TRH pretreatment, 5-HT inhibits GABA-ergic synaptic transmission in all DMV neurons, including those which were previously unresponsive to 5-HT. Such a disfacilitation of GABA-ergic inputs increases the action potential firing frequency of DMV neurons and could thus account for the synergistic interaction observed *in vivo* on gastric motility and acid secretion.[44,53,54,70,71] Electrophysiological studies have indicated that such synergism does not occur at the level of the DMV neuron itself[16] but rather at the level of the synaptic inputs from the NTS to the DMV.[69] By inhibiting the GABA-ergic input from NTS to gastric-projecting DMV neurons, TRH and 5-HT increase DMV neuronal action potential firing frequency and induce a disinhibition of parasympathetic outflow from the DMV. Although neither TRH nor the cAMP-PKA agonists increased the magnitude of the 5-HT-induced inhibition of synaptic transmission to individual neurons, they did increase the number of neurons to which 5-HT inhibited synaptic transmission. This relatively modest reduction in the inhibition of DMV neurons results in a massive increase of cholinergic (excitatory) input to the stomach with a several fold increase in gastric motility and acid secretion.[44,53,54,70] While keeping in mind the possibility that in the in vitro slice preparation the levels of neuronal activation and GABA-ergic inputs into DMV might be lower than in vivo, such a dramatic increase in gastric function in response to a moderate reduction in the GABA-ergic input implies that the NTS plays a vital role in depressing the efferent output from DMV. Indeed, recent in vivo experiments have shown that microinjection of the GABA$_A$ antagonist, bicuculline, increases gastric motility and tone, suggesting that the tonic GABA-ergic inhibition is a predominant influence on rat DMV neurons.[72]

DMV neurons are spontaneously active[13,41,47] and, since their resting membrane potential is close to the threshold for action potential firing, it is feasible that minute changes in their membrane potential would allow a dramatic increase in action potential firing. By consequence, the cholinergic (excitatory) output to the stomach would be greatly enhanced with a resultant massive increase in gastric function. Indeed, following an increase in intracellular cAMP, just as would be obtained with TRH, perfusion with 5-HT increased significantly the firing rate (and, by consequence, the cholinergic output) of DMV neurons previously unresponsive to 5-HT.[63] In the rat, under normal conditions, a tonic GABA-ergic input acts as a brake on DMV output.[72] If our hypothesis that a minimal reduction in this GABA-ergic inhibitory input results in an amplification of cholinergic excitatory tone to the gastrointestinal tract, then a projection from the raphe nuclei has the potential to over-ride or counteract vago-vagal reflexes which tend to attenuate cholinergic excitatory outputs. TRH has a principal role in the regulation of metabolic and autonomic responses to cold stress.[73] The resultant release of thyrotropin induces an increase in metabolic rate and heat production.[74] As a secondary effect, the TRH-induced increase in gastrointestinal function would also act to increase core heat production as well as stimulate feeding as a protective mechanism to counteract cold exposure.[74]

It is likely that similar types of synergism resulting in long-term modulation of synaptic transmission occur with other neurotransmitters and may represent an important mechanism for the integration and regulation of neuronal behavior.

CONCLUSIONS

In conclusion, the evidence discussed above points toward a highly arranged viscerotopic organization within those areas of the DVC that provide modulation of gastrointestinal functions. The challenge for the future, then, will be to elucidate the circuitry underlying the specific synapses between DMV and NTS and their modulation by other brainstem or higher nuclei such as the medullary raphe nuclei, the area postrema, the hypothalamus and Barrington's nucleus, whose inputs to the DVC have been identified but have not been investigated as to the specificity of their cellular target(s).

ACKNOWLEDGMENTS

The Authors would like to thank NIH (DK-55530 and DK-29975) and NSF (# 9816662) for their support.

REFERENCES

1. Fox EA, Powley TL. Longitudinal columnar organization within the dorsal motor nucleus represents separate branches of the abdominal vagus. Brain Res 1985;341:269–282.
2. Shapiro RE, Miselis RR. The central organization of the vagus nerve innervating the stomach of the rat. J Comp Neurol 1985;238:473–488.
3. Laughton WB, Powley TL. Localization of efferent function in the dorsal motor nucleus of the vagus. Am J Physiol 1987;252:R13–R25.
4. Powley TL, Fox EA, Berthoud HR. Retrograde tracer technique for assessment of selective and total subdiaphragmatic vagotomies. Am J Physiol 1987;253:R361–R370.
5. Norgren R, Smith GP. Central distribution of subdiaphragmatic vagal branches in the rat. Journal of Comparative Neurology 1988;273:207–223.
6. Berthoud HR, Carlson NR, Powley TL. Topography of efferent vagal innervation of the rat gastrointestinal tract. Am J Physiol 1991;260:R200–R207.
7. Fox EA, Powley TL. Morphology of identified preganglionic neurons in the dorsal motor nucleus of the vagus. J Comp Neurol 1992;322:79–98.
8. Huang X, Tork I, Paxinos G. Dorsal motor nucleus of the vagus nerve: a cyto- and chemoarchitectonic study in the human. J Comp Neurol 1993;330:158–182.
9. Fogel R, Zhang X, Renehan WE. Relationships between the morphology and function of gastric and intestinal distention-sensitive neurons in the dorsal motor nucleus of the vagus. J Comp Neurol 1996;364;78–91.
10. Jarvinen MK, Powley TL. Dorsal motor nucleus of the vagus neurons: a multivariate taxonomy. J Comp Neurol 1999;403:359–377.
11. Browning KN, Renehan WE, Travagli RA. Electrophysiological and morphological heterogeneity of rat dorsal vagal neurons which project to specific areas of the gastrointestinal tract. J Physiol 1999;517:521–532.

12. Sah P, McLachlan EM. Potassium currents contributing to action potential repolarization and the afterhyperpolarization in rat vagal motoneurons. J Neurophysiol 1992;68:1834–1841.
13. Travagli RA, Gillis RA, Vicini S. Effects of thyrotropin-releasing hormone on neurons in rat dorsal motor nucleus of the vagus, in vitro. Am J Physiol 1992;263:G508–G517.
14. Sah P, McLachlan EM. Differences in electrophysiological properties between neurons of the dorsal motor nucleus of the vagus in rat and guinea pig. J Auton Nerv Syst 1993;42:89–98.
15. Travagli RA, Gillis RA. Hyperpolarization-activated currents I_H and I_{KIR}, in rat dorsal motor nucleus of the vagus neurons in vitro. J Neurophysiol 1994;71:1308–1317.
16. Travagli RA, Gillis RA. Effects of 5-HT alone and its interaction with TRH on neurons in rat dorsal motor nucleus of the vagus. Am J Physiol 1995;268;G292–G299.
17. Dean JB, Huang RQ, Erlichman JS, et al. Cell-cell coupling occurs in dorsal medullary neurons after minimizing anatomical-coupling artifacts. Neuroscience 1997;80:21–40.
18. Bertolino M, Wang XD, Vicini S, Gillis RA. Differences between the firing pattern of neurons located in the medial portion and lateral portion of the rat dorsal motor nucleus of the vagus (DMV). Soc Neurosci 1997;23 (Abstract).
19. Henneman E, Somjen G, Carpenter DO. Functional significance of cell size in spinal motoneurons. J Neurophysiol 1965;28:560–580.
20. Hunt JN. Mechanisms and disorders of gastric emptying. Annu Rev of Med 1983;34:219–229.
21. Szurszewski JH. Electrical basis for gastrointestinal motility. In LR Johnson (ed), Physiology of the Gastrointestinal Tract, 2nd edition. New York: Raven Press, 1987;383–422.
22. Hall KE, El Sharkawy TY, Diamant DE. Vagal control of migrating motor complex. Am J Physiol 1982;243:276–281.
23. Kubek MJ, Rea MA, Hodes ZI, Aprison MH. Quantitation and characterization of thyrotropin-releasing hormone in vagal nuclei and other regions of the medulla oblongata of the rat. J Neurochem 1983;40:1307–1313.
24. Armstrong DM, Manley L, Haycock JW, Hersh LB. Co-localization of choline acetyltransferase and tyrosine hydroxylase within neurons of the dorsal motor nucleus of the vagus. J Chem Neuroanat 1990;3:133–140.
25. Krowicki ZK, Hornby PJ. Hindbrain neuroactive substances controlling gastrointestinal function. In TS Gaginella (ed), Regulatory Mechanism in Gastrointestinal Function. Boca Raton: CRC Press, 1995;277–319.
26. Lynn RB, Hyde TM, Cooperman RR, Miselis RR. Distribution of bombesin-like immunoreactivity in the nucleus of the solitary tract and dorsal motor nucleus of the rat and human: colocalization with tyrosine-hydroxylase. J Comp Neurol 1996;369:552–570.
27. Krowicki ZK, Sharkey KA, Serron SC, et al. Distribution of nitric oxide synthase in rat dorsal vagal complex and effects of microinjection of NO compounds upon gastric motor function. J Comp Neurol 1997;377:49–69.
28. Ritchie TC, Westlund KN, Bowker RM, et al. The relationship of the medullary catecholamine containing neurones to the vagal motor nuclei. Neuroscience 1982;7:1471–1482.
29. Gwyn DG, Ritchie TC, Coulter JD. The central distribution of vagal catecholaminergic neurons which project into the abdomen in the rat. Brain Res 1985;328:139–144.
30. Manier M, Mouchet P, Feuerstein C. Immunohistochemical evidence for the coexistence of cholinergic and catecholaminergic phenotypes in neurones of the vagal motor nucleus in the adult rat. Neurosci Lett 1987;80:141–146.
31. Tayo EK, Williams RG. Catecholaminergic parasympathetic efferents within the dorsal motor nucleus of the vagus in the rat: a quantitative analysis. Neurosci Lett 1990;90:1–5.
32. Willing AE, Berthoud HR. Gastric distension-induced c-fos expression in catecholaminergic neurons of rat dorsal vagal complex. Am J Physiol 1997;272:R59–R67.
33. Rinaman L, Verbalis JG, Stricker EM, Hoffman GE. Distribution and neurochemical phenotypes of caudal medullary neurons activated to express cFos following peripheral administration of cholecystokinin. J Comp Neurol 1993;338:475–490.
34. Zheng ZL, Rogers RC, Travagli RA. Selective gastric projections of nitric oxide synthase-containing vagal brainstem neurons. Neuroscience 1999;90:685–694.
35. Berthoud HR. Anatomical demonstration of vagal input to nicotinamide acetamide dinucleotide phosphate diaphorase-positive (nitrergic) neurons in rat fundic stomach. J Comp Neurol 1995;358:428–439.

36. Rogers RC, Hermann GE, Travagli RA. Brainstem pathways responsible for oesophageal control of gastric motility and tone in the rat. J Physiol 1999;514:369–383.
37. Takahashi T, Owyang C. Characterization of vagal pathways mediating gastric accomodation reflex in rats. J Physiol 1997;504:479–488.
38. Glavin GB, Murison R, Overmier JB, et al. The neurobiology of stress ulcers. Brain Res Rev 1991;16:301–343.
39. Guo J, Browning KN, Rogers RC, Travagli RA. Catecholaminergic neurons in rat dorsal motor nucleus of vagus project selectively to gastric corpus. Am J Physiol 2001;280: G361–G367.
40. Fukuda A, Minami T, Nabekura J, Oomura Y. The effects of noradrenaline on neurones in the rat dorsal motor nucleus of the vagus, in vitro. J Physiol 1987;393:213–231.
41. Travagli RA, Gillis RA, Rossiter CD, Vicini S. Glutamate and GABA-mediated synaptic currents in neurons of the rat dorsal motor nucleus of the vagus. Am J Physiol 1991;260:G531–G536.
42. Willis A, Mihalevich M, Neff RA, Mendelowitz D. Three types of postsynaptic glutamatergic receptors are activated in DMNX neurons upon stimulation of NTS. Am J Physiol 1996;271:R1614–R1619
43. Palkovits M, Mezey E, Eskay RL, Brownstein MJ. Innervation of the nucleus of the solitary tract and the dorsal vagal nucleus by thyrotropin-releasing hormone-containing raphe neurons. Brain Res 1986;373:246–251.
44. McCann MJ, Hermann GE, Rogers RC. Dorsal medullary serotonin and gastric motility: enhancement of effects by thyrotropin-releasing hormone. J Auton Nerv Syst 1988;25:35–40.
45. Hornby PJ, Rossiter CD, Pineo SV, et al. TRH: immunocytochemical distribution in vagal nuclei of the cat and physiological effects of microinjection. Am J Physiol 1989; 257:G454–G462.
46. McCann MJ, Hermann GE, Rogers RC. Nucleus raphe obscurus (nRO) influences vagal control of gastric motility in rats. Brain Res 1989;486:181–184.
47. McCann MJ, Hermann GE, Rogers RC. Thyrotropin-releasing hormone: effects on identified neurons of the dorsal vagal complex. J Auton Nerv Syst 1989;26:107–112.
48. Hornby PJ, Rossiter CD, White RL, et al. Medullary raphe: a new site for vagally mediated stimulation of gastric motility in cats. Am J Physiol 1990;258:G637–G647.
49. Tache Y, Yang H, Kaneko H. Caudal raphe-dorsal vagal complex peptidergic projections: role in gastric vagal control. Peptides 1995;16:431–435.
50. Spencer S, Talman W. Central modulation of gastric pressure by substance P: a comparison with glutamate and acetylcholine. Brain Res 1986;385:371–374.
51. Krowicki ZK, Hornby PJ. Opposing gastric motor responses to TRH and substance P upon their microinjection into the nucleus raphe obscurus of the rat. Am J Physiol 1993;248:1–33.
52. Tache Y, Yang H. Brain regulation of gastric secretion by peptides. Site and mechanism of action. Ann N Y Acad Sci 1989;597:128–145.
53. Yoneda M, Tache Y. Serotonin enhances gastric acid response to TRH analogue in dorsal vagal complex through 5-HT2 receptors in rats. Am J Physiol 1995;269:R1–R6.
54. Varanasi S, Chi J, Stephens RL Jr. 5-CT or DOI augments TRH analog-induced gastric acid secretion at the dorsal vagal complex. Am J Physiol 1997;273:1607–1611.
55. Manaker S, Verderame HM. Organization of serotonin 1A and 1B receptors in the nucleus of the solitary tract. J Comp Neurol 1990;301:535–553.
56. Thor KB, Blitz-Siebert A, Helke CJ. Autoradiographic localization of 5-HT$_1$ binding sites in autonomic areas of the rat dorsomedial medulla oblongata. Synapse 1992;10:217–227.
57. Harfstrand A, Fredholm B, Fuxe K. Inhibitory effects of neuropeptide Y on cyclic AMP accumulation in slices of the nucleus tractus solitarius region of the rat. Neurosci Lett 1987;76:185–190.
58. Wright DE, Seroogy KB, Lundgren KH, et al. Comparative localization of serotonin 1A, 1C, and 2 receptor subtype mRNAs in rat brain. J Comp Neurol 1995;351:357–373.
59. Steward LJ, West KE, Kilpatrick GJ, Barnes NM. Labelling of 5-HT3 receptor recognition sites in the rat brain using the agonist radioligand [3H]meta-chlorophenylbiguanide. Eur J Pharmacol 1993;243:13–18.
60. Wang Y, Ramage AG, Jordan D. In vivo effects of 5-hydroxytryptamine receptor activation on rat nucleus tractus solitarius neurones excited by vagal C-fibre afferents. Neuropharmacology 1997;36:489–498.

61. Albert AP, Spyer KM, Brooks PA. The effect of 5-HT and selective 5-HT receptor agonists and antagonists on rat dorsal vagal preganglionic neurones in vitro. Br J Pharmacol 1996;119:519–526.
62. Wang Y, Ramage AG, Jordan D. Mediation by $5-HT_3$ receptors of an excitatory effect of 5-HT on dorsal vagal preganglionic neurones in anaesthetized rats: an ionophoretic study. Br J Pharmacol 1996;118:1697–1704.
63. Browning KN, Travagli RA. Characterization of the in vitro effects of 5-hydroxytryptamine (5-HT) on identified neurones of the rat dorsal motor nucleus of the vagus (DMV). Br J Pharmacol 1999;128:1307–1315.
64. Wang Y, Jones JF, Ramage AG, Jordan D. Effects of 5-HT and $5-HT_{1A}$ receptor agonists and antagonists on dorsal vagal preganglionic neurones in anaesthetized rats: an ionophoretic study. Br J Pharmacol 1995;116:2291–2297.
65. Rinaman L, Card JP, Schwaber JS, Miselis RR. Ultrastructural demonstration of a gastric monosynaptic vagal circuit in the nucleus of the solitary tract in rat. J Neurosci 1989;9:1985–1996.
66. Rinaman L, Miselis RR. Thyrotropin-releasing hormone-immunoreactive nerve terminals synapse on the dendrites of gastric vagal motoneurons in the rat. J Comp Neurol 1990;294:235–251.
67. Livingston CA, Berger AJ. Response of neurons in the dorsal motor nucleus of the vagus to thyrotropin-releasing hormone. Brain Res 1993;621:97–105.
68. Rogers RC, McCann MJ. Effects of TRH on the activity of gastric inflation-related neurons in the solitary nucleus in the rat. Neurosci Lett 1989;104:71–76.
69. Browning KN, Travagli RA. The peptide TRH uncovers the presence of presynaptic $5-HT_{1A}$ receptors via activation of a second messenger pathway in the rat dorsal vagal complex. J Physiol 2001;531:425–435.
70. McTigue DM, Rogers RC, Stephens RL Jr. Thyrotropin-releasing hormone analogue and serotonin interact within the dorsal vagal complex to augment gastric acid secretion. Neurosci Lett 1992;144:61–64.
71. Shockley RA, Lepard KJ, Stephens RL Jr. Fluoxetine pretreatment potentiates intracisternal TRH-analogue-stimulated gastric acid secretion in rats. Regul Pept 1992;38:121–128.
72. Sivarao DV, Krowicki ZK, Hornby PJ. Role of $GABA_A$ receptors in rat hindbrain nuclei controlling gastric motor function. Neurogastroenterol Motil 1998;10:305–313.
73. Rogers RC, McTigue DM, Hermann GE. Vagovagal reflex control of digestion: afferent modulation by neural and "endoneurocrine" factors. Am J Physiol 1995;268:G1–G10.
74. Kraly FS, Blass EM. Increased feeding in rats in a low ambient temperature. In D Novin, W Wyrwocka, GA Bray (eds), Hunger: Basic Mechanism and Clinical Implications. New York: Raven Press,1976;77–88.

PART II

Gastrointestinal Dysfunction in Neurological Disease: The Neurological Perspective

Chapter 3

An Overview of Gastrointestinal Dysfunction in Diseases of Central and Peripheral Nervous Systems

Michael Camilleri and Adil E. Bharucha

The nervous system modulates normal gut function through the extrinsic neural supply and the enteric nervous system of the gastrointestinal tract. Disorders of the autonomic nervous system affecting gastrointestinal tract function are manifested primarily as abnormalities in motor rather than absorptive or secretory functions or other digestive processes. This chapter will review the normal neural-gut interactions, common clinical presentations of gut dysmotility encountered in autonomic disorders, and the diagnosis and treatment of neurologic diseases affecting the gut.

INTERACTIONS BETWEEN THE AUTONOMIC NERVOUS SYSTEM AND THE GUT[1]

Normal motility and transit through the gastrointestinal tract result from an intricately balanced series of control mechanisms (Figure 3.1): extrinsic pathways (sympathetic and parasympathetic nervous systems); control by the intrinsic nervous system through chemical transmitters such as acetylcholine, biogenic amines, gastrointestinal neuropeptides and nitric oxide; and the electrical and contractile properties of the smooth muscle cell. The neuropeptides may act as circulating hormones or at the site of their release (paracrine).

The electrical properties of gut smooth muscle result from transmembrane fluxes of ions; as in other excitable tissues, these fluxes alter the membrane potential and result in muscle contraction. Infiltrative or degenerative processes that affect the excitability of the smooth muscle cells of the gut prevent normal contractions, resulting in gastrointestinal dysmotility.

In the mammalian digestive tract, the intrinsic, or enteric, nervous system contains about 100 million neurons, approximately the same number of neurons present in the spinal cord. This integrative system is organized in ganglionated plexi (Figure 3.2), and is separate from the sympathetic and parasympathetic portions of the autonomic nervous system. It has several components: sensory mechanoreceptors and chemoreceptors; interneurons that process sensory input and control

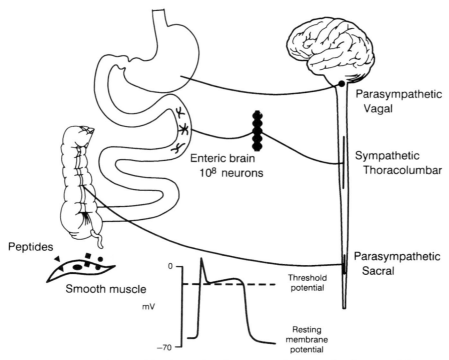

Figure 3.1. Control of gut motility: interactions between extrinsic neural pathways and the "enteric brain" (intrinsic nervous system) modulate contractions of gastrointestinal smooth muscle. Interactions between transmitters (e.g., peptides, amines) and receptors alter muscle membrane potentials by stimulating bidirectional ion fluxes. In turn, membrane characteristics dictate whether or not the muscle cell contracts. (From Camilleri M, Phillips SF: Disorders of small intestinal motility. Gastroenterol Clin NA 1989;18:405, by permission of Mayo Foundation.)

effector (motor and secretory) units; and effector motor neurons involved in motor function of the gut. Preprogrammed synaptic circuits within the enteric nervous system serve to integrate motor function within and between different regions, and thereby control certain coordinated functions in the entire gastrointestinal tract, such as the peristaltic reflex and probably the interdigestive migrating motor complex (Figure 3.2). Synaptic pathways in the gut wall are capable of autonomous adjustment in response to sensory input from the lumen (via chemo or osmo receptors) or the wall (via mechanoreceptors); they can also be modulated by the extrinsic nervous system, such as excitation by vagal preganglionic fibers, or inhibition by sympathetic pathways.

The vagus conveys parasympathetic fibers to the stomach, small intestine and proximal colon, while sacral (S2,3,4) nerves enter the distal colon and subsequently ascend in retrograde fashion to supply the mid-distal colon. Sympathetic fibers originate from the intermediolateral column of the spinal cord, between the levels of the fifth thoracic and third lumbar segments, and synapse in the prevertebral celiac, superior mesenteric, and inferior mesenteric ganglia; sympathetic fibers follow the respective arterial trunks.

The vagus is composed of preganglionic cholinergic fibers that synapse with preprogrammed circuits in the ganglionated enteric plexuses. These enteric neurons

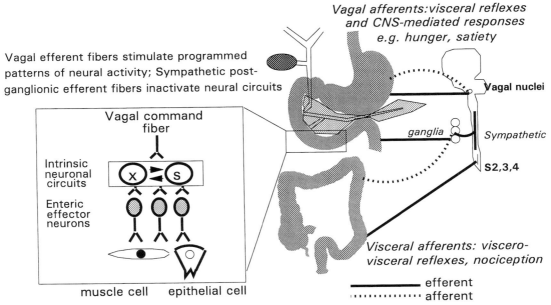

Figure 3.2. Overall function of extrinsic afferent and efferent fibers. The left half shows models of the classic and current concepts of interaction between extrinsic and enteric plexuses. According to the classic concept, which is incorrect, preganglionic cholinergic fibers synapse with a small number of enteric neurons; according to the current concept, vagal command fibers synapse with preprogrammed circuits with "hard-wired" functions. In the right half of the figure, note the major functions of vagal afferents (reflexes and CNS-mediated responses) and splanchnic visceral afferents (reflexes and nociception).

include myenteric cholinergic neurons, which in turn excite smooth muscle cells to produce contraction, or surface epithelial cells which absorb or secrete fluids and electrolytes. Since there is a great disparity between the limited number of extrinsic nerve fibers and the millions of enteric plexus neurons, it is currently believed that the enteric programmed circuits that facilitate motor or secretory behavior of the gut are controlled by command vagal preganglionic or sympathetic postganglionic fibers. Thus, there are approximately 40,000 preganglionic vagal fibers (many of which are afferent, not efferent) at the level of the diaphragm; in contrast, 100 million neurons populate the enteric nervous system. The sympathetic supply inactivates neural circuits that generate motor activity while allowing intrinsic inhibitory innervation by the enteric nerves. Extrinsic vagal fibers also synapse with nonadrenergic inhibitory intramural neurons in the gut which produce transmitters such as nitric oxide, vasoactive intestinal peptide (VIP) and somatostatin. Loss of the sympathetic inhibitory supply ("the brake") results in excessive or uncoordinated phasic pressure activity in the gut.

Extrinsic nerves are intimately involved in controlling the pharynx, the striated muscle portion of the esophagus, pelvic floor, and the external anal sphincter. Cortical pathways to the swallowing musculature and anal sphincter are represented in each hemisphere with inter-hemispheric asymmetry.[2,3] Although the smooth muscle portion of the gut can function fairly normally without the extrinsic nerves, the latter modulate the intrinsic neural circuits, integrate activity in widely separated regions of the gastrointestinal tract (often through reflexes that synapse in prevertebral ganglia), and appear to influence greater control in certain regions (for example, the stomach and distal portion of the colon) than in others (such as the small bowel).

Visceral Afferent Function

Gastrointestinal afferents are thought to be predominantly unmyelinated C afferent fibers that respond to low threshold, polymodal stimulation.[4] These fibers travel towards the central nervous system in the company of splanchnic sympathetic fibers. It is currently thought that nociceptors do not exist in the gut and that the sensation of gut pain arises from higher intensity stimulation of naked nerve endings that act as mechanoreceptors in the mucosa, muscle or surrounding structures. These nerve endings convey a train of impulses predominantly along C fibers to produce the dull, ill-localized sensation characteristic of abdominal pain. As with C afferent fiber stimulation in the somatic nervous system, this train of impulses is conducted through the classic three neurons whose cell bodies are in the dorsal root ganglion, the dorsal horn of the spinal cord, and either the brain stem reticular formation or the thalamus. C afferent stimulation is associated with the affective motivational (discomfort, fear, anger) components of pain sensation and may reflexively stimulate autonomic responses (e.g., change in pulse and blood pressure). Afferent input to central sensory nuclei also stimulates the descending modulation signals from the cerebral cortex, hypothalamus or reticular formation. Thus, descending pathways serve to modulate incoming afferent signals by inhibition or facilitation of dorsal horn neurons. Somatic and visceral afferents converge on the same neurons in lamina V of the dorsal horn; this "convergence" explains such processes as referred pain (e.g., shoulder tip pain in response to diaphragmatic irritation) or the reduction of pain by counter-irritation (since afferent stimulation in the receptive field of a dorsal horn neuron blocks ["gate control"] sensation of a train of noxious impulses arising anywhere else in the receptive field of the same neuron).

Clearly, disorders at several levels of the neural axis (e.g., dysautonomias or autonomic neuropathies affecting peripheral pathways, spinal cord transection, multiple sclerosis, or strokes) may alter the ascending afferent functions or descending modulation of visceral sensation arising from the gastrointestinal tract.

GASTROINTESTINAL MANIFESTATIONS

Dysphagia

Oropharyngeal or transfer dysphagia is characterized by an inability to initiate the swallow or propel the food bolus from the mouth to the esophagus[5,6] and typically occurs in neurologic disorders affecting the cerebral cortex, lower cranial nerves, neuromuscular junction or muscle. Patients with oropharyngeal dysphagia often complain of a hold-up in the cervical area. Nasoendoscopy of the pharynx is useful to exclude a malignancy. A videofluoroscopic swallowing study may provide additional clues to etiology of dysfunction, quantify severity of swallowing dysfunction, and suggest which compensatory maneuvers will ameliorate dysfunction. Videofluoroscopy will unequivocally demonstrate if there is aspiration; aspiration probably predicts the risk of pneumonia. Patients with distal esophageal obstruction, attributable to benign or malignant narrowing of the esophagus or a motility disorder such as idiopathic achalasia, may also experience the sensation of hold-up in the neck or retrosternal area; thus, cervical hold-up is not specific for oropharyngeal dysphagia.

Achalasia is an intrinsic disorder characterized by progressive degeneration and loss of inhibitory nerves containing nitric oxide (NO) and VIP and failure of the lower esophageal sphincter to relax fully during deglutition. The same process involves the esophageal body, causing simultaneous esophageal contractions, and a common cavity phenomenon.

Gastroparesis

Motor dysfunction resulting in delayed gastric emptying is a common gastrointestinal manifestation of autonomic neuropathies such as diabetes mellitus.[7,8] Symptoms range from vague postprandial abdominal discomfort to recurrent postprandial emesis resulting in weight loss and malnutrition. There may be a succussion splash on physical examination. It is essential to exclude gastric outlet obstruction by a barium study or gastroscopy. Appropriately conducted scintigraphic gastric emptying tests confirm the impaired emptying of solids from the stomach[9,10] and may be extended over time to assess small bowel transit, also. Gastric stasis may result from abnormal motility of the stomach or small bowel,[11] and intubated studies of pressure profiles by manometry or solid state pressure transducers placed in the distal stomach and small bowel can help identify these motor dysfunctions (Figure 3.3A), differentiate neuropathic from myopathic processes (Figure 3.3B), and exclude mechanical obstruction that may have been missed on previous radiographic studies of the small bowel.[12,13]

However, many patients with diabetes and gastrointestinal symptoms have normal gastric and small bowel transit. It is conceivable that long-standing diabetic vagal neuropathy with degeneration of visceral afferent fibers may cause exaggerated perception of luminal stimuli. This hypothesis requires testing in future studies akin to the ones that showed abnormal colonic sensory function in diabetic patients.[14]

Currently available therapeutic options include the use of a more easily digestible diet (low in fat and fiber), anti-emetic agents preferably on an as-needed basis, and i.v. erythromycin (3 mg/kg q 8h for 72 h) to treat acute exacerbation of gastroparesis. Infrequently, a venting gastrostomy with a feeding enterostomy is required; these tubes are placed percutaneously, either by endoscopy or by open/laparoscopic surgery. In patients with previous gastric surgery, a total gastrectomy with esophago-Roux-Y-jejunostomy may be necessary. In our practice, low dose antidepressants (e.g., nortriptyline, 10 mg qhs) may relieve the nausea experienced by patients with diabetes and normal gastric emptying. The prokinetic agent, cisapride, is available only in a company-sponsored research protocol, since it is associated with EKG abnormalities including prolonged Q-T interval. Life-threatening ventricular arrhythmias have been reported rarely. In small open-label studies, gastric electrical stimulation improved symptoms and accelerated gastric emptying. Placebo-controlled trials of gastric electrical stimulation and a newer serotonin 5-HT$_4$ receptor agonist, tegaserod, for gastroparesis are in progress.

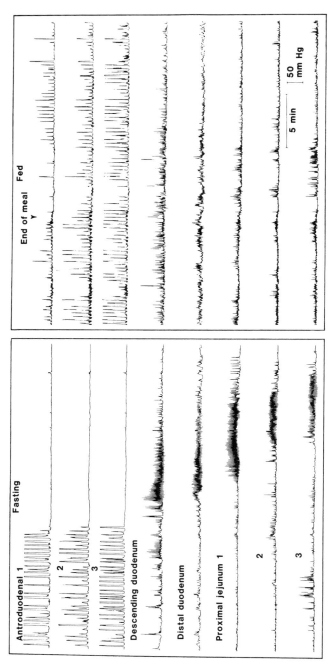

Figure 3.3. A. Tracing showing normal upper gastrointestinal motility in the fasting and fed states. The fasting tracing shows phase III of the interdigestive migrating motor complex. (From Malagelada J-R, Camilleri M, Stanghellini V. Manometric Diagnosis of Gastrointestinal Motility Disorders. New York: Thieme, 1986, by permission of Mayo Foundation.)

Figure continued on opposite page

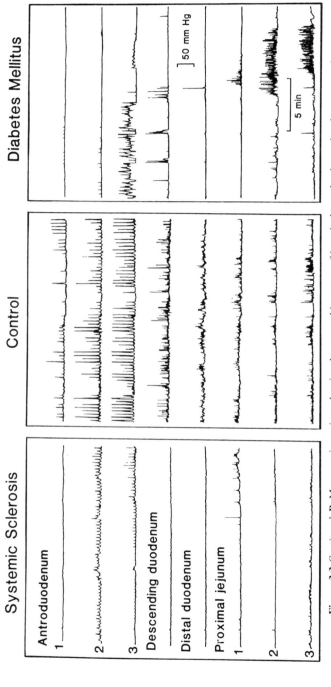

Figure 3.3 *Continued.* **B.** Manometric tracings showing the myopathic pattern of intestinal pseudo-obstruction due to systemic sclerosis (*left panel*). Note the low amplitude of phasic pressure activity compared to control (*middle panel*). A manometric example of neuropathic intestinal pseudo-obstruction in diabetes mellitus. Note the absence of antral contractions and persistence cyclical fasting-type motility in the postprandial period (*right panel*). (Reproduced by permission from Camilleri M. Medical treatment of chronic intestinal pseudo-obstruction. Practical Gastroenterol 1991;15:10–22.)

Chronic Intestinal Pseudo-Obstruction

Chronic intestinal pseudo-obstruction is a syndrome characterized by nausea, vomiting, early satiety, and abdominal discomfort, suggestive of intestinal obstruction in the absence of a mechanical cause. It may be associated with weight loss and, in some patients, either diarrhea (secondary to bacterial overgrowth) or constipation. These symptoms are the consequence of abnormal intestinal motility rather than mechanical obstruction. The syndrome may result (Table 3.1) from a number of neurologic diseases extrinsic to the gut (e.g., disorders at any level of the brain-neural axis), from a dysfunction of neurons in the myenteric plexus,[7] or from degeneration of smooth muscle.

The pathophysiology of these diseases can be broadly subdivided into a myopathic variety (e.g., infiltrative amyloidosis, hollow visceral myopathy, or muscular dystrophies) and a neuropathic variety (see Table 3.1).

The clinical features may suggest the presence of an underlying disease process, features that suggest autonomic dysfunction including postural dizziness, difficulties in visual accommodation on exposure to bright lights, and sweating abnormalities. Alternatively, recurrent urinary infections and difficulty emptying the bladder suggest genitourinary involvement by a generalized visceral neuromyopathic disorder, and associated peripheral sensory or motor symptoms suggest an associated peripheral neuropathy. Patients should be questioned about the use of phenothiazines, antihypertensive agents such as clonidine, tricyclic antidepressants which have anticholinergic effects, and calcium channel blockers.

On physical examination, we pay particular attention to pupillary reflexes to light and accommodation, measurement of the blood pressure and pulse in the lying and standing positions, and search for abdominal distention or a succussion splash.

Table 3.1. Causes of Chronic Intestinal Pseudo-obstruction

	Myopathic	Neuropathic
Infiltrative	PSS Amyloidosis	Early PSS Amyloidosis
Familial	Familial visceral myopathies (autosomal dominant or recessive)	Familial visceral neuropathies
General neurologic diseases	Myotonic and other dystrophies	Diabetes mellitus
		Porphyria, heavy metal poisoning Brain stem tumor, Parkinson's Multiple sclerosis Spinal cord transections
Infectious		Chagas' disease Cytomegalovirus
Drug-induced		Tricyclic antidepressants Narcotic bowel
Neoplastic		Paraneoplastic (bronchial small cell carcinoma or carcinoid)
Idiopathic	Hollow visceral myopathy	Chronic intestinal pseudo-obstruction (? myenteric plexopathy)

PSS-progressive systemic sclerosis.

Abdominal radiographs and barium follow-through examinations are often non-specific; dilatation of the small intestine is identified in about 60% of patients with chronic idiopathic intestinal pseudo-obstruction,[15] but it is probably less frequent in disorders associated with extrinsic neuropathies. Thus, contrast studies of the small bowel are important to exclude mechanical obstruction, but they rarely lead to an etiologic diagnosis. Motility studies (Figure 3.3A and B) are helpful to differentiate myopathic and neuropathic processes and may also suggest the presence of mechanical obstruction; this diagnosis should be considered even in the presence of an underlying neuromuscular disorder.[13] A motility tracing that is suggestive of a neuropathic process does not differentiate extrinsic from intrinsic (enteric) neuropathy; hence, autonomic function tests, serology and imaging of the brain and spinal cord should be performed to identify the cause of the autonomic neuropathy or cerebrospinal disease (see below).[16]

The principles of treatment of chronic intestinal pseudo-obstruction include the restoration of hydration and nutrition (preferably orally or enterally; alternatively parenterally), stimulation of intestinal propulsion, suppression of bacterial overgrowth, and relief of pain associated with dilatation by venting decompression or surgery. Bacterial overgrowth can be suppressed by a rotating course of antibiotics for 7 days every month. Options include norfloxacin (400 mg b.i.d), amoxicillin-clavulanic acid (500 mg t.i.d), doxycycline (100 mg, b.i.d on day 1, then 100 mg daily), and metronidazole (250 mg, t.i.d). The cholinesterase inhibitor neostigmine facilitates cholinergic neurotransmission in the myenteric plexus and neuromuscular junction. An initial dose of 1–2 mg i.v., administered with monitoring of heart rate and blood pressure, is effective in acute colonic pseudo-obstruction and, according to anecdotal reports, also for acute exacerbations of chronic intestinal pseudo-obstruction. Cholinergic side effects of neostigmine, e.g., abdominal pain, excessive salivation, vomiting, bradycardia, and syncope, can be reversed if necessary by atropine. The 5-HT$_4$ agonist, cisapride, improved gastric emptying and small bowel transit of solids, but symptoms in patients with chronic intestinal pseudo-obstruction were not significantly improved over placebo. The long-acting somatostatin analog, octreotide, induces small intestinal activity fronts, which may accelerate transit if they are propagated. In an uncontrolled study of 6 patients, octreotide (50 μg qhs) improved GI symptoms in scleroderma.

Surgical therapy should be restricted to patients who need venting, or an entrostomy for severe persistent intestinal distention, or to provide access for enteral nutritional support. Localized pseudo-obstruction is very rare and may be amenable to resection or bypass of the affected segment.

Constipation

Constipation is a common complaint and may be perceived by the patient as infrequent, incomplete evacuation or excessively hard stools. Most causes of constipation are easily identifiable, such as inadequate fiber intake or lack of exercise, which may be important in inactive patients with neurologic disorders such as Parkinson's disease or paraplegia. Other factors contributing to constipation in neurologic disorders are lack of rectal sensation of stool resulting in an absence of the urge to defecate. As in patients without neurologic disorders, constipation may be due to obstructing lesions which are identified by barium x-ray or colonoscopy, altered colonic motility, or disordered defecation.[17] Anatomic abnormalities such as tumors, megacolon, megarectum, volvulus, occult mucosal prolapse, and rectoceles can be effectively ruled out by barium enema, including defecation proctography, if clinically indicated.

The coexistence of incontinence and lack of rectal sensation suggests a pudendal neuropathy, and is common among patients with diabetic neuropathy. The presence of blood in the stool or anemia necessitate further tests to exclude colonic mucosal lesions such as polyps or cancer, or perianal conditions such as hemorrhoids.

Colon transit studies using radiopaque markers[18] or radioscintigraphy[19] will detect abnormally prolonged transit; however, pelvic floor dysfunction as might occur in paraplegic patients with pudendal neuropathy may result in outlet obstruction and secondarily prolonged colonic transit. Hence, anorectal manometry, evaluation of rectal emptying (e.g., by testing the ability to expel a balloon) and rectal sensation, as well as measurements of the anorectal angle during defecation proctography in selected cases are useful in assessing patients with disorders of defecation. These principles are reviewed elsewhere[20] (see Chapter 13).

Fecal Incontinence

Major incontinence with loss of formed stool is frequently due to neurologic damage to the pelvic nerves which denervate the pelvic floor musculature and the external anal sphincter.[17] Sympathetic denervation results in weakness of the internal anal sphincter and manifests as nocturnal incontinence. Stretching of the pudendal nerves with repetitive prolonged straining may complicate disorders of colonic transit and, hence, may be secondary to a primary disease process that causes delayed colonic transit. Incontinence occurring only at night time suggests internal anal sphincter dysfunction (as in diabetic autonomic neuropathy or due to muscle weakness due to systemic sclerosis); stress incontinence during coughing, sneezing, or laughing suggests loss of external sphincter control, typically from pudendal nerve or S2, 3 or 4 root lesions, as in cauda equina syndrome.

In evaluating such patients, it is important to first exclude overflow incontinence due to fecal impaction. Excessive use of laxatives or other medications causing diarrhea, such as magnesium-containing antacids, may result in reversible incontinence. Examination of the incontinent patient should include inspection of the anus with and without straining to detect rectal prolapse, a digital rectal exam to exclude impaction or mucosal disease, and proctoscopy and barium enema or colonoscopy to exclude mucosal lesions. If these fail to identify the cause for incontinence, further tests may be necessary. These tests include anorectal manometry and assessment of rectal sensation for anal sphincter weakness and sensory deficits. The ability to expel a balloon from the rectum, anorectal angle, and emptying during simulated defecation by defecating proctography assess the defecation process. External anal sphincter and puborectalis muscle EMG are necessary in selected cases. Pudendal nerve conduction studies (terminal motor latency) are operator dependent, and lack sensitivity and specificity for identifying nerve damage.

Initial treatment of patients with denervation-induced incontinence includes care of the perianal skin, use of incontinence pads, and anti-diarrheal agents for patients with diarrhea (loperamide [Imodium A-D; 2 mg, 30 minutes before meals, up to 8 tablets/day]). Biofeedback therapy is of limited efficacy for patients with severe weakness of anal musculature, complete loss of rectal sensation, or cognitive impairment.[21] A colostomy may provide a more manageable solution to chronic incontinence. Sacral nerve stimulation is approved by the FDA for treating urge urinary incontinence, and is being evaluated for the treatment of fecal incontinence. It is important to exclude mucosal prolapse in association with incontinence since surgical correction of the prolapse may permit better function of the external sphincter and at least temporarily improve continence.[22]

EXTRINSIC NEUROLOGICAL DISORDERS CAUSING GUT DYSMOTILITY

It is possible to distinguish the disorders that affect the gut muscle ("myopathic disorders"), those of the myenteric plexus, and diseases of the extrinsic pathways that supply the gut. Some diseases affect both intrinsic and extrinsic neural control.[16] This review concentrates on neurologic diseases of extrinsic neural control and smooth muscle that affect gut motility. Diseases affecting the enteric nervous system are reviewed elsewhere.[23]

Brain Diseases

Cerebrovascular Accident

At least one-third of patients have some degree of dysphagia after a stroke. Swallowing recovers, together with increased pharyngeal representation within the unaffected cerebral hemisphere, in most patients within a few weeks,[2] suggesting nervous system plasticity after the stroke. Colonic pseudo-obstruction occurs rarely.[24] Placement of a percutaneous endoscopic gastrostomy is usually the most effective method to provide nutrition without interfering with rehabilitation; feedings can be given in the form of boluses or by nighttime infusion. Not infrequently, patients subsequently recover sufficient oropharyngeal coordination to resume oral feeding and for the gastrostomy tube to be removed.

Parkinsonism

Patients with prolonged Parkinson's disease or progressive supranuclear palsy may also have oropharyngeal dysfunction with impaired swallowing[25] and mild to moderate malnutrition. In the absence of severe malnutrition or significant aspiration, conservative treatment with attention to the consistency of food (thickened liquids) and ensuring adequate caloric content of meals will suffice. Feeding through a percutaneous gastrostomy is an appropriate alternative for severe symptoms.

Constipation is common in patients with Parkinsonism[25] and may be the result of slow colonic transit or pelvic floor[26] or anal sphincter dysfunction.[27] Gastrointestinal hypomotility, generalized hypokinesia, associated autonomic dysfunction, and the effects of various anticholinergic and dopamine agonist medications may all play a role. The bioavailability of other medications can be affected by delayed gut transit and impaired delivery of medications to the small bowel for absorption.

Head Injury

Immediately following moderate to severe head injury, most patients develop transient delays in gastric emptying. The underlying mechanism is unknown, although correlations exist between the severity of injury, increased intracranial pressure, and severity of the gastric stasis. These patients frequently require parenteral nutrition to meet their increased metabolic demands. Enteral nutrition can often be introduced within two to three weeks as the gastric emptying improves.[28]

Autonomic Epilepsy and Migraine

Autonomic epilepsy and migraine are infrequent causes of nausea, vomiting, or abdominal pain.

Amyotrophic Lateral Sclerosis

Patients with amyotrophic lateral sclerosis (ALS) and progressive bulbar palsy have predominant weakness of the muscles supplied by the glossopharyngeal and vagus nerves.[29] Dysphagia is a frequent complaint, and patients may have respiratory difficulty while eating as a result of aspiration or respiratory muscle fatigue. Rarely, patients with vagal dysfunction will show features of a chronic intestinal pseudo-obstruction syndrome.[30]

Barium swallow of liquids and solids evaluates swallowing, determines whether aspiration occurs, and guides decisions regarding nutritional support: oral or via gastrostomy. Cervical esophagostomy or cricopharyngeal myotomy have been performed in selected cases for significant cricopharyngeal muscle dysfunction that aggravates the transfer dysphagia.

Post-polio Dysphagia

Individuals with post-polio syndrome with bulbar involvement frequently have dysphagia and aspiration. Attention to the position of the patient's head during swallowing and changing food consistency to semisolid food can decrease the incidence of choking and aspiration.[31]

Brainstem Tumors

Brainstem lesions can present with isolated gastrointestinal motor dysfunction. In the absence of increased intracranial pressure, symptoms likely result from direct effects of the mass in the brainstem with distortion of the vomiting center on the floor of the 4th ventricle. Motor dysfunction is typically evident on manometric or radionuclide studies of the stomach and small bowel.[32] Although most reports are associated with vomiting, colonic or anorectal dysfunction have also been described.[33] The presence of autonomic neuropathy in a patient with a motility disorder necessitates a search for a structural lesion in the central nervous system, particularly if the tests suggest a preganglionic sympathetic lesion. Magnetic resonance imaging is considered preferable to CT for detecting brainstem lesions.[32]

Autonomic System Degenerations

Pandysautonomia or Selective Dysautonomias

Pandysautonomias are characterized by preganglionic or postganglionic lesions affecting both sympathetic and parasympathetic nerves. Vomiting, paralytic ileus, constipation, or a chronic pseudo-obstruction syndrome have been reported in acute, subacute, or familial dysautonomias.[16] Motor dysfunctions have been documented in the esophagus, the stomach, and the small bowel. Selective cholinergic dysautonomia affects parasympathetic nerves and sympathetic nerves to sweat glands, and may also impair upper and lower gastrointestinal motor activity. This picture may follow a viral infection, such as infectious mononucleosis.[34]

Idiopathic Orthostatic Hypotension

Idiopathic orthostatic hypotension is sometimes associated with motor dysfunction of the gut, such as esophageal dysmotility, gastric stasis, alteration in bowel movements, and fecal incontinence.[35,36] Cardiovascular abnormalities usually precede gut involvement. The precise site of the lesion causing the gut dysmotility is unknown.

Multiple System Atrophy

Constipation and fecal incontinence were among the classic features of the original description by Shy and Drager.[37] Reports have documented substantial reduction in fasting and postprandial antral and small bowel motility. Abnormal esophageal motility has been demonstrated by videofluoroscopy and simultaneous low-amplitude waves on esophageal manometry.[35]

Spinal Cord Lesions

Spinal Cord Injury

Ileus is a frequent but transient complication after spinal cord injury. In the chronic phase, disorders of upper gastrointestinal motility are uncommon; on the other hand, colonic and anorectal dysfunction are common and result from interruption of supraspinal control of the sacral parasympathetic supply to the colon, pelvic floor, and anal sphincters.[38,39] There is a decrease in colonic compliance and an absence of postprandial colonic motor and myoelectric activity in patients with thoracic spinal cord injury.[40] While the latter are predictable from altered extrinsic neural control, the mechanism for the altered compliance is unclear.

The loss of voluntary control of defecation may be the most significant disturbance in patients who rely on reflex rectal stimulation for stool evacuation. Loss of control of the external anal sphincter with fecal incontinence is the most common chronic gastrointestinal problem in spinal cord injury patients. This is usually managed with a combination of bulk agents and scheduled enemas. Computerized stimulation of the sacral anterior roots has been proposed as a method to restore normal function to the pelvic colon and anorectal sphincters[41]; however, the long-term efficacy is unclear.

Multiple Sclerosis

Severe constipation frequently accompanies urinary bladder dysfunction in patients with advanced multiple sclerosis.[42] In one study, colonic transit of radiopaque markers was prolonged in 14 of 16 patients with multiple sclerosis and urinary bladder involvement; 10 patients also had evidence of fecal incontinence, and 5 had spontaneous rectal contractions. The studies performed to date have not been sufficiently detailed to assess the relative contributions of the sympathetic and parasympathetic denervation. Pelvic colon dysfunction is probably due to impaired supraspinal or spinal control affecting the sacral parasympathetic supply to the colon. Further studies need to address the mechanism of impaired gut transit in multiple sclerosis which, as with spinal cord injury, results more frequently in dysmotility of the lower than the upper gut.[43]

Peripheral Neuropathy

Gastrointestinal dysfunction in association with autonomic peripheral neuropathy is discussed in greater detail in Chapter 5.

Acute Peripheral Neuropathy

Autonomic dysfunction accompanied by nausea, vomiting, abdominal cramps, and constipation, may occur in acute peripheral neuropathic syndromes seen with the Guillain-Barré syndrome, herpes zoster, Epstein-Barr virus,[34] botulism B, and cytomegalovirus.[44] HIV-induced diarrhea may be another manifestation of autonomic dysfunction (see below), but the data require confirmation.

Chronic Peripheral Neuropathy

Chronic peripheral neuropathy is the most commonly encountered extrinsic neurologic disorder that results in gastrointestinal motor dysfunction.

Diabetes Mellitus

Diabetic autonomic neuropathy of the gut has been studied extensively and has been reviewed elsewhere.[45] Gastrointestinal symptoms are very common (up to 76% of patients) in diabetics seen at tertiary care centers.[46] However, the occurrence and spectrum of gastrointestinal symptoms in middle-aged community subjects with insulin- and noninsulin-dependent diabetes mellitus do not differ from those of the general population[47,48] except for constipation in insulin-dependent diabetes mellitus.[48] Gastroparesis is most consistent with an "autovagotomy"[49]; the role of hyperglycemia itself is being investigated. During the early stages of diabetes, gastric emptying of liquids is accelerated, but this has little impact on glycemic control.[50]

Constipation is a frequent, although often unreported, symptom in patients with diabetes. It is associated with an absent myoelectric response of the colon to meal ingestion[51] leading to slow colonic transit with abnormalities of the rectal evacuation process.[52] In many diabetic patients, constipation is associated with medication use, e.g., calcium channel blockers.[48] Diarrhea or fecal incontinence (or both) may result from several mechanisms (reviewed in detail[53]): dysfunction of the anorectal sphincter or abnormal rectal sensation, steatorrhea due to bacterial overgrowth, or rapid transit from uncoordinated small bowel motor activity. Rarely, an associated gluten-sensitive enteropathy or pancreatic exocrine insufficiency may be present. The diagnostic algorithm used in our practice is shown in Figure 3.4.

Peripheral cholinergic and $5HT_4$ agonists (such as metoclopramide, bethanechol, and cisapride) and alpha-2-adrenergic agonists (such as clonidine) have been respectively used to treat gastric stasis and diarrhea secondary to diabetic gut neuropathy.[54] Available therapeutic options have resulted in only transient relief. Erythromycin (i.v.) is useful during the acute phase, but few patients tolerate it beyond two weeks.[55] Macrolides should not be combined with cisapride because of the risk of cardiac tachyarrhythmias. Pancreas transplantation is reported to restore gastric emptying towards normal in patients with diabetic gastroparesis.[56] However, long-term results are not yet available. We have observed gastric stasis in those with autonomic neuropathy that persisted after the pancreas transplantation.

Paraneoplastic Neuropathy

Gastrointestinal symptoms (from achalasia to pseudo-obstruction) have been reported in association with small cell carcinoma of the lung (>95% cases), kidney cancer, or pulmonary carcinoid.[57] A circulating IgG antibody (called ANNA-1 or anti-Hu) directed against enteric neuronal nuclei[58] has been detected, suggesting that the enteric plexus is the major target of this immune paraneoplastic process. However, several patients also have evidence of extrinsic visceral neuropathies,[57,59] suggesting a more extensive neuropathologic process. The chest x-ray is frequently negative and a chest CT scan is indicated when the syndrome is suspected, typically in middle-aged smokers with recent onset of nausea, vomiting, or feeding intolerance. ANNA-1 is associated with paraneoplastic neuropathies; 14% being restricted to GI manifestations.[60]

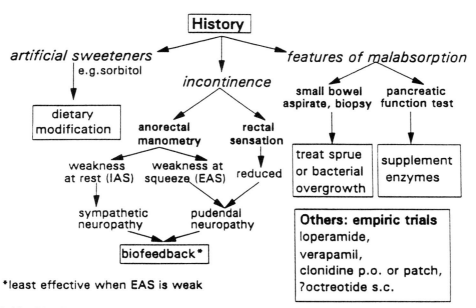

Figure 3.4. Algorithm for management of diarrhea in patients with diabetes mellitus.

Amyloid Neuropathy

Familial or acquired amyloid neuropathy may lead to constipation,[61] diarrhea, or steatorrhea. Intestinal myoelectric disturbances in amyloidosis[35] mimic those of ganglionectomy.[62]

Chronic Sensory and Autonomic Neuropathy of Unknown Cause

This is a rare, nonfamilial progressive neuropathy affecting a number of autonomic functions.[63] Patients may have only a chronic autonomic disturbance (e.g., abnormal sweating or blood pressure control or gastrointestinal dysfunction) manifesting for many years before the peripheral sensory symptoms become apparent. This may account for a subset of patients who present with features suggesting the irritable bowel syndrome.[64] A review of the Mayo Clinic experience of 27 patients with idiopathic autonomic neuropathy identified gastrointestinal involvement in 19 patients.[65] A recent study suggested that antibodies to nicotinic cholinergic receptors in autonomic ganglia identified patients with an autoimmune neuropathy and distinguished these patients from other types of dysautonomia. Rarely, these antibodies were associated with idiopathic gastrointestinal dysmotility. Levels of these antibodies decreased in patients who had clinical improvement.[66]

Others have reported familial cases of intestinal pseudo-obstruction with degeneration of the myenteric plexus and evidence of sensory or motor neuropathies affecting peripheral or cranial nerves.[23]

Porphyria

Acute intermittent porphyria and hereditary coproporphyria may present with abdominal pain, nausea, vomiting, and constipation.[67,68] Porphyric polyneuritis is characterized by demyelination of peripheral and autonomic nerves; dilatation and impaired motor function may be seen in any part of the intestinal tract, and is likely the result of extrinsic autonomic dysfunction since disturbances of the enteric nervous system have not been described to date.

Human Immunodeficiency Virus Infection

Neurological disease may manifest at any phase of the infection with HIV-1 virus; autonomic dysfunction may be associated with chronic diarrhea, possibly as a result of increased extrinsic parasympathetic activity to the gut,[69] or damage to the enteric plexuses.[70] Further studies are needed to characterize these abnormalities; it is, of course, important to exclude gut infections or infestations in patients with HIV or AIDS and diarrhea.

IDENTIFICATION OF NEUROLOGIC DISEASE IN PATIENTS WITH GASTROINTESTINAL DYSMOTILITY

As discussed above, patients with lesions at virtually any level of the nervous system may have symptoms of gastrointestinal motor dysfunction. Therefore, the diagnostic evaluation of disordered gastrointestinal function necessitates a search for autonomic dysfunction, as this may help identify the cause of the gut symptoms

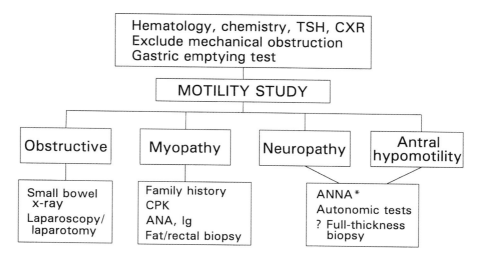

ANNA *- Antineuronal enteric antibody

Figure 3.5. Algorithm for the investigation of patients with suspected gastrointestinal dysmotility. (Reproduced by permission from Camilleri M. Study of human gastroduodenojejunal motility. Applied physiology in clinical practice. Dig Dis Sci 1993;38:785–794.)

(Figure 3.5). It is here that the paths of the neurologist and gastroenterologist with interest in motility disorders meet. Patients should undergo further testing, particularly if they have clinical features suggestive of autonomic or peripheral nerve dysfunction or a known underlying neuromuscular disorder. It is essential to stop all medications that influence gut motility or autonomic tests prior to performing formal tests.

Gastrointestinal motility and transit measurements confirm the disturbance in the motor function of the gut and help to distinguish between neuropathic and myopathic disorders. Tests of autonomic function are useful for identifying the presence of other visceral denervation and localizing the anatomic level of the disturbance in extrinsic neural control.[16] There is generally good agreement between tests of abdominal vagal dysfunction, including the plasma pancreatic polypeptide response to modified sham feeding (Figure 3.6), and cardiovagal dysfunction in patients with diabetes.[71] This suggests that these tests may provide a good evaluation of the overall function of the autonomic supply to the viscera, including the gastrointestinal tract. Table 3.2 lists the autonomic investigations, normal values at Mayo Clinic, and interpretation of abnormal tests.[16] In addition, spectral analysis of heart rate variability reveals low and high frequency components.[72] Abnormalities in the high frequency component, which reflects parasympathetic tone, correlate well with other indices of an autonomic neuropathy.[73]

When a defect of the sympathetic nervous system is identified, the effect of intravenous edrophonium on plasma norepinephrine levels assesses the integrity of postganglionic sympathetic nerves (Figure 3.7), many of which supply the digestive tract.[74,75] Thus, the digestive tract also provides target organs whose integrity can be used as a means to appraise the extrinsic autonomic nerves to viscera in general. Superior mesenteric blood flow measured by doppler ultrasound provides a measure of abdominal sympathetic neuropathy.[76]

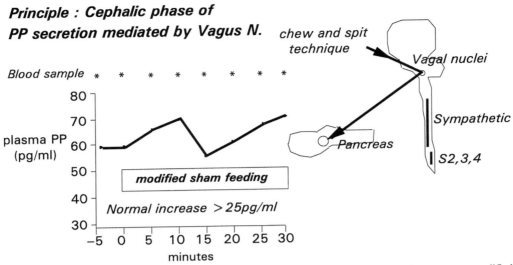

Figure 3.6. Assessment of abdominal vagal function by the plasma pancreatic polypeptide (PP) response to modified sham feeding by chewing and spitting a toasted bacon and cheese sandwich.

Once visceral autonomic neuropathy is identified, further tests are needed to identify the cause of the neuropathy; examples include lung tumors (CT chest), porphyria (uroporphyrinogen-1-synthase and coproporphyrinogen oxidase in erythrocytes) or amyloidosis (special protein studies in blood and urine, fat aspirate or rectal biopsy). Imaging of the brain and spinal cord is needed when autonomic tests indicate a central lesion, such as when a thermoregulatory sweat test is abnormal,

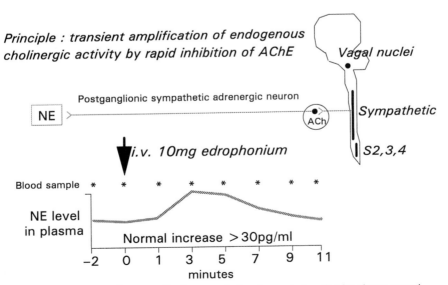

Figure 3.7. Assessment of postganglionic sympathetic adrenergic function by plasma norepinephrine (NE) response to IV edrophonium, a short-acting anticholinesterase.

Table 3.2. Interpretation of Results of Autonomic Function Tests

Test of Autonomic Function	Normal Value	Abnormal Results Imply Dysfunction of
Pupillary tests		
Response to light		
Latency	0.2-0.3 s	P
Constriction	2.0-4.0 mm	P
Pharmacologic tests		
0.125% Pilocarpine	0-0.5 mm constriction	P
0.1% Epinephrine	No change	PG, S
5% Cocaine	>1.5 mm dilation	S
Blood pressure reduction on tilt to 80°		
Systolic	<25 mm Hg	S
Diastolic	<15 mm Hg	S
Valsalva ratio	>1.5	S or P
Pulse rate change with deep breathing	Age related, 6-18 beats/min	P
Thermoregulatory sweat test		S
% surface area of anhidrosis	M: 0%	
	F: <3%	
Quantitative sudomotor axon reflex test		PG, S
Sweat output (µL/cm^3)		
Forearm	M: 0.76-5.51	
	F: 0.34-1.33	
Foot	M: 0.92-5.73	
	F: 0.25-1.95	
Latency (min)		
Forearm	M: 1.0-2.4	
	F: 0.9-1.9	
Foot	M: 1.0-2.7	
	F: 1.0-2.8	
Plasma norepinephrine		
Patient supine	70-750 pg/ml	PG, S
Patient standing	200-1,700 pg/ml	S
Response to IV edrophonium	>35% increase above baseline within 2-8 min	PG, S

P-parasympathetic; PG-postganglionic; S-sympathetic.
From Camilleri M. Disorders of gastrointestinal motility in neurologic diseases. Mayo Clin Proc 1990;65:825–846. With permission of the Mayo Foundation.

but tests of postganglionic nerves (e.g., the quantitative sudomotor axon reflex test, or plasma norepinephrine response to edrophonium) are normal.[53] This situation is quite rare in clinical practice, but it provides the basis for selecting patients for brain and spinal cord imaging.

SUMMARY AND CONCLUSIONS

Gastrointestinal motor dysfunctions result when extrinsic autonomic nerves are diseased and are unable to modulate the motor functions of the digestive tract, which depend on the enteric nervous system and the automaticity of the smooth muscles. Gut motor dysfunction may result from disorders at all anatomic levels of the extrinsic neural control and degeneration of gut smooth muscle and illustrates the important modulation of gut motor function by the nervous system. Although much emphasis in the literature is laid on dysphagia and constipation in neurologic disorders, more recent studies have highlighted other important symptoms, such as incontinence, vomiting, and abdominal distention. Strategies that evaluate the motor functions of the digestive tract and the extrinsic neural control are available and aid in selection of rational therapies for these patients. These include physical therapy and biofeedback training (e.g., dysphagia, incontinence), prokinetic agents (for neuropathic forms of gastroparesis, chronic intestinal dysmotility, or slow transit colonic disorders), and nutritional support using the enteral or parenteral route. Electrical stimulation of the stomach or sacral roots may offer novel methods to improve symptoms of gastroparesis and continence respectively.

REFERENCES

1. Camilleri M. Autonomic regulation of gastrointestinal motility. In PA Low (ed), Clinical Autonomic Disorders: Evaluation and Management. Boston: Little, Brown and Company, 1992;125–132.
2. Hamdy S, Aziz Q, Rothwell JC, et al. Recovery of swallowing after dysphagic stroke relates to functional reorganization in the intact motor cortex. Gastroenterology 1998;115:1104–1112.
3. Turnbull GK, Hamdy S, Aziz Q, et al. The cortical topography of human anorectal musculature. Gastroenterology 1999;117:32–39.
4. Mayer EA, Gebhart GF. Basic and clinical aspects of visceral hyperalgesia. Gastroenterology 1994;107:271–293.
5. Anonymous. American Gastroenterological Association medical position statement on management of oropharyngeal dysphagia. Gastroenterology 1999;116:452–454.
6. Cook IJ, Kahrilas PJ. AGA technical review on management of oropharyngeal dysphagia. Gastroenterology 1999;116:455–478.
7. Colemont L, Camilleri M. Chronic intestinal pseudo-obstruction: diagnosis and treatment. Mayo Clin Proc 1989;64:60–70.
8. Read NW, Houghton LA. Physiology of gastric emptying and pathophysiology of gastroparesis. In A Ouyang (ed), Gastroenterology Clinics of North America. Philadelphia: WB Saunders, 1989; vol. 18, 359–374.
9. Camilleri M, Zinsmeister AR, Greydanus MP, et al. Towards a less costly but accurate test of gastric emptying and small bowel transit. Dig Dis Sci 1991;36:609–615.
10. Tougas G, Eaker EY, Abell TL, et al. Assessment of gastric emptying using a low fat meal: establishment of international control values. Am J Gastroenterol 2000;95:1456–1462.
11. Camilleri M, Malagelada J-R. Abnormal intestinal motility in diabetics with gastroparesis. Eur J Clin Invest 1984;14:20–27.
12. Camilleri M. Medical treatment of chronic intestinal pseudo-obstruction. Practical Gastroenterology 1991;15:10–22.
13. Frank JW, Sarr MG, Camilleri M. Use of gastroduodenal manometry to differentiate mechanical and functional intestinal obstruction: an analysis of clinical outcome. Am J Gastroenterology 1994;89:339–344.
14. Sarno S, Erasmus LP, Haslbeck M, Hölzl R. Visceral perception and gut changes in diabetes mellitus. Neurogastroenterol Motil 1994;6:85–94.
15. Stanghellini V, Camilleri M, Malagelada J-R. Chronic idiopathic intestinal pseudo-obstruction: clinical and intestinal manometric findings. Gut 1987;28:5–12.
16. Camilleri M. Disorders of gastrointestinal motility in neurologic diseases. Mayo Clin Proc 1990;65:825–846.
17. Pemberton JH, Phillips SF. Constipation and diarrhea. In FG Moody (ed), Surgical Treatment of Digestive Diseases. Chicago: Year Book Medical Publishers, 1990;39–52.
18. Metcalf AM, Phillips SF, Zinsmeister AR, et al. Simplified assessment of segmental colonic transit. Gastroenterology 1987;92:40–47.
19. Stivland T, Camilleri M, Vassallo M, et al. Scintigraphic measurement of regional gut transit in idiopathic constipation. Gastroenterology 1991;101:107–115.

20. Wald A. Colonic transit and anorectal manometry in chronic idiopathic constipation. Arch Intern Med 1986;146:1713–1716.
21. Bielefeldt K, Enck P, Wienbeck M. Diagnosis and treatment of fecal incontinence. Dig Dis Sci 1990;8:179–188.
22. Leighton JA, Valdovinos MA, Pemberton JH, et al. Anorectal dysfunction and rectal prolapse in progressive systemic sclerosis. Dis Colon Rectum 1993;36:182–185.
23. Krishnamurthy S, Schuffler MD. Pathology of neuromuscular disorders of the small intestine and colon. Gastroenterology 1987;93:610–639.
24. Reynolds BJ, Eliasson SG. Colonic pseudoobstruction in patients with stroke. Ann Neurol 1977;1:305.
25. Edwards LL, Pfeiffer RF, Quigley EMM, et al. Gastrointestinal symptoms in Parkinson's disease. Mov Disord 1991;6:151–156.
26. Kupsky WJ, Grimes MM, Sweeting J, et al. Parkinson's disease and megacolon: concentric hyaline inclusions (Lewy bodies) in enteric ganglion cells. Neurology 1987;37:1253–1265.
27. Mathers SE, Kempster PA, Law PJ, et al. Anal sphincter dysfunction in Parkinson's disease. Arch Neurol 1989;46:1061–1064.
28. Ott L, Young B, Phillips R, et al. Altered gastric emptying in the head-injured patient: relationship to feeding intolerance. J Neurosurg 1991;74:738–742.
29. Hillel AD, Miller RM. Management of bulbar symptoms in amyotrophic lateral sclerosis. Adv Exp Med Biol 1987;209:201–221.
30. Camilleri M, Balm RK, Low PA. Autonomic dysfunction in patients with chronic intestinal pseudo-obstruction. Clin Auton Res 1993;3:95–100.
31. Sonies BC, Dalakas MC. Dysphagia in patients with the post-polio syndrome. N Engl J Med 1991;324:1162–1167.
32. Wood JR, Camilleri M, Low PA, Malagelada J-R. Brainstem tumor presenting as an upper gut motility disorder. Gastroenterology 1985;89:1411–1414.
33. Weber J, Denis P, Mihout B, et al. Effect of brainstem lesion on colonic and anorectal motility: study of three patients. Dig Dis Sic 1985;30:419–425.
34. Vassallo M, Camilleri M, Caron BL, Low PA. Gastrointestinal motor dysfunction in acquired selective cholinergic dysautonomia associated with infectious mononucleosis. Gastroenterology 1991;100:252–258.
35. Camilleri M, Malagelada J-R, Stanghellini V, et al. Gastrointestinal motility disturbances in patients with orthostatic hypotension. Gastroenterology 1985;88:1852–1859.
36. Thatcher BS, Achkar E, Fouad FM, et al. Altered gastroesophageal motility in patients with idiopathic orthostatic hypotension. Cleve Clin J Med 1987;54:77–82.
37. Shy GM, Drager GA. A neurological syndrome associated with orthostatic hypotension: a clinical-pathologic study. Arch Neurol 1960;2:511–527.
38. Stone JM, Nino-Murcia M, Wolfe VA, Perkash I. Chronic gastrointestinal problems in spinal cord injury patients: a prospective analysis. Am J Gastroenterol 1990;85:114–119.
39. Sun WM, Read NW, Donnelly TC. Anorectal function in incontinent patients with cerebrospinal disease. Gastroenterology 1990:1372–1379.
40. Meshkinpour H., Nowroozi F, Glick ME. Colonic compliance in patients with spinal cord injury. Arch Phys Med Rehabil 1983;64:111–112.
41. MacDonagh RP, Sun WM, Smallwood R, et al. Control of defecation in patients with spinal injuries by stimulation of sacral anterior nerve roots. BMJ 1990;300:1494–1497.
42. Weber J, Grise P, Roquebert M, et al. Radiopaque marker transit and anorectal monometry in 16 patients with multiple sclerosis and urinary bladder dysfunction. Dis Colon Rectum 1987;30:95–100.
43. Caruana BJ, Wald A, Hinds JP, Eidelman BH. Anorectal sensory and motor function in neurogenic fecal incontinence. Comparison between multiple sclerosis and diabetes mellitus. Gastroenterology 1991;100:465–470.
44. Sonsino E, Mouy R, Foucaud P, et al. Intestinal pseudoobstruction related to cytomegalovirus infection of the myenteric plexus (letter to the editor). N Engl J Med 1984;311:196–197.
45. von der Ohe M, Camilleri M., Zimmerman BR. Management of diabetic enteropathy. The Endocrinologist 1993;3:400–408.
46. Feldman M, Schiller LR. Disorders of gastrointestinal motility associated with diabetes mellitus. Ann Intern Med 1983;98:378–384.

47. Janatuinen E, Pikkarainen P, Laakso M., Pyorala K. Gastrointestinal symptoms in middle-aged diabetic patients. Scand J Gastroenterol 1993;28:427–432.
48. Maleki D, Camilleri M, Zinsmeister AR, et al. Prevalence of gastrointestinal symptoms in insulin-(IDDM) and noninsulin-dependent diabetes mellitus (NIDDM) in a U.S. community. Dig Dis Sci 1996;41:1900.
49. Feldman M, Corbett DB, Ramsey EJ, et al. Abnormal gastric function in long-standing insulin-dependent diabetic patients. Gastroenterology 1979;77:7–12.
50. Frank JW, Saslow SB, Camilleri M, et al. Mechanism of accelerated gastric emptying of liquids and hyperglycemia in patients with type II diabetes mellitus. Gastroenterology 1995;109:755–765.
51. Battle WM, Snape WJ Jr, Alavi A, et al. Colonic dysfunction in diabetes mellitus. Gastroenterology 1980;79:1217–1221.
52. Maleki D, Camilleri M, Burton DD, et al. Pilot study of pathophysiology of constipation among community diabetics. Dig Dis Sci 1998;43:2373–2378.
53. Valdovinos MA, Camilleri M, Zimmerman BR. Chronic diarrhea in diabetes mellitus: mechanisms and an approach to diagnosis and treatment. Mayo Clin Proc 1993;68:691–702.
54. Camilleri M. A guide to the treatment of GI motility disorders. Drug Therapy 1991;21:15–28.
55. Camilleri M. The current role of erythromycin in the clinical management of gastric emptying disorders (editorial). Am J Gastroenterol 1993;88:169–171.
56. Murat A, Pouliquen B, Cantarovich D, et al. Gastric emptying improvement after simultaneous pancreas and kidney transplantation. Transplant Proc 1992;24:855.
57. Chinn JS, Schuffler MD. Paraneoplastic visceral neuropathy as a cause of severe gastrointestinal motor dysfunction. Gastroenterology 1988;95:1279–1286.
58. Lennon VA, Sas DF, Busk MF, et al. Enteric neuronal autoantibodies in pseudoobstruction with small-cell lung carcinoma. Gastroenterology 1991;100:137–142.
59. Sodhi N, Camilleri M., Camoriano JK, et al. Autonomic function and motility in intestinal pseudoobstruction caused by paraneoplastic syndrome. Dig Dis Sci 1989;34:1937–1942.
60. Lucchinetti CF, Kimmel DW, Lennon VA. Paraneoplastic and oncologic profiles of patients seropositive for type 1 antineuronal nuclear autoantibodies. Neurology 1998;50:652–657.
61. Battle WM, Rubin MR, Cohen S, Snape WJ Jr. Gastrointestinal-motility dysfunction in amyloidosis. N Engl J Med 1979;301:24–25.
62. Marlett JA, Code CF. Effects of celiac and superior mesenteric ganglionectomy on interdigestive myoelectric complex in dogs. Am J Physiol 1979;237:E432–E436.
63. Okajima T, Yamamura S, Hamada K, et al. Chronic sensory and autonomic neuropathy. Neurology 1983;33:1061–1064.
64. Camilleri M, Fealey RD. Idiopathic autonomic denervation in eight patients presenting with functional gastrointestinal disease: A causal association? Dig Dis Sci 1990;35:609–616.
65. Suarez GA, Fealey RD, Camilleri M, Low PA. Idiopathic autonomic neuropathy: clinical, neurophysiologic, and follow-up studies in 27 patients. Neurology 1994;44:1675–1682.
66. Vernino S, Low PA, Fealey RD, et al. Autoantibodies to ganglionic acetylcholine receptors in autoimmune autonomic neuropathies. N Engl J Med 2000;343:847–855.
67. Berlin L, Cotton R. Gastro-intestinal manifestations of porphyria. Am J Dig Dis 1950;17:110–114.
68. Stein JA, Tschudy DP. Acute intermittent porphyria. Medicine 1970;49:1–16.
69. Coker RJ, Horner P, Bleasdale-Barr K, et al. Increased gut parasympathetic activity and chronic diarrhoea in a patient with the acquired immunodeficiency syndrome. Clin Auton Res 1992;2:295–298.
70. Griffin GE, Miller A, Bateman P, et al. Damage to jejunal intrinsic autonomic nerves in HIV infection. AIDS 1988;2:79–82.
71. Buysschaert M, Donckier J, Dive A, et al. Gastric acid and pancreatic polypeptide responses to sham feeding are impaired in diabetic subjects with autonomic neuropathy. Diabetes 1985;34:1181–1185.
72. Anonymous. Heart rate variability: standards of measurement, physiological interpretation and clinical use. Task Force of the European Society of Cardiology and the North American Society of Pacing and Electrophysiology. Circulation 1996;93:1043–1065.

73. Howorka K, Pumprla J, Schabmann A. Optimal parameters of short-term heart rate spectrogram for routine evaluation of diabetic cardiovascular autonomic neuropathy. J Auton Nerv Sys 1998;69:164–172.

74. Gemmill JD, Venables GS, Ewing DJ. Noradrenaline response to edrophonium in primary autonomic failure: distinction between central and peripheral damage. Lancet 1988;i:1018–1021.

75. Leveston SA, Shah SD, Cryer PE. Cholinergic stimulation of norepinephrine release in man. Evidence of a sympathetic postganglionic axonal lesion in diabetic adrenergic neuropathy. J Clin Invest 1979;64:374–380.

76. Fujimura J, Camilleri M, Low PA, et al. Effect of perturbations and a meal on superior mesenteric artery flow in patients with orthostatic hypotension. J Auton Nerv Sys 1997;67:15–23.

may be due to a delayed or absent pharyngeal swallow response, impaired tongue control, or a variety of other less frequent problems.[56] Aspiration is common in these individuals,[56] with a rate of over 40%,[55] and rehabilitation may take longer.[54]

Delayed gastric emptying may occur following traumatic brain injury.[57] The impairment is typically, but not invariably, transient and may respond to treatment with prokinetic agents such as metoclopramide[58] and cisapride.[59] The anatomic or pathologic basis for the dysfunction is unknown.

Inadvertent intracranial placement of nasogastric tubes is an iatrogenic GI-related complication following traumatic brain injury that is reported with surprising frequency.[60–66] Stress ulcers with consequent GI hemorrhage may also develop following traumatic brain injury, especially in the setting of steroid administration in an effort to control intracranial hypertension.[67–69]

DISORDERS AFFECTING BASAL GANGLIA

Parkinson's Disease

In recent years the occurrence and importance of GI dysfunction in Parkinson's disease (PD) has been increasingly recognized and characterized. However, credit for the initial description of such GI dysfunction must go to James Parkinson himself who, in his seminal 1817 monograph, provided a surprisingly detailed description of virtually all of the currently recognized GI features of PD. He describes *disordered swallowing*: "the saliva fails of being directed to the back part of the fauces, and hence it is continually draining from the mouth"; *dysphagia*: "food is with difficulty retained in the mouth until masticated; and then as difficultly swallowed"; *constipation:* "the bowels which all along had been torpid, now in most cases, demand stimulating medications of very considerable power"; and *difficult defecation*: "the expulsion of the feces from the rectum sometimes requiring mechanical aid."[70]

Following Parkinson's initial description, little attention was subsequently paid to this aspect of PD until Eadie and Tyrer in 1965 provided an analysis of GI dysfunction in 107 patients with parkinsonism (49 with idiopathic PD), compared to a comparably aged control group of persons with "acute orthopedic" disorders.[71] They found chewing difficulty, drooling of saliva, dysphagia, frequent heartburn, and constipation to be present more frequently in persons with PD than in control subjects. Edwards and colleagues revisited this issue 26 years later in a survey of 98 individuals with PD and 50 comparably aged spousal controls.[72] In this and a subsequent series of papers these authors have identified and further characterized five features of GI dysfunction in PD: disordered salivation, dysphagia, nausea, constipation, and defecatory dysfunction.[73–75] Pfeiffer and Quigley have subsequently provided more recent reviews of this same topic.[76–80]

Disordered Salivation

Individuals with PD often describe a sense of increased saliva in the mouth and may experience drooling. The drooling may range in severity from a mere tendency to wet the pillow at night to prominent drooling during the daytime that forces the individual to have a handkerchief constantly in hand or in shirt pocket. Disordered salivation was noted in 78% of PD patients by Eadie and Tyrer[71] in their survey, while Edwards and colleagues documented it in 70% of PD patients, compared to 6% of controls.[72]

While it has often been assumed that the tendency of patients with PD to drool is a reflection of increased salivary production, quite the opposite has been the case when salivary secretion has actually been measured. Eadie measured resting salivary secretion in both PD patients and controls and found no significant difference between the two.[81] Bateson and colleagues also compared salivary secretion in PD patients to that in controls, and further subdivided the PD patients into those who described drooling and those who noted a dry mouth.[82] They found no difference in salivary flow between the dry-mouthed and drooling PD patients, and documented that both groups produced less saliva than controls. Korczyn, in a review of autonomic dysfunction in PD, refers to some of his unpublished data in which the amount of saliva produced by individuals with PD was normal.[83] More recent studies have again noted diminished saliva production in PD patients.[84] Thus, it appears that saliva production is decreased, or at best normal, in PD and that drooling is, then, a consequence of impaired swallowing, with pooling of saliva in the mouth, rather than the result of actual excess saliva production.

This, in turn, has several implications for treatment. Oral anticholinergic medications have traditionally been utilized in this situation to reduce saliva production. However, since saliva production is already normal or diminished in PD, reducing secretion further by employing systemic anticholinergic therapy is potentially problematic, and Korczyn notes that such drugs may actually aggravate the problem by making the saliva more viscous, further impeding swallowing.[85] Potent oral anticholinergic agents such as trihexyphenidyl, moreover, are also prone to produce significant toxicity in elderly individuals. Recently, a potential pathway around these problems has been reported in that sublingual application of a 1% atropine ophthalmic solution twice daily may safely and effectively reduce drooling in persons with PD.[86] Marsden notes that radiation of the salivary glands to reduce salivary secretion is generally an unsatisfactory approach to this problem.[87] Levodopa administration may be helpful, presumably by improving swallowing,[83,85] and the use of the mucolytic agent, bromhexine, has been reported to be useful.[83] Simply asking the patient to chew gum or suck on hard candy, especially during social occasions where drooling might be particularly embarrassing, is a "low-tech" but often effective approach to the problem of drooling, probably because it temporarily converts the act of swallowing to a more conscious action.

Intraparotid injections of botulinum toxin have also recently been effectively employed in alleviating parkinsonian drooling. Subjective improvement was noted by 75% of individuals and objective reduction of saliva formation was documented in 62.5%.[88] A potential risk of this treatment approach in the form of pharyngeal muscular weakness needs to be borne in mind.

Dysphagia

Swallowing is a very complex act that requires precisely coordinated action of a multitude of muscles, mixing both voluntary and reflex actions that are mediated at both brainstem and cortical levels. It should not be surprising then, that such an exquisitely choreographed motor action should become impaired in PD; and indeed, such is the case.

The reported frequency of dysphagia in PD varies considerably from study to study, depending partly upon the method of ascertainment. In the large survey studies of Edwards and colleagues and of Eadie and Tyrer, where patients reported symptoms of dysphagia, frequencies of 52% and 50% respectively were described (vs. 6% and 12% in controls).[71,72] Leopold and Kagel reported an even higher frequency of 82% and attributed this higher number to the detailed nature of their questionnaire.[89] When disordered swallowing is studied by objective techniques, such as the modified barium swallow (MBS) test, the number of patients with abnormalities of the oral or pharyngeal phases of swallowing is in the 75–95% range.[90,91]

Correlation between subjective symptoms and objective findings of dysphagia in individuals with PD is surprisingly low. Patients with objective swallowing abnormalities—sometimes severe—may have no symptoms at all, while other persons may describe very troublesome swallowing difficulty, but have completely normal radiographic and other swallowing studies. Bushman and colleagues noted a variety of abnormalities (see below) on MBS in 75% of the 20 patients they studied, but only 35% actually reported swallowing complaints.[90] Similarly, Logemann and colleagues detailed abnormalities on MBS in 95% of their study sample of PD patients, while less than 20% reported symptoms of dysphagia.[91] In contrast, in a study of 13 patients with PD by Edwards and colleagues, 77% experienced dysphagia while only 38% were found to have abnormalities on blinded analysis of videoesophagrams.[75]

Dysphagia severe enough to produce aspiration can occur in a significant number of individuals with PD and the aspiration may be completely silent. Bushman and colleagues noted true (tracheal) aspiration in 15% of their study subjects; none had symptoms of aspiration.[90] They noted an additional 35% to have vestibular aspiration, in which the vocal cords were not penetrated. In a study of 6 patients with PD, all with disordered swallowing demonstrated on MBS, Robbins and colleagues noted aspiration in two—both were without symptoms.[92] Ali and colleagues utilized simultaneous videoradiography and pharyngeal manometry to study 19 individuals with PD, 12 of whom had symptomatic dysphagia.[93] They found aspiration in 33% of subjects with dysphagia and in 14% of those without. Utilizing videofluoroscopy, Stroudley and Walsh studied 24 PD patients with symptomatic dysphagia and found tracheal aspiration in 46%.[94] Thus, it appears that aspiration is a significant—and potentially life-threatening—complication of PD that may be amenable to treatment if discovered.

In the large survey studies, the presence of symptomatic dysphagia appeared to correlate with increasing severity of PD.[71,72] This correlation, however, has not been so clear when objective measurements of dysphagia are employed.[90,93] On rare occasions, dysphagia may actually be the presenting clinical feature of PD.[95,96]

The pathophysiologic mechanisms responsible for dysphagia in PD appear to lie at multiple levels. While oral and pharyngeal abnormalities have been studied most thoroughly, it is quite clear that dysfunction in all three phases of swallowing—oral, pharyngeal, and esophageal—occurs in PD. Patients with PD experiencing dysphagia typically localize the site of dysfunction to the back of the throat.[72,97] However, this does not seem to accurately predict the site of abnormality on objective testing.[75]

Since the tongue and other oral muscles are typical striated muscles, it should not be surprising they would be affected in PD, and that rigidity and bradykinesia of these muscles might produce functional impairment. This, indeed, appears to be so. Logemann and her colleagues were among the earliest to report abnormalities of lingual control in PD.[98,99] Bushmann and colleagues described decreased tongue and oral mobility in some of their study subjects, along with disturbed lingual peristalsis and increased oral transit time.[90] They also noted that repetitive tongue pumping was employed by some individuals to move the food bolus into the pharynx. Robbins and her colleagues also noted this.[92] Silbiger and colleagues described hesitancy in initiating swallowing and difficulty with bolus formation in their study subjects[100]; reduced bolus control was also noted by Stroudley and Walsh.[94] Tongue tremor also occurs in PD and is present in some individuals with dysphagia.[92,93] Indeed, Ali and colleagues found lingual tremor to be significantly more frequent in PD patients with dysphagia than in those without.[93]

Pharyngeal abnormalities also contribute to dysphagia in PD. Delayed swallowing reflex, decreased pharyngeal peristalsis, abnormal pharyngeal wall motion, decreased laryngeal elevation, vallecular stasis, vallecular and pyriform sinus residue, and pharyngeal and vallecular wall coating have all been described.[90,92–94] Therefore, impaired pharyngeal bolus transport has been suggested to be a major determinant of dysphagia in persons with PD.[77,93] In contrast, Calne and colleagues found no abnormality of pharyngeal deglutition in a study of 19 subjects with PD.[101] The reason for this divergent result was not clear to the investigators, although they suggested that their patients may have had less severe PD.

Cricopharyngeal dysfunction has also been linked to dysphagia in PD. Palmer rather boldly suggested that in PD the basis for difficulty swallowing "is almost always hypopharyngeal dysphagia" due to either delayed opening or premature closing of the cricopharyngeus muscle as the food bolus descends, and that cricopharyngeal sphincterotomy is the treatment of choice.[102] Many other investigators, however, make no mention of cricopharyngeal dysfunction in their study subjects.[90,92,94,101] In more recent studies, cricopharyngeal dysfunction has been documented in a relatively small percentage of individuals with PD and dysphagia. Byrne and colleagues noted this in 22% of 23 subjects with PD evaluated for dysphagia, specifically describing the presence of Zenker's diverticula and cricopharyngeal bars in these patients.[103] In a subsequent report, Born and colleagues describe these five patients—two with a Zenker's diverticulum and three with cricopharyngeus muscle dysfunction—with PD and dysphagia.[104] Cricopharyngeal myotomy (with Zenker's diverticolotomy when present) was performed in four of the five subjects with subsequent improvement in or resolution of dysphagia, confirming that in at least some patients with PD, cricopharyngeal dysfunction is responsible for dysphagia. Ali and colleagues demonstrated diminished upper esophageal sphincter opening in patients with PD and dysphagia, and noted this to be multifactorial in its mechanism.[93] In some instances it was due to incomplete sphincter relaxation, but more often it was the result of diminished pharyngeal propulsive forces. Quigley has, therefore, suggested that three basic, possibly interrelated, factors are responsible for the development of dysphagia in PD: lingual tremor (or festination), pharyngeal peristaltic dysfunction, and impaired opening of the upper esophageal sphincter.[76,77]

While it has received considerably less attention than oropharyngeal dysfunction, esophageal dysmotility clearly occurs in some individuals with PD and dysphagia. Exactly how often it occurs, however, is an unsettled matter. In 1942 Penner and Druckerman provided an early description of segmental esophageal spasms in two individuals with PD, but did not study the frequency of this abnormality in the PD population.[105] Subsequently, Eadie and Tyrer noted the radiographic presence of segmental esophageal spasms in 5% of 72 patients with PD,[106] and Gibberd and colleagues documented abnormal esophageal peristalsis in 25% of the 37 subjects with PD (not selected for GI symptoms) they studied.[107] Blonsky and colleagues noted slowing of the esophageal transit of food bolus in 86% of the 100 PD patients they studied, in contrast to 10% of controls and 10% of subjects with essential tremor.[99] More recently, Byrne and colleagues described esophageal abnormalities in 65% of the 23 patients with PD and dysphagia that they studied.[103] In adding some possible perspective to these figures, however, Edwards and colleagues noted that while 69% of the 13 PD subjects they studied demonstrated dysmotility of the esophageal body on esophagography, so did 43% of their 7 age-matched control subjects.[75]

That esophageal function might be impaired in PD should not be surprising, since the proximal one-third of the esophagus is composed exclusively of striated muscle, and in the middle one-third striated and smooth muscle interdigitate. The rigidity and bradykinesia characteristic of PD might be expected to compromise muscle function here, just as elsewhere. Degeneration of the dorsal motor nucleus of the vagus, which clearly occurs in PD,[108] might be responsible for esophageal dysfunction in PD. In fact, neuronal loss and Lewy body formation isolated to the dorsal motor nucleus of the vagus have been described in individuals presenting clinically with dysphagia and no other PD features.[109] Peripheral pathologic mechanisms, which could account for esophageal dysfunction in PD separate from any CNS pathology, have also been described. Myenteric plexus pathology, with Lewy body formation, has been documented in PD.[110] The pathologic changes and Lewy body formation were noted at all levels of the esophagus, and were actually more prominent distally. A role for dopamine in esophageal function and the presence of dopamine receptors in the esophageal wall have been proposed by Mukhopadhyay and Weisbrodt, based on studies in the opossum.[111] Moreover, in this study bilateral cervical vagotomy did not alter the esophageal response to intravenous dopamine administration.

Esophageal dysfunction in PD may assume several forms and its mechanism is uncertain. As noted above, segmental esophageal spasm was first described in PD over 60 years ago[105] and later noted in 5% of patients studied radiographically.[106] Bramble and colleagues, however, did not record esophageal spasm in any of the 20 patients they studied manometrically, despite prolonged recording.[112] Lieberman and his colleagues demonstrated the presence of nonpropulsive tertiary contractions in the esophagus of both patients they studied; pharyngeal abnormalities were also present in both.[113] In 16% of 37 PD patients studied by Gibberd and colleagues, esophageal dilatation was present, but only one patient (3%) experienced symptomatic dysphagia.[107] Kempster and colleagues described two individuals with PD who experienced prominent and distressing belching that was primarily confined to "off" periods when levodopa effectiveness was lost.[114] Barium fluoroscopic studies demonstrated abnormal esophageal motility, with ineffective or tertiary contractions and air trapping in both patients and esophageal dilatation in one. Both the belching and the fluoroscopic abnormalities completely resolved following apomorphine administration, leading the authors to suggest that central dopaminergic mechanisms are responsible for esophageal dysmotility in PD. Bramble and colleagues, in contrast, suggested that cholinergic, rather than dopaminergic, mechanisms are of foremost importance in the control of swallowing in PD, since atropine disrupted esophageal peristalsis when given intravenously.[112] They also noted no significant difference in lower esophageal sphincter pressure between PD patients and controls.

Gastroesophageal reflux may develop in individuals with PD. Blonsky and colleagues noted radiographic evidence of reflux in 25% of their PD patients, compared to 10% of comparably-aged controls.[99] Byrne and colleagues described reflux symptoms in 26% of the 43 patients with PD referred to them for evaluation of GI problems.[103] Advanced reflux disease and esophagitis may develop; treatment with appropriate antireflux measures may lead to significant improvement in symptomatic dysphagia.[77,103]

Gastroparesis

Delayed gastric emptying is a common GI manifestation of autonomic neuropathy, and is characterized by a variety of symptoms that may include postprandial abdominal discomfort or fullness, early satiety, nausea, vomiting, weight loss, and even malnutrition.[57] Some,[115,116] although not all,[117] investigators have noted a reduction in gastric emptying rate with aging. Since individuals with PD tend to be elderly, this information by itself is of potential significance. More importantly, Djaldetti and colleagues, utilizing a radionuclide gastric emptying technique, have reported that gastric emptying is slowed in PD compared to control subjects.[118] This interpretation, however, is clouded by the fact that the mean age of their control group was almost 20 years younger than the mean age of their PD patients. Harada and colleagues reported similar findings while employing an acetaminophen absorption method of measurement of gastric emptying.[119] Age of patients and controls was not mentioned in this abstract. More recent studies have also confirmed the development of impaired gastric emptying in PD.[120]

Individuals with PD may display symptoms that suggest the presence of gastroparesis. Edwards and colleagues noted an increased frequency of nausea in patients with PD that could not be explained simply on the basis of medication toxicity,[72,74] and suggested that at least in some instances this nausea might be a manifestation of gastroparesis. Marsden adds postprandial fullness and vomiting as PD symptoms attributable to abnormalities of gastric emptying.[87]

Investigators utilizing electrogastrography (EGG) have also documented abnormalities in persons with PD, even in untreated individuals. The clinical significance of these abnormalities, however, is still uncertain.[121,122]

Delayed gastric emptying, if present, also has important implications in the pharmacologic management of PD. Levodopa is primarily absorbed from the small intestine.[123–125] If release of levodopa from the stomach is delayed, intestinal absorption will be also. Indeed, "trapping" of levodopa in the stomach with delayed or erratic release has been proposed to play a role in the development of at least some of the motor fluctuations that can occur with levodopa therapy, especially the "delayed-on" and "no-on" phenomena, in which patients experience either prolonged latency from the time of levodopa ingestion until onset of clinical efficacy ("delayed-on"), or no response at all from a given levodopa dose ("no-on").[118,126,127] Random fluctuations of parkinsonian mobility have also been ascribed to erratic gastric emptying.[128] Motor fluctuations of these types can be improved by the employment of prokinetic agents that improve gastric emptying, such as cisapride,[129,130] and by constant duodenal levodopa infusion, which totally bypasses the stomach.[128,131] Domperidone has also been shown to improve gastric emptying in persons with PD, although its effect on motor fluctuations was not assessed.[132]

The mechanism by which gastric emptying might be impaired in PD is not certain. Traditional doctrine would look to the CNS as the source of the dysfunction, perhaps via vagally-mediated mechanisms. Increasing evidence is accumulating, however, that suggests that enteric nervous system involvement is an integral part of the PD process and may be responsible for GI dysfunction independent from any CNS factors.[74] The discovery by Wakabayashi and colleagues of Lewy bodies in both myenteric and submucosal plexuses in the stomach of individuals with PD further supports this suggestion.[133]

For the pharmacologic management of PD, prolonged gastric retention of administered levodopa may also lead to additional consequences. Aromatic amino acid decarboxylase is present in the gastric mucosa.[116,118] Prolonged gastric retention of levodopa can, thus, result in increased decarboxylation of the levodopa to dopamine, which renders it inaccessible to the CNS and further reduces dose efficacy. The dopamine formed within the stomach may then actually retard gastric emptying still further,[134,135] perhaps via stimulation of gastric dopamine receptors that promote receptive relaxation of the stomach and inhibit gastric motility,[136] thus initiating a potentially vicious circle of events that may lead to erratic and suboptimal dose-response patterns.

Gastric secretion may also be reduced in PD.[81] The clinical importance of this observation is unclear, especially since it is excessive gastric acidity that can slow gastric emptying and interfere with levodopa efficacy.[137] Magnesium-containing antacid therapy promotes gastric motility through the action of gastrin[138] and, thus, may improve levodopa response, presumably by accelerating gastric emptying.[137] Excessive use of antacids, however, may also result in incomplete carbidopa/levodopa tablet dissolution with reduced efficacy.[139]

Small Intestine Dysmotility

Because of its relative inaccessibility, the small intestine has received slight attention in the setting of PD, and little is known of its function or dysfunction in patients with PD. Several studies have shown no effect of aging on small intestinal function,[117,140,141] although Anuras and Sutherland did demonstrate reduced postprandial jejunal motility in individuals aged 65–85.[142] Bozeman and colleagues described abnormalities in small intestinal motor patterns in PD subjects studied with manometry,[143] but did not report whether these changes were associated with clinical symptoms. Dilatation of the small intestine has also been reported in PD.[144]

In the clinic, patients are occasionally encountered who experience a sensation of abdominal tightness and bloating, which can be excruciatingly uncomfortable. These individuals usually are suffering fluctuations in motor performance as a consequence of levodopa therapy, and the episodes of subjective abdominal bloating and tightness occur virtually exclusively during "off" periods when the patients are rigid and immobile. They may unbutton trousers in an attempt to relieve the sense of tightness (even though the trousers may already be very loose) and may become agitated or even panicky because of the subjective discomfort. The physiologic basis for this phenomenon is uncertain. Tightness or rigidity of abdominal musculature is one possible explanation, but dilatation of small intestine could conceivably also be responsible.

The pathophysiology of small intestine dysfunction in PD is uncertain. As with dysfunction at other levels of the GI tract, both central and enteric nervous system mechanisms are possible. Studies by Eaker and colleagues with MPTP in rats have demonstrated disruption of the MMC in the jejunum.[145] The authors suggested that the effect of the MPTP was mediated at an ENS, rather than CNS, level.

Since levodopa is primarily absorbed from the proximal small intestine,[123–125] it should not be surprising that processes that affect the absorption sites at this level can alter levodopa efficacy. The competition between protein (specifically large neutral amino acids) and levodopa for both GI and blood-brain barrier transport is widely recognized.[146] A more unusual example of levodopa malabsorption is the case report by Gatto and colleagues describing loss of levodopa efficacy due to *Strongyloides stercoralis*-induced duodenitis.[147] Appropriate antiparasitic treatment restored levodopa efficacy.

Constipation and Defecatory Dysfunction

Difficulty with bowel function is probably the most widely recognized GI manifestation of PD. It is not unusual for PD patients to rank difficulty with bowel movements as a greater source of discomfort and aggravation than the traditional motor features of PD, much to the subsequent discomfort of their neurologist, who may feel ill-prepared to provide advice on this "non-neurological" aspect of PD.

It has become evident that bowel dysfunction in PD may actually assume two forms. Decreased frequency of bowel movements may be present. Alternatively, patients may experience difficulty with the actual act of defecation, finding it necessary to strain excessively in order to expel the stool; at times complete evacuation cannot be achieved. The term constipation is typically utilized when decreased frequency is the problem, while the term defecatory dysfunction is employed for the constellation of straining and incomplete evacuation. Of course, individuals may experience both facets of bowel dysfunction simultaneously.

In their 1965 survey, Eadie and Tyrer noted that 51% of their subjects did not have daily bowel movements, compared to 13% of controls.[71] Furthermore, 52% were using laxatives regularly. They did not assess defecatory dysfunction. Earlier, Schwab and England had found constipation to be present in two-thirds of their patients.[148] Pallis also reported that constipation is very common in parkinsonism, especially in more severe cases.[149] Edwards and colleagues queried their patients regarding both constipation and defecatory dysfunction and, to their surprise, found that defecatory dysfunction was actually the more common of the two problems.[72] Using a more contemporary definition of constipation as having a bowel movement less than three times weekly, they found this to be the case with 29% of their PD subjects, compared to 10% of their spousal controls. Meanwhile, 67% of the subjects experienced defecatory dysfunction, along with 28% of controls.

Decreased bowel movement frequency in PD is generally ascribed to slowed transit of fecal material through the colon. Prolonged colon transit times in PD patients have been documented both by Jost[150,151] and by Edwards[75] and their colleagues, with mean transit times ranging from 44–90 hours.

Impaired colonic function in PD is also reflected in multiple case reports of megacolon in individuals with parkinsonism.[144,152–154] The older reports contain a mixture of PD, postencephalitic parkinsonism, and multiple system atrophy cases, but it is quite clear that megacolon is seen in individuals with parkinsonism with a higher than expected frequency. Megacolon by itself can produce the picture of pseudoobstruction and may result in bowel perforation.[77] Volvulus, especially in the sigmoid region, can also develop as a complication of megacolon in PD and produce frank mechanical obstruction.[71,152,153] Sigmoid volvulus, once it occurs, has a predilection to recur and may have fatal consequences with an overall mortality rate of 25%.[155] Surgical management may be required.

While a variety of factors, such as physical inactivity, antiparkinson medication (especially anticholinergic drugs), inadequate fluid intake, and deficient abdominal and diaphragmatic muscle function, have been invoked as being responsible for, or at least contributory to, colonic dysfunction in PD,[144,148,149,152] it is becoming increasingly evident that enteric nervous system involvement as an integral part of the PD process itself may be at least partially, if not largely, responsible. Edwards and colleagues found no correlation of diet or physical activity with GI dysfunction in PD,[72] and Kupsky and colleagues demonstrated the presence of Lewy bodies in colonic myenteric and submucosal plexuses from a patient with PD and megacolon.[154] In a series of reports, Wakabayashi and colleagues have detailed the occurrence of Lewy bodies throughout the GI tract in PD and have noted that, in contrast to the CNS, the ENS Lewy bodies are primarily in VIP-containing neurons.[133,156–159] More recently, Singaram and colleagues have demonstrated a marked deficiency of dopaminergic neurons in colonic myenteric plexus from patients with PD and constipation; 9 of the 11 PD patients studied also had megacolon.[160] Importantly, this dopaminergic depletion was not present in patients with idiopathic constipation without PD. The investigators also confirmed the presence of Lewy bodies in VIP-containing neurons.

The vexing problem of defecatory dysfunction in PD has been the focus of increasing interest and study. The act of defecation requires rather precisely coordinated action of a number of muscles in order to proceed smoothly; both reflex and voluntary mechanisms are operative. Fecal continence is normally maintained by contraction of the internal anal sphincter, which is under autonomic control, and the external anal sphincter and puborectalis muscles, which are under voluntary control, with the internal sphincter shouldering the primary responsibility.[161] Formation of an "anorectal angle," produced by anterior pull of the puborectalis muscle, has been felt by some to be an important element in maintaining continence,[162] although others have questioned its importance.[161] During defecation, these muscles relax while the glottic, diaphragmatic, and abdominal wall muscles contract simultaneously, elevating intra-abdominal pressure; colonic pressure waves also may occur.[163,164]

Mathers and colleagues have documented that some individuals with PD and constipation display a disturbed pattern of muscle activity in which there is paradoxical contraction of the external anal sphincter and puborectalis muscles during attempted defecation, producing functional outlet obstruction.[163,164] They suggested that this represented a focal dystonic phenomenon. More recently, Bassotti and colleagues confirmed the presence of pelvic floor dysynergia in over 60% of individuals with PD, utilizing anorectal manometry to document the abnormality.[165] Edwards and colleagues noted altered puborectalis muscle function, with failure to relax and widen the anorectal angle during straining, in 31% of the 13 PD patients they studied with defecography; none of their seven control subjects displayed this pattern.[75] However, incomplete evacuation was noted in comparable percentages of PD patients and controls (54% vs. 57%). In the same study, anorectal manometry revealed several distinctive abnormalities in the PD subjects. Lower basal sphincter pressure was noted, as was an inability to maintain a sustained increase in sphincter pressure.[75] This decay in sphincter sustained squeeze pressure and squeeze duration (squeeze index) is probably analogous to the fatigue that is frequently evident during other skeletal muscle activity in PD, which may be a component of parkinsonian akinesia.[166] Additionally, prominent phasic contractions of the sphincter muscle were evident during the squeeze maneuver in 77% of the PD patients, compared to 14% of controls. Perhaps the most striking abnormality, however, was the presence of a hyper-contractile response on testing of the rectosphincteric reflex, instead of the expected relaxation of the sphincter. This abnormality was seen in no control subjects. In a follow-up study utilizing simultaneous anorectal manometry and electromyography, Ashraf and colleagues demonstrated that this hyper-contractile response originates in the external anal sphincter and puborectalis muscles.[167] Furthermore, they demonstrated definite deterioration in anorectal function during "off" periods, paralleling the deterioration seen in other facets of motor function. Improvement in both defecographic and anorectal manometric abnormalities was documented following apomorphine administration by Edwards and colleagues.[168] Since the subjects had been pretreated with the peripheral dopamine antagonist, domperidone, prior to apomorphine administration, a CNS localization for the effect of apomorphine on anorectal function was suggested. Mathers and colleagues noted similar improvement in defecographic abnormalities following apomorphine administration in the PD patients they studied.[164] Ashraf and colleagues have also reinforced recognition that the pattern of abnormalities detailed in the aforementioned studies is specific for PD and not simply a general reflection of constipation. In a study in which 15 PD patients, 9 persons with chronic idiopathic constipation, and 8 control subjects were evaluated with anorectal manometry, they found no significant differences between the control and idiopathic constipation groups, while the PD group again demonstrated abnormalities noted in previous studies.[169]

Fecal incontinence may also occur in PD. Byrne and colleagues described incontinence in 24% of the 33 PD patients with symptoms of bowel dysfunction that they studied.[103] The incontinence was attributed to overflow around fecal impaction and usually resolved with treatment of the constipation.

Multiple System Atrophy

The term multiple system atrophy (MSA), originally introduced by Graham and Oppenheimer,[170] has now become the generally accepted terminology for a multi-faceted, sporadic, neurodegenerative disease process that may feature either a predominantly parkinsonian or a predominantly cerebellar syndrome, usually with associated progressive autonomic failure; degenerative cell loss occurs at multiple sites in cerebrum, brainstem, and spinal cord.[171–174] It encompasses the entities previously referred to as Shy-Drager syndrome, striatonigral degeneration, and the sporadic form of olivopontocerebellar atrophy.

Although other features of autonomic failure, especially orthostatic hypotension and genitourinary dysfunction, have received the most attention, GI difficulties also regularly occur in MSA. In many respects the GI abnormalities mirror those of PD; however, differences exist and postprandial hypotension, in particular, is more frequent in MSA.

Salivary gland dysfunction may occur in MSA and produce xerostomia,[175] although this is relatively uncommon.[176] When parkinsonian features are prominent, impaired swallowing ability can result in excess saliva accumulation in the mouth.

Dysphagia is quite common in MSA and may even be episodic in the early stages of the illness.[177] Smith and Bryan described feeding difficulties in 50% of the 10 patients they studied,[178] and Mathias notes that, while symptoms suggestive of aspiration (coughing, choking) may occur, the swallowing abnormalities seen on testing may be clinically silent.[176] While oropharyngeal dysfunction appears to be the principal localization for dysphagia in MSA,[176,178] abnormalities in esophageal motility have also been described.[179] Botulinum toxin injections, sometimes utilized for treating cervical dystonia in MSA, may also precipitate dysphagia.[180]

Postprandial fullness, suggesting impaired gastric emptying, may occur in MSA but is uncommon.[176] However, gastric emptying and small intestine function have not been extensively studied in MSA.

A more significant GI problem for individuals with MSA is the development of postprandial hypotension, which occurs as a result of vasodilatation in the splanchnic circulation that is not counterbalanced by compensatory cardiovascular changes because of the sympathetic dysfunction present in MSA.[176] The blood pressure usually falls within 15 minutes of food ingestion and hypotension may then persist for as long as three hours.[181,182] Carbohydrates are most prone to produce postprandial hypotension, lipids less so, and protein least likely.[183] Alcohol will accentuate the hypotension.[176] Treatment approaches include smaller and more frequent meals, reduced carbohydrate content of meals, avoidance of alcohol, and employment of pharmacological measures such as indomethacin, caffeine, and octreotide.[176,184,185]

Constipation and fecal incontinence were included by Shy and Drager in their original description of what now is called MSA.[186] Constipation actually occurs in the majority of individuals with MSA and may become severe.[176] Sigmoid volvulus has also been described.[153] Anal sphincter EMG studies have delineated a characteristic abnormality in MSA, consisting of a pattern of denervation and reinnervation.[187,188] The urethral sphincter is similarly involved, and it is suspected that the sphincter abnormalities are the consequence of neuronal degeneration in Onuf's nucleus in the sacral spinal cord.[176,187,188] These abnormalities have been suggested to be of diagnostic value in the clinical evaluation of individuals with suspected MSA,[189] but the reliability and specificity of this abnormality has been questioned.[190–194]

Progressive Supranuclear Palsy

Progressive supranuclear palsy (PSP) was first described in 1964, and dysphagia was noted by Steele and colleagues to be a frequent clinical feature.[195] In a subsequent report, Steele also described drooling and symptoms of aspiration along with dysphagia in some individuals with PSP.[196] Others have confirmed the occurrence of dysphagia in PSP.[197–199] Golbe and colleagues suggest that dysphagia is almost invariably present in advanced PSP.[200] In a recent study, Johnston and colleagues studied seven patients with PSP, utilizing modified barium swallow (MBS) and esophageal manometry.[201] Slow mastication and delayed initiation of swallowing were noted on MBS in four of the six patients tested, while diffuse esophageal spasm was noted on manometry in 29% of the patients, and inadequate relaxation of the upper esophageal sphincter during swallowing in 43%. Similar oral phase abnormalities were noted by Sonies in a videofluoroscopic study of 22 patients with PSP.[202] Leopold and Kagel also documented a rather extensive array of abnormalities in individuals with PSP undergoing videofluoroscopy.[198] Unlike PD, the severity of dysphagia experienced by PSP patients correlated well with the radiographic abnormalities.[201,202] For patients with PSP, eating difficulties may be compounded by difficulty with inferior gaze and by neck extension, both making it harder to see the plate.

Other aspects of GI function have not been extensively studied in PSP, although abnormalities on anal sphincter EMG were noted in 42% of 12 patients studied by Valldeoriola and colleagues.[203]

Huntington's Disease

Gastrointestinal dysfunction is not a striking feature of Huntington's disease, but dysphagia can occur and primarily involves the oropharyngeal phase of swallowing.[204] In a study of 35 patients, Kagel and Leopold demonstrated a variety of oral and pharyngeal abnormalities on videofluoroscopy, including oral-stage retention, delayed lingual transfer, pharyngeal dysmotility, and laryngeal incoordination.[205] Esophageal dysfunction was also noted in 31%.

SUMMARY

Gastrointestinal dysfunction can be found in a broad array of disorders affecting the cerebral hemispheres. In this chapter, several of these disorders have been highlighted to serve as illustrations of the diversity and complexity of interactions that exist between the nervous and gastrointestinal systems. The increasing recognition of the role played by the enteric nervous system in at least some of these neurological disorders adds another layer of intricacy to the web of interaction. In this group of neurological diseases, gastrointestinal problems are not just a minor curiosity. They occur frequently and have important ramifications for both patient safety and comfort. Prompt recognition of and attendance to these problems is vital and the skills of both neurologist and gastroenterologist are often necessary to manage the patient optimally.

ACKNOWLEDGMENT

The superb secretarial assistance of Stacey Fifer and Sharon Williams is gratefully appreciated.

REFERENCES

1. Livingston S. Abdominal pain as a manifestation of epilepsy (abdominal epilepsy) in children. J Pediatr 1951;38:687–675.
2. Douglas EF, White PT. Abdominal epilepsy—a reappraisal. J Pediatr 1971;78:59–67.
3. Babb RR, Echman PB. Abdominal epilepsy. JAMA 1972;222:65–66.
4. Peppercorn MA, Herzog AG, Dichter MA, Mayman CI. Abdominal epilepsy. JAMA 1978; 2450–2451.
5. Mitchell WG, Greenwood RS, Messenheimer JA. Abdominal epilepsy. Cyclic vomiting as the major symptom of simple partial seizures. Arch Neurol 1983;40:251–252.
6. Gastaut H, Poirier F. Experimental, or "reflex," induction of seizures. Report of a case of abdominal (enteric) epilepsy. Epilepsia 1964;5:256–270.
7. Mulder DW, Daly D, Bailey AA. Visceral epilepsy. Arch Int Med 1954;93:481–493.
8. Jacome DE, Fitzgerald R. Ictus emeticus. Neurology 1982;32:209–212.
9. Kramer RE, Lüders H, Goldstick LP, et al. Ictus emeticus: an electroclinical analysis. Neurology 1988;38:1048–1052.
10. Devinsky O, Frasca J, Pacia SV, et al. Ictus emeticus: Further evidence of nondominant temporal involvement. Neurology 1995;45:1158–1160.
11. Gastaut H. Les troubles du comportement alimentaire chez les epileptiques psychomoteurs. Rev Neurol 1955;92:55–62.
12. Fisher CM. Hunger and the temporal lobe. Neurology 1994;44:1577–1579.

13. Penfield WG, Jasper H. Epilepsy and the Functional Anatomy of the Human Brain. Boston: Little, Brown & Company, 1954.
14. Gordon C, Langton-Hewer R, Wade D. Dysphagia in acute stroke. Br Med J 1987;295: 411–414.
15. Teasell R, Foley N, Fisher J, Finestone H. The incidence, management, and complications of dysphagia in patients with medullary strokes admitted to a rehabilitation unit. Dysphagia 2002;17:115–120.
16. Horner J, Massey EW, Riski JE, et al. Aspiration following stroke: clinical correlates and outcome. Neurology 1988;38:1359–1362.
17. Robbins J, Levine RL, Maser A, et al. Swallowing after unilateral stroke of the cerebral cortex. Arch Phys Med Rehabil 1993;74:1295–1300.
18. Baer DH. The natural history and functional consequences of dysphagia after hemispheric stroke. J Neurol Neurosurg Psychiatry 1989;52:236–241.
19. Wong EH, Pullicino PM, Benedict R. Deep cerebral infarcts extending to the subinsular region. Stroke 2001;32:2272–2277.
20. Aziz Q, Rothwell JC, Hamdy S, et al. The topographic representation of esophageal motor function on the human cerebral cortex. Gastroenterology 1996;111:855–862.
21. Hamdy S, Aziz Q, Rothwell JC, et al. The cortical topography of human swallowing musculature in health and disease. Nat Med 1996;2:1217–1224.
22. Hamdy S, Aziz Q, Rothwell JC, et al. Explaining oropharyngeal dysphagia after unilateral hemispheric stroke. Lancet 1997;350:686–692.
23. Hamdy S, Aziz Q, Rothwell JC, et al. Recovery of swallowing after dysphagic stroke relates to functional reorganization in the intact motor cortex. Gastroenterology 1998;115: 1104–1012.
24. Ullman T, Reding M. Gastrointestinal dysfunction in stroke. Semin Neurol 1996;16: 269–275.
25. Veis S, Logemann J. Swallowing disorders in persons with cerebrovascular accident. Arch Phys Med Rehabil 1985;66:372–375.
26. Wang Y, Lim LL, Levi C, et al. A prognostic index for 30-day mortality after stroke. J Clin Epidemiol 2001;54:766–773.
27. Sharma JC, Fletcher S, Vassallo M, Ross I. What influences outcome of stroke—pyrexia or dysphagia? Int J Clin Pract 2001;55:17–20.
28. Celifacrco A, Gerard G, Faegenburg D, Burakoff R. Dysphagia as the sole manifestation of bilateral strokes. Am J Gastroenterol 1990;85:610–613.
29. Buchholz DW. Neurogenic dysphagia: What is the cause when the cause is not obvious? Dysphagia 1994;9:245–255.
30. Chiti-Batelli S, Delap T. Lateral medullary infarct presenting as acute dysphagia. Acta Otolaryngol 2001;121:419–420.
31. Alberts JJ, Horner J, Gray L, Brazer MJ. Aspiration after stroke: Lesion analysis by brain MRI. Dysphagia 1992;7:170–173.
32. Perlman AL, Booth BM, Grayhack JP. Videofluoroscopic predictors of aspiration in patients with oropharyngeal dysphagia. Dysphagia 1994;9:90–95.
33. Finestone HM, Green Finestone LS, Wilson ES, Teasell RW. Malnutrition in stroke patients on the rehabilitation service and at follow-up: prevalence and predictors. Arch Phys Med Rehabil 1995;76:310–316.
34. Horner J, Buoyer FG, Alberts MJ, Helms MJ. Dysphagia following brainstem stroke. Arch Neurol 1991;48:1170–1173.
35. Perlman AL. Dysphagia in stroke patients. Semin Neurol 1996;16:341–348.
36. Perry L, Love CP. Screening for dysphagia and aspiration in acute stroke: a systematic review. Dysphagia 2001;16:7–18.
37. Schmidt J, Holas M, Halvorson K, Reding M. Videofluoroscopic evidence of aspiration predicts pneumonia and death but not dehydration following stroke. Dysphagia 1994;9:7–11.
38. Langmore SE. Dysphagia in neurologic patients in the intensive care unit. Semin Neurol 1996;16:329–340.
39. Whelan K. Inadequate fluid intakes in dysphagic acute stroke. Clin Nutr 2001;20:423–428.
40. Davalos A, Ricart W, Gonzalez-Huix F, et al. Effect of malnutrition after acute stroke on clinical outcome. Stroke 1996;27:1028–1032.

41. Brooks FP. Brain-stomach interactions: an overview. In Y Tache, D Wingate (eds), Brain-Gut Interactions. Boca Raton: CRC Press, 1991;163–168.
42. Crome P, Rizeq M, George S, et al. Drug absorption may be delayed after stroke: results of the paracetamol absorption test. Age Ageing 2001;30:391–393.
43. Reynolds BJ, Eliasson SG. Colonic pseudo obstruction in patients with stroke. Ann Neurol 1977;1:305.
44. Johanson JF, Sonnenberg A, Koch TR, McCarty DJ. Association of constipation with neurologic diseases. Dig Dis Sci 1992;37:179–186.
45. Sonnenberg A, Tsou VT, Muller AD. The "institutional colon": a frequent colonic dysmotility in psychiatric and neurologic disease. Am J Gastroenterol 1994;89:62–66.
46. Andrew J, Nathan P. Lesions of the anterior frontal lobes and disturbances of micturition and defaecation. Brain 1964;87:233–261.
47. White HH. Brain stem tumors occurring in adults. Neurology 1963;13:292–300.
48. Bray PF, Carter S, Taveras JM. Brain stem tumors in children. Neurology 1958;8:1–7.
49. Paritch HS, Berg BO. Brain stem tumors of childhood and adolescence. Am J Dis Child 1970;119:465–472.
50. Wood JR, Camilleri M, Low PA, Malagelada JR. Brainstem tumor presenting as an upper gut motility disorder. Gastroenterology 1985;89:1411–1414.
51. Morgan AS, Mackay LE. Causes and complications associated with swallowing disorders in traumatic brain injury. J Head Trauma Rehabil 1999;14:454–461.
52. Cherney LR, Halper AS. Recovery of oral nutrition after head injury in adults. J Head Trauma Rehabil 1989;4:42–50.
53. Weinstein CJ. Neurogenic dysphagia: frequency, progression, and outcome in adults following head injury. Phys Ther 1983;12:1992–1993.
54. Cherney LR, Halper AS. Swallowing problems in adults with traumatic brain injury. Semin Neurol 1996;16:349–353.
55. Mackay LE, Morgan AS, Bernstein BA. Swallowing disorders in severe brain injury: risk factors affecting return to oral intake. Arch Phys Med Rehabil 1999;80:365–371.
56. Lazarus CL, Logemann JA. Swallowing disorders in closed head trauma patients. Arch Phys Med Rehabil 1987;68:79–84.
57. Camilleri M, Bharucha AE. Gastrointestinal dysfunction in neurologic disease. Semin Neurol 1996;16:203–216.
58. Jackson MD, Davidoff G. Gastroparesis following traumatic brain injury and response to metoclopramide therapy. Arch Phys Med Rehabil 1989;70:553–555.
59. Altmayer T, O'Dell MW, Jones M, et al. Cisapride as a treatment for gastroparesis in traumatic brain injury. Arch Phys Med Rehabil 1996;77:1093–1094.
60. Cornett MA, Paris A Jr, Huang TY. Case report: intracranial penetration of a nasogastric tube. Am J Emerg Med 1993;11:94–96.
61. Estebe JP, Fleureaux O, Lenaoures A, Malledant Y. Intracranial insertion of a nasogastric tube in a patient with severe head injuries. Ann Fr Anesth Reanim 1994;13:843–845.
62. Casagli S, Malacarne P, Tosi G, Biancofiore G. Accidental introduction of a naso-gastric tube into the cranial cavity in a patient with non-severe cranial and facial trauma. Minerva Anestesiol 1994;60:277–279.
63. Katz MI, Faibel M. Inadvertent intracranial placement of a nasogastric tube. AJR Am J Roentgenol 1994;163:222.
64. Gianelli Castiglione A, Bruzzone E, Burrello C, et al. Intracranial insertion of a nasogastric tube in a case of homicidal head trauma. Am J Forensic Med Pathol 1998;19:329–334.
65. Ferreras J, Junquera LM, Garcia-Consuegra L. Intracranial placement of a nasogastric tube after severe craniofacial trauma. Oral Surg Oral Med Oral Pathol Oral Radiol Endod 2000;90:564–566.
66. Arslantas A, Durmaz R, Cosan E, Tel E. Inadvertent insertion of a nasogastric tube in a patient with head trauma. Childs Nerv Syst 2001;17:112–114.
67. Kelly DF. Steroids in head injury. New Horiz 1995;3:453–455.
68. Lu WY, Rhoney DH, Boling WB, et al. A review of stress ulcer prophylaxis in the neurosurgical intensive care unit. Neurosurgery 1997;41:416–425.
69. Alderson P, Roberts I. Corticosteroids for acute traumatic brain injury. Cochrane Database Syst Rev 2000;2:CD000196.

70. Parkinson J. An Essay on the Shaking Palsy. London: Whittingham and Rowland, 1817.
71. Eadie MJ, Tyrer JH. Alimentary disorders in parkinsonism. Aust Ann Med 1965;14:13–22.
72. Edwards LL, Pfeiffer RF, Quigley EMM, et al. Gastrointestinal symptoms in Parkinson's disease. Mov Disord 1991;6:151–156.
73. Edwards L, Quigley EMM, Hofman R, Pfeiffer RF. Gastrointestinal symptoms in Parkinson's disease: 18-month follow-up study. Mov Disord 1993;8:83–86.
74. Edwards LL, Quigley EMM, Pfeiffer RF. Gastrointestinal dysfunction in Parkinson's disease: Frequency and pathophysiology. Neurology 1992;42:726–732.
75. Edwards LL, Quigley EMM, Harned RK, et al. Characterization of swallowing and defecation in Parkinson's disease. Am J Gastroenterol 1994;89:15–25.
76. Quigley EMM. Epidemiology and pathophysiology of gastrointestinal manifestations of parkinson's disease. In E Corazziari (ed), NeuroGastroenterology. Berlin: deGruyter, 1996;167–178.
77. Quigley EMM. Gastrointestinal dysfunction in Parkinson's disease. Semin Neurol 1996;16:245–250.
78. Pfeiffer RF. Gastrointestinal dysfunction in Parkinson's disease. Clin Neurosci 1998;5:136–146.
79. Pfeiffer RF, Quigley EMM. Gastrointestinal motility problems in patients with Parkinson's disease. Epidemiology, pathophysiology and guidelines for management. CNS Drugs 1999;11:435–448.
80. Quigley EMM. Gastrointestinal features. In SA Factor, WJ Weiner (eds), Parkinson's Disease. Diagnosis and Clinical Management. New York: Demos, 2002;87–93.
81. Eadie MJ. Gastric secretion in parkinsonism. Aust Ann Med 1963;12:346–350.
82. Bateson MC, Gibberd FB, Wilson RSE. Salivary symptoms in Parkinson's disease. Arch Neurol 1973;29:274–275.
83. Korczyn AD. Autonomic nervous system disturbances in parkinson's disease. In MB Streifler, AD Korczyn, E Melamed, MBH Youdim (eds), Parkinson's Disease: Anatomy, Pathology and Therapy (Advances in Neurology, Vol 53). New York: Raven Press, 1990;463–468.
84. Bagheri H, Damase-Michel C, Lapeyre-Mestre M, et al. A study of salivary secretion in Parkinson's disease. Clin Neuropharmacol 1999;22:213–215.
85. Korczyn AD. Autonomic nervous system screening in patients with early parkinson's disease. In H Przuntek, P Riederer (eds), Early Diagnosis and Preventive Therapy in Parkinson's Disease. Vienna: Springer Verlag, 1989;41–48.
86. Hyson HC, Jog MS, Johnson A. Sublingual atropine for sialorrhea secondary to parkinsonism. Parkinsonism Relat Disord 2001;7(Supplement):P-TU-194(abst).
87. Marsden CD. Gastrointestinal manifestations of movement disorders. In E Corazziari (ed), NeuroGastroenterology. Berlin: deGruyter, 1996;161–165.
88. Pal PK, Calne DB, Calne S, Tsui JKC. Botulinum toxin A as treatment for drooling saliva in PD. Neurology 2000;54:244–247.
89. Leopold NA, Kagel MC. Prepharyngeal dysphagia in Parkinson's disease. Dysphagia 1996;11:14–22.
90. Bushmann M, Dobmeyer SM, Leeker L, Perlmutter JS. Swallowing abnormalities and their response to treatment in Parkinson's disease. Neurology 1989;39:1309–1314.
91. Logemann JA, Blonsky ER, Boshes B. Dysphagia in parkinsonism. JAMA 1975;231:69–70.
92. Robbins JA, Logemann JA, Kirshner HS. Swallowing and speech production in Parkinson's disease. Ann Neurol 1986;19:283–287.
93. Ali GN, Wallace KL, Schwartz R, et al. Mechanisms of oral-pharyngeal dysphagia in patients with Parkinson's disease. Gastroenterology 1996;110:383–392.
94. Stroudley J, Walsh M. Radiological assessment of dysphagia in Parkinson's disease. Brit J Radiol 1991;64:890–893.
95. Thomas M, Haigh RA. Dysphagia, a reversible cause not to be forgotten. Postgrad Med J 1995;71:94–95.
96. Croxson SCM, Pye I. Dysphagia as the presenting feature of Parkinson's disease. Geriatric Medicine 1988;August:16.
97. Johnston BT, Li Q, Castell JA, Castell DO. Swallowing and esophageal dysfunction in Parkinson's disease. Am J Gastroenterol 1995;90:1741–1746.

98. Logemann J, Blonsky ER, Boshes B. Lingual control in Parkinson's disease. Trans Am Neurol Assoc 1973;98:276–278.

99. Blonsky ER, Logemann JA, Boshes B, Fisher HB. Comparison of speech and swallowing function in patients with tremor disorders and in normal geriatric patients: a cinefluorographic study. J Gerontol 1975;30:299–303.

100. Silbiger ML, Pikielny RT, Donner MW. Neuromuscular disorders affecting the pharynx. Cineradiographic analysis. Invest Radiol 1967;2:442–448.

101. Calne DB, Shaw DG, Spiers ASD, Stern GM. Swallowing in parkinsonism. Br J Radiol 1970;43:456–457.

102. Palmer ED. Dysphagia in parkinsonism. JAMA 1974;229:1349.

103. Byrne KG, Pfeiffer R, Quigley EMM. Gastrointestinal dysfunction in Parkinson's disease. A report of clinical experience at a single center. J Clin Gastroenterol 1994;19:11–16.

104. Born LJ, Harned RH, Rikkers LF, et al. Cricopharyngeal dysfunction in Parkinson's disease: Role in dysphagia and response to myotomy. Mov Disord 1996;11:53–8.

105. Penner A, Druckerman LJ. Segmental spasms of the esophagus and their relation to parkinsonism. Am J Dig Dis 1942;9:282–286.

106. Eadie MJ, Tyrer JH. Radiological abnormalities of the upper part of the alimentary tract in parkinsonism. Aust Ann Med 1965;14:23–27.

107. Gibberd FB, Gleeson JA, Gossage AAR, Wilson RSE. Oesophageal dilation in Parkinson's disease. J Neurol Neurosurg Psychiatry 1974;37:938–940.

108. Eadie MJ. The pathology of certain medullary nuclei in parkinsonism. Brain 1963; 86:781–792.

109. Jackson M, Balsitis M, Lennox G, Lowe J. Lewy body dysphagia. Ann Neurol 1994;36:274.

110. Qualman SJ, Haupt HM, Yang P, Hamilton SR. Oesophageal Lewy bodies associated with ganglion cell loss in achalasia. Gastroenterology 1984;87:848–856.

111. Mukhopadhyay AK, Weisbrodt N. Effect of dopamine on esophageal motor function. Am J Physiol 1977;232:E19–E24.

112. Bramble MG, Cunliffe J, Dellipani AW. Evidence for a change in neurotransmitter affecting oesophageal motility in Parkinson's disease. J Neurol Neurosurg Psychiatry 1978; 41:709–712.

113. Lieberman AN, Horowitz L, Redmond P, et al. Dysphagia in Parkinson's disease. Am J Gastroenterol 1980;74:157–160.

114. Kempster PA, Lees AJ, Crichton P, et al. Off-period belching due to a reversible disturbance of oesophageal motility in Parkinson's disease and its treatment with apomorphine. Mov Disord 1989;4:47–52.

115. Evans MA, Triggs EJ, Cheung M, et al. Gastric emptying rate in the elderly: Implications for drug therapy. J Am Geriatr Soc 1981;29:201–205.

116. Evans MA, Broe GA, Triggs EJ, et al. Gastric emptying rate and the systemic availability of levodopa in the elderly parkinsonian patient. Neurology 1981;31:1288–1294.

117. Fich A, Camilleri M, Phillips SF. Effect of age on human gastric and small bowel motility. J Clin Gastroenterol 1989;11:416–420.

118. Djaldetti R, Baron J, Ziv H, Melamed E. Gastric emptying in Parkinson's disease: Patients with and without response fluctuations. Neurology 1996;46:1051–1054.

119. Harada T, Orita R, Hiwaki C, et al. Evaluation of gastric emptying in Parkinson's disease affect of l-dopa treatment. Can J Neurol Sci 1993;20(suppl 4):S119(abst).

120. Hardoff R, Sula M, Tamir A, et al. Gastric emptying time and gastric motility in patients with Parkinson's disease. Mov Disord 2001;16:1041–1047.

121. Krygowska-Wajs A, Lorens K, Thor P, et al. Gastric electromechanical dysfunction in Parkinson's disease. Funct Neurol 2000;15:41–46.

122. Soykan I, Lin Z, Bennett JP, McCallum RW. Gastric myoelectrical activity in patients with Parkinson's disease: evidence of a primary gastric abnormality. Dig Dis Sci 1999; 44:927–931.

123. Wade DN, Mearrick PT, Morris J. Active transport of l-dopa in the intestine. Nature 1973; 242:463–465.

124. Sasahara K, Nitanai J, Habara T, et al. Dosage from design for improvement of bioavailability of levodopa: absorption and metabolism of levodopa in intestinal segment of dogs. J Pharm Sci 1981;70:1157–1160.

Chapter 5
The Autonomic Neuropathies

Phillip A. Low

Peripheral nerve is made up of nerve fibers that vary in diameter from 1 μm (unmyelinated) to 11–12 μm (large myelinated).[1] Most neuropathies involve large myelinated fibers (>6 μm), and these patients have a loss of touch, vibration, and proprioception. A less common group of neuropathies involve small nerve fibers. These fibers are small myelinated (2 to 5 μm) fibers or are unmyelinated. The autonomic neuropathies are one group of neuropathies with disproportionate involvement of small fibers. The small myelinated fibers are preganglionic, sympathetic, or parasympathetic. The unmyelinated fibers are autonomic "C" fibers: one subpopulation is sympathetic adrenergic, supplying the arterioles, smaller arteries, and splanchic-mesenteric bed; the other is sympathetic sudomotor, supplying eccrine sweat glands; these fibers are either affected disproportionately or in isolation in the autonomic neuropathies. The preganglionic synapse is cholinergic. The postganglionic parasympathetic fiber is cholinergic, while the corresponding sympathetic fiber is adrenergic, except for the sudomotor fibers, which are cholinergic.

This traditional concept has been helpful but incomplete, and in some situations, inaccurate. For instance, the neurotransmitter responsible for erection is nitric oxide, with a lesser role for vasoactive intestinal polypeptide. The neurotransmitters in the adrenergic system include neuropeptide Y (NPY), endothelin, and certain prostaglandins. For a definitive description of the autonomic neuropathies, the reader is referred to recent reviews.[2–6]

This description will comprise a practical classification in the following outline, followed by more detailed description, and finally, by an approach to the evaluation of the patient with suspected autonomic neuropathy.

THE CLINICAL DISORDERS

The Acute Autonomic Neuropathies

Acute Autonomic Neuropathy

Acute Pandysautonomia. Acute pandysautonomia is better designated as acute panautonomic neuropathy.

PERSPECTIVE.   It was well recognized as a rare but characteristic syndrome with absolute specificity for the autonomic nervous system. Experience over the past 2 decades has rendered this view untenable.[7] There is instead a group of presumably immune-mediated, often post viral acute autonomic neuropathies, which might be limited in distribution (acute autonomic neuropathy), limited to the cholinergic system (acute cholinergic neuropathy), associated with substantial somatic involvement (Guillan-Barré syndrome), or with widespread sympathetic and parasympathetic failure (panautonomic neuropathy). When the latter is associated with a neoplasm, the term paraneoplastic is added.

CLINICAL FEATURES.   The core features of acute autonomic neuropathy are the acute or subacute onset of an autonomic neuropathy with relative or complete sparing of somatic nerve fibers. There is an antecedent viral infection occurring in about 50% of patients.[7] Somatic symptoms are common as parasthesias, itching, or acral pain, but the examination of large fiber function is typically normal.[7] Infrequently, overt distal small fiber involvement is present.

The term acute panautonomic neuropathy is best reserved for cases with widespread and severe sympathetic and parasympathetic failure. Fully-developed acute panautonomic neuropathy is rare but highly characteristic.[5] Previously healthy individuals develop the acute or subacute onset of widespread sympathetic failure with orthostatic hypotension, anhidrosis, and parasympathetic failure with dry eyes, dry mouth, and disturbances of bowel and bladder function. Abdominal pain, often colicky, is common and early satiety, bloating, nausea, vomiting, diarrhea, or alternating constipation-diarrhea may persist for years. Patients will usually have a fixed heart rate and pupils.

Neurologic examination in the fully-developed case confirms the presence of orthostatic hypotension, a fixed heart rate, and fixed dilated pupils. The skin is dry. Urine retention is usually present. Strength and sensation are typically normal. Occasionally, there may be some distal impairment of pain and temperature perception. Pruritus is not uncommon as an early symptom.

Acute autonomic neuropathies with more restricted expression of dysautonomia are much more common. In a recent review of the Mayo experience,[7] based on 27 cases, many patients had restricted rather than "pan" autonomic neuropathy. The restricted neuropathy can result in distinctive autonomic syndromes. Involvement might be selectively cholinergic, with a fixed heart rate, widespread anhidrosis, paralytic ileus, neurogenic bladder, and obstinate constipation. A length-dependent autonomic neuropathy with peripheral adrenergic failure and intact cardiac innervation results in orthostatic tachycardia, the postural tachycardia syndrome (POTS). Involvement is sometimes selectively adrenergic (acute adrenergic neuropathy). Another pattern is a restrictive gastrointestinal neuropathy, presenting as an intestinal psuedo-obstruction syndrome.

INVESTIGATIONS.   Nerve conduction studies are typically normal, and the majority of patients who have neuropathic sensory symptoms have normal studies. The motor unit potentials are normal, or show only minor abnormalities. Computer assisted sensory examination may occasionally show impairment of temperature or pain perception. Sural nerve biopsy may show perivascular round cell infiltration, and the C potential may be reduced or absent.[1] The autonomic reflex screen, which evaluates the severity and distribution of postganglionic sudomotor, cholinergic, and adrenergic failure,[2-4] and the thermoregulatory sweat test (TST), are markedly abnormal. The lesion is typically postganglionic. Widespread adrenergic failure is manifest as orthostatic hypotension on tilt-up, with a collapse of pulse pressure associated with a fixed heart rate, and the alterations in beat-to-beat BP recordings to the Valsalva maneuver show the pattern indicative of combined peripheral and cardiac adrenergic denervation. Salivation test is usually reduced, and Schirmer test confirms reduced tear secretion. Gastrointestinal motility is markedly abnormal, and cystometrogram shows detrusor denervation. Supine plasma norepinephrine determination shows the pattern of widespread postganglionic adrenergic denervation, with a reduced supine plasma norepinephrine, which fails to rise upon standing. The sural nerve biopsy findings may be negative or may show a reduction of unmyelinated and small myelinated fibers and an absence of the C potential in in vitro compound nerve action potential recordings.

DIFFERENTIAL DIAGNOSIS.   The main differential diagnoses are: 1) paraneoplastic pandysautonomia; 2) the acute cholinergic neuropathies; and 3) Guillan-Barré syndrome.

There are 3 criteria for the diagnosis of acute autonomic neuropathy. The elements are: 1) acute onset; 2) significant autonomic involvement; and 3) absence of other causes of acute autonomic failure. The neuropathy should have evolved, from onset to peak disability, within 8 weeks. There should be significant objective evidence of autonomic failure. This evidence is best obtained in an autonomic laboratory (see below). Significant objective clinical evidence includes the presence of orthostatic hypotension, neurogenic bladder, widespread anhidrosis, or paralytic ileus. It is necessary to exclude other causes of autonomic neuropathy. A neoplastic, especially pulmonary, neoplasm is excluded by imaging studies (roentgen, computed tomography, magnetic resonance imaging) of the chest, and anti-neuronal antibody determination. It is also necessary to exclude the other entities listed under acute autonomic neuropathy in the following outline (medications, toxins and drugs, porphyria, and botulism):

I. The Acute Autonomic Neuropathies
   A. Acute autonomic neuropathy
      1. Panautonomic neuropathy (pandysautonomia)
      2. Acute paraneoplastic pandysautonomia
      3. Acute cholinergic neuropathy
      4. Guillain-Barré syndrome
   B. Botulism
   C. Porphyria
   D. Drug-induced acute autonomic neuropathies (cisplatinum, vincristine, Vacor, amiodarone)
   E. Toxic acute autonomic neuropathies (heavy metals; thallium, arsenic, mercury, organic solvents, acrylamide)
II. The Chronic Peripheral Autonomic Neuropathies
   A. Distal sympathetic neuropathies
      1. Idiopathic distal small fiber neuropathy (DSFN)
      2. Peripheral neuropathies with DSFN
   B. Pure cholinergic neuropathies
      1. Lambert-Eaton myasthenic syndrome (LEMS)
      2. Chronic idiopathic anhidrosis (CIA)
      3. Idiopathic cholinergic neuropathy
      4. Adies' syndrome
      5. Chagas' disease
   C. Pure adrenergic neuropathy

III. Combined Sympathetic and Parasympathetic Failure—autonomic dysfunction clinically *important*
   A. Amyloid
   B. Diabetic autonomic neuropathy (DAN)
   C. Sensory neuropathy with autonomic failure
   D. Pure autonomic failure (PAF; idiopathic orthostatic)
   E. Familial dysautonomia
   F. Fabry's disease
   G. Tangier disease
IV. Paroxysmal or Intermittent Dysautonomia

Acute Paraneoplastic Pandysautonomia.   Acute autonomic neuropathy may be indistinguishable from paraneoplastic dysautonomia until serologic tests (antineuronal antibody) are positive or a neoplasm is found. Paraneoplastic panautonomic neuropathy can be acute or subacute, but very rapidly evolving cases (over 1 to 2 days) are likely to be post viral or idiopathic.

Acute Cholinergic Neuropathy.   The acute cholinergic neuropathies do not have adrenergic failure and therefore do not have significant orthostatic hypotension. This disorder is probably a restricted expression of acute panautonomic neuropathy with abnormalities confined to the postganglionic cholinergic neuron.[5] Patients have alacrima, xerostomia, anhidrosis, constipation, urinary retention, and blurred vision, but do not have orthostatic hypotension. Gastrointestinal complaints are very common, with ileus during the early stages and abdominal pain, gastroparesis, and constipation during the chronic phase. In some patients motility abnormalities may dominate the clinical picture.[8]

Guillain-Barré Syndrome.   The core features of Guillain-Barré syndrome are the acute onset of an ascending, predominantly motor polyradiculoneuropathy, and autonomic involvement is not a requirement for diagnosis. Autonomic over/under activity is not uncommon. Autonomic dysfunction is relatively common in some series.[5] Patients may have tachycardia, and orthostatic hypotension may alternate with hypertension. Bladder or bowel involvement tends to be mild compared to somatic involvement, but can occur. Some patients with Guillain-Barré syndrome will have life-threatening dysautonomia, occurring most frequently in the acute evolving phase of the disease. The dysautonomia tends to correlate with the severity of somatic involvement, and is especially common in patients with respiratory failure, although this relationship is inconsistent. In addition to orthostatic hypotension, hypertensive episodes can occur. They are usually paroxysmal, but may occasionally be sustained. Microneurographic evidence of sympathetic overactivity has been described, and subsides with recovery from the neuropathy.[9] Sinus tachycardia may occur in over 50% of patients with severe Guillain-Barré syndrome. Less common or less troublesome autonomic symptoms include constipation, rectal incontinence, gastroparesis, ileus, erectile failure, and pupillary abnormalities.
   INVESTIGATIONS.   Tests of autonomic function are often abnormal. Orthostatic hypotension, impaired cardiovagal, sudomotor, and adrenergic vasomotor function have been described. Abnormalities of cardiac rhythm include sinus tachycardia and bradyarrhythmias. Heart block or even asystole has been described and may necessitate a cardiac pacemaker. Sinus arrest may occur following vagal stimulation, as might occur with tracheal suction.

ETIOLOGY OR MECHANISMS. The etiology of this disorder is unknown, but many or most cases are likely to be immune-mediated. The evidence is based on the sural nerve biopsy finding of perivascular round cell infiltration, the frequent antecedent viral infection, the selectivity of involvement by fiber type and autonomic level, and the merging of cases with Guillain-Barré.

COURSES AND PROGNOSIS. Most cases have had only partial improvement.[5,7] We recently reviewed and followed up the course of 27 patients with acute autonomic neuropathy at Mayo.[7] The impression is that it runs a chronic debilitating course with significant residual deficits in the majority of patients. Patients seem to improve substantially over the first year, followed by a slower rate of improvement over the subsequent 4 years. Approximately one third of patients make a good functional recovery.

MANAGEMENT. Patients with autonomic instability require close monitoring of heart rate and BP. Paroxysmal hypertension may alternate with hypotension and patients may be supersensitive to hypotensive and other agents. For these patients, the use of hypotensive agents is usually best avoided. When sustained hypertension develops, combined alpha and beta adrenergic blockade has been suggested, and bradyarrhythmias are probably best treated by the use of a demand pacemaker.

Beyond the intensive case unit, the management of autonomic failure assumes great importance. Meticulous attention should be paid to maintaining an adequate blood volume, since the denervated vascular bed is extremely sensitive to volume depletion. Also important is the need to prevent deconditioning. The head of the bed should be elevated about 4 to 6 inches at all times, and the patient should be mobilized as soon as possible to prevent the reduced orthostatic tolerance of prolonged bed rest.

The mainstay of treatment is supportive for the management of orthostatic hypotension, and bowel and bladder symptoms. Since there is suggestive evidence of an immune-mediated process, treatment with prednisone, plasma exchange, or intravenous gamma globulin could be considered in patients seen within the first 8 weeks. Should these treatments be used, it is important to quantitate the neurologic and autonomic status before and with treatment. Plasma exchange is given as 3 exchanges a week for 2 weeks. Intravenous gamma globulin is given as .4 g/kg (over 4 hours) thrice weekly for 2 weeks. Reports of marked improvement in autonomic function following gamma globulin therapy, with autonomic laboratory documentation, have appeared.[10,11]

Botulism

CLINICAL FEATURES. The core features are the acute development of cholinergic neuropathy, ptosis, and bulbar weakness following the ingestion of home-canned foods contaminated by *Clostridium botulinum* spores. Symptoms of nausea and vomiting are common. Neurologic symptoms consist of ptosis, extraocular muscle palsy, involvement of other cranial nerves, and weakness, which may progress to generalized neuromuscular paralysis.[12,13] Autonomic symptoms consist of severe cholinergic failure with anhidrosis, dry eyes and mouth, paralytic ileus, and urinary retention.[13] Gastrointestinal symptoms, including paralytic ileus and gastric dilatation, are relatively common.[13,14] Orthostatic hypotension may also occur,[15] but is less common. Typically, symptoms begin 12 to 36 hours after the ingestion of contaminated food. The frequency, severity, and duration of autonomic failure may relate to the type of botulism.

INVESTIGATIONS.   Cardiovagal tests are abnormal, and orthostatic hypotension may be present.[15] Orthostatic hypotension recovers before parasympathetic function, and the neuromuscular transmission deficit recovers last of all.[15] Esophageal manometry may demonstrate marked reduction in peristaltic amplitude.[13] Schirmer test may confirm impaired tear secretion, and salivation is reduced.[16]

DIAGNOSIS AND MANAGEMENT.   The diagnosis rests on clinical grounds. It can be confirmed by identification of the toxin in the food or serum.[12] If available, contaminated food can be suspended in saline and injected intraperitoneally in mice. The animal dies within 24 hours of botulism (the mouse test). Management is mainly supportive with early tracheotomy and ventilatory support in patients with respiratory failure. The role of antitoxins is uncertain. Guanidine may be effective in some cases[16] but not others.

Porphyria

Dysautonomia is common in acute intermittent porphyria, and autonomic over-activity predominates over autonomic failure, although both are present, and often coexist. Symptoms of sympathetic over-activity include abdominal colic, hypertension, and tachycardia.[17] Porphyria is consistently associated with obstinate constipation.[18] Dysautonomia may also occur in variegate porphyria. Persistent tachycardia may be an early feature of an attack, and may also precede the onset of neuropathy. Other clinical features of autonomic neuropathy include abdominal pain, nausea and vomiting, constipation, diarrhea, bladder distension, and disordered sweating, both anhidrosis and hyperhidrosis.[18,19]

Drug-induced Autonomic Neuropathies

Cisplatinum.   Cisplatinum (cis-dichlorodiammineplatinum) is neurotoxic and side-effects include retrobulbar neuritis, and peripheral neuropathy. Neuropathy, when present, has usually developed in patients who received a cumulative dose of 210 to 825 mg/m^2, typically corresponding to 3 or 4 courses of therapy.[22] Autonomic symptoms include progressive orthostatic hypotension, dry mouth, and poikilothermia.[22]

Vincristine.   Vincristine, used in the treatment of lymphoma, leukemia, and some other malignancies, causes an axonal peripheral neuropathy.[23] Its neurotoxicity is dose-related and cumulative with repeated dosing; the drug needs to be stopped after a cumulative dose of 30 to 50 mg.[24] Autonomic symptoms include postural hypotension, constipation, abdominal pain, paralytic ileus, and urinary retention.[23–25]

Vacor.   Vacor (N-3-pyridylnethyl-N'-p-nitrophenyl urea; PNU) is a rodenticide that antagonizes nicotinamide metabolism. Ingestion may be deliberate (suicidal or homicidal) or accidental. Quantities ingested have usually been between 0.39 and 7 g, and ingestion results in acute hyperglycemic ketoacidosis, along with a combined somatic and autonomic neuropathy. Autonomic manifestations include orthostatic hypotension and gastrointestinal hypomotility.[26,27] Parenteral nicotinamide, especially if administered early, may be beneficial.[27]

Amiodarone.   Amiodarone, an antiarrhythmic agent, causes a sensorimotor neuropathy in about 10% of patients in most series.[28,29] Sural nerve neuropathologic changes involve both unmyelinated and myelinated fibers, with fiber loss, mixed demyelination, and axonal degeneration; lamellated lysosomal inclusions are characteristic.[30] Autonomic failure with severe orthostatic hypotension may occur,[31] but detailed autonomic studies have not been published. Improvement in neuropathy occurs with cessation of the drug.

Toxic Autoimmune Neuropathies

Heavy Metal Poisoning.   There have been very few cases of heavy metal poisoning in which autonomic function has been adequately studied. In thallium poisoning, tachycardia and hypertension have been reported in association with peripheral neuropathy.[32] In arsenical poisoning, excessive sweating and impairment of sweating on the extremities have been described.[33,34] Subacute, or chronic, inorganic mercury poisoning causes acrodynia, which occurs mainly in children and includes among its manifestations, tachycardia, hypertension, pain and redness of the fingers, toes, and ears (hence Pink disease and acrodynia), and profuse sweating.[35] Treatment with ganglion-blocking agents and chelation has been recommended.[36]

Organic Solvents.   Hexacarbon neuropathy occurs through industrial exposure or through inhalant abuse. Inhalation of n-hexane and methyl-n-butyl-ketone may result in a rapidly progressive polyneuropathy associated with autonomic features of excessive or impaired sweating, vasomotor alterations, postural hypotension, and impotence.[37]

The Chronic Peripheral Autonomic Neuropathies

Distal Sympathetic Neuropathies

Idiopathic Distal Small Fiber Neuropathy.
    CLINICAL FEATURES.   Distal small fiber neuropathy (DSFN) is characterized by distal dysesthesias and postganglionic sympathetic dysfunction occurring in the absence of significant somatic neuropathy. Symptoms include superficial burning and deeper aching pain. The pain is most common in the sole and toe-pads, with later involvement of the dorsum. Troublesome allodynia, where light touch or firm pressure, as with weight bearing, causes pain, is common. Sympathetic dysfunction is manifest as vasomotor changes, with pallor, sometimes alternating with rubor (with accentuation of pain-erythromelalgia), cyanosis, and mottling being common. Sudomotor dysfunction, manifest as excessive sweating or as anhidrosis, is also common.
    Distal small fiber neuropathy may be a manifestation of neuropathies such as diabetes—inherited, immune-mediated, or related to AIDS. However, the majority of instances of distal small fiber neuropathy are idiopathic and run a benign course. The neurologic examination in idiopathic DSFN is usually unremarkable. Strength is normal. Sensation may be mildly impaired, especially for sharp-dull discrimination and temperature perception, or it is normal. Reflexes are usually normal. Electromyography and nerve conduction studies are normal or unremarkable. The most sensitive diagnostic test is QSART or TST showing distal anhidrosis.[38]
    INVESTIGATIONS.   The majority of patients with distal small fiber neuropathy will have abnormalities of QSART in the distal lower extremities.[38] The diagnostic yield is enhanced if multiple recording sights are used.[4] QSART shows normal sweat

volume in the forearm and anhidrosis in the lower extremities, maximal distally. PASP is positive in a minority of patients.[39] Computer assisted examination for small fiber function may be helpful.[40] Jamal and colleagues found abnormalities in sensory testing in 25/25 patients. However, the actual sensitivity is uncertain, since these patients were selected into the study on the basis of impaired sensory examinations.[40]

Peripheral Neuropathies with Distal Small Fiber Neuropathy.   The majority of chronic peripheral neuropathies are associated with some distal axonal degeneration. In general, the demyelinating neuropathies, such as chronic inflammatory demyelinating polyradiculoneuropathy and monoclonal gammopathy associated neuropathies, are associated with less postganglionic autonomic failure than the axonal neuropathies such as arsenical neuropathies.[38,41] Those neuropathies with prominent diffuse autonomic failure are covered separately.

Pure Cholinergic Neuropathies

Chronic Idiopathic Anhidrosis.
   CLINICAL FEATURES.   The core features are acquired widespread anhidrosis in the absence of generalized adrenergic and cardiovagal failure. These patients have total or subtotal anhidrosis and are heat intolerant, becoming hot, flushed, dizzy, dyspneic, and weak when the ambient temperature is high, or when they exercise. Distal vasomotor changes may be present, but orthostatic hypotension or other evidence of generalized adrenergic failure, or symptomatic somatic neuropathy, are absent. Pupillary abnormalities may be present. This disorder is important to recognize, since it is relatively common and often confused with the more malignant autonomic disorders, such as multiple system atrophy, pure autonomic failure, and the autonomic neuropathies. Chronic idiopathic anhidrosis probably is comprised of a heterogeneous group of disorders with restricted autonomic failure. Segmental anhidrosis with Adie's pupil (Ross syndrome) is well recognized,[42] and is often one type of chronic idiopathic anhidrosis, although rare cases of Ross syndrome are associated with more widespread autonomic failures. The prognosis appears to be distinctly better than the progressive autonomic disorders. The sweating deficit may remain stable, progress, or, infrequently, regress. The great majority of patients do not subsequently develop adrenergic failure.
   INVESTIGATIONS.   These patients have widespread anhidrosis on thermoregulatory sweat tests. The majority of cases are associated with postganglionic impairment.[43] Orthostatic hypotension is absent, and cardiovascular heart rate tests, supine and standing plasma, norepinephrine and beat-to-beat BP responses to tilt, and the Valsalva maneuver show no evidence of autonomic failure.
   TREATMENT.   Treatment is focused on the avoidance of heat stress. These patients should live in an air-conditioned environment. Some patients seem to have an altered comfort zone, setting their home thermostats to relatively lower temperatures (often in the low 60s). They should avoid vigorous exercise in a hot environment, since they are more prone to heat injury, including heat exhaustion and heat stroke.

Adie's Syndrome.   The typical tonic pupil is a large pupil that does not react to direct light. It is due to a postganglionic parasympathetic lesion. Because of denervation super-sensitivity, the pupil constricts to sub-threshold concentrations of parasympathetic agents, such as pilocarpine 0.125% or methacholine 2.5%, whereas the normal pupil would be unaffected. The pupillary abnormality may be unilateral or bilateral, and may occur in isolation or in association with more widespread neurologic or autonomic abnormalities. Adie's syndrome refers to the combination of a tonic pupil with areflexia.[44] Widespread sympathetic failure is uncommon but is well documented.[45,44] Another combination is tonic pupil and segmental anhidrosis, sometimes referred to as Ross syndrome.[42] This syndrome is important to recognize, since the widespread anhidrosis does not indicate a progressive autonomic disorder.[43] Yet another combination is tonic pupil(s) with chronic inflammatory demyelinating polyradiculoneuropathy (CIDP). Another combination is tonic pupil(s) with a sensory neuropathy as part of Sjögren's syndrome. These patients have widespread autonomic failure with anhidrosis, orthostatic hypotension, impairment of cardiovagal function, and keratoconjunctivities sicca and xerostomia.[46] Adie's pupil may also occur as part of the autonomic paraneoplastic neuropathy. The site of the lesion is likely in the ciliary ganglion and degenerative changes have been described in autopsy tissue.[47]

Chagas' Disease. Chagas' disease is caused by *Trypanosoma cruzi*, an intracellular protozoan. *T cruzi* is found only in the Americas, from the southern United States to southern Argentina. Acute Chagas' disease is rare in the United States, and chronic Chagas', which develops years to decades after primary infection, is seen in increasing numbers in South American immigrants, especially Salvadoran, Nicaraguan, and Mexican. The most commonly affected organs are the heart, resulting in biventricular cardiomegaly and conduction defects, and the gastrointestinal tract.[48] An autonomic syndrome is manifest as a chronic cholinergic megaesophagus, megaduodenum, and megacolon, and patients complain of increasing dysphagia and constipation. Other parts of the gastrointestinal and urinary tracts, gall bladder, and salivary glands may be affected.[48]

Autonomic function tests may be abnormal. There may be orthostatic hypotension, baroreflex abnormalities, impaired heart rate response to standing, and Valsalva maneuver.[50,51] Plasma norepinephrine may be reduced.[52] Cardiac nerves undergo degeneration.[53] Multifocal inflammatory lesions associated with demyelination are present in the peripheral nervous system in humans and in the murine experimental model.[54] Multifocal inflammatory lesions associated with demyelination are present in the peripheral nervous system in humans and in the murine experimental model.[54] There is evidence that the destruction of the peripheral and sympathetic nervous systems has an autoimmune basis, T-lymphocytes and possibly humoral factors being responsible for an attack on neural elements. Antigenic determinants may be shared by the parasite and the host. A recent placebo-controlled clinical trial of mixed gangliosides has demonstrated improved blood pressure control with treatment, possibly due to an indirect neurotropic effect.[55] The disease may be transmitted in endemic areas in South America by the bite of a reduviid bug. Transmission may also occur via blood transfusions, a more likely mode of infection within the United States. The diagnosis of chronic Chagas' disease is made by detecting antibodies to *T cruzi* using complement fixation, immunofluorescence, or ELISA assay. A false positive test may occur with Leishmaniasis. When one test is positive, the test is usually confirmed by two additional tests.[56]

Pure Adrenergic Neuropathy

Pure adrenergic neuropathy is uncommon. It may occur as part of an unusual immune-mediated acute or chronic autonomic adrenergic neuropathy. Pure autonomic failure and multiple system atrophy may also occur as pure adrenergic failure, with orthostatic hypotension but normal thermoregulatory sweat tests and tests of cardio-vagal function. The combination is uncommon, occurring in less than 10% of patients with multiple system atrophy and pure autonomic failure.

Another pure adrenergic neuropathy is an adrenergic neuropathy due to an inherited absence of the enzyme dopamine β-hydroxylase.[57,58] Patients are unable to convert dopamine to norepinephrine. The disorder is characterized by early onset, severe orthostatic hypotension, an absence of plasma norepinephrine, and excessive dopamine. The disorder responds to treatment with threo-DOPS, which can be converted to norepinephrine.

Combined Sympathetic and Parasympathetic Failure

Amyloid Neuropathy

Sporadic Systemic Amyloid Neuropathy.

CLINICAL FEATURES.   Sporadic systemic amyloid neuropathy is characterized by the onset in middle- to old-age of a generalized small fiber neuropathy with a predominant loss of pain and temperature sensation,[59] autonomic failure, and weight loss. The diagnosis is confirmed by the demonstration of amyloid deposits in tissues. Autonomic failure is an early and prominent cause of symptoms. Orthostatic hypotension with presyncope and syncope is common,[60] and is of serious prognostic significance.[60] Dysphagia is common and is due to amyloid infiltration of the lower esophagus.[61] Diarrhea, constipation, or alternating constipation with diarrhea, is common and is due to infiltration of the myenteric (Auerbach) and submucosal (Meissner) plexi. At a later stage, vomiting and abdominal distention may be a problem. Impotence is common in males. Anhidrosis is usually widespread.

DIAGNOSIS AND PROGNOSIS.   The diagnosis is made from the gestalt of a small fiber and autonomic neuropathy, with confirmation of amyloid deposition in tissue by nerve, rectal, or subcutaneous fat biopsy. Conjunctival biopsy is positive in at least 80% of patients.[62] Amyloid may also be identified in muscle biopsies by its presence at perivascular sites and in intramuscular nerve bundles.[63] Amyloidosis may mimic the effect of achalasia on the lower esophageal sphincter. Esophageal manometry has occasionally demonstrated a hypertensive sphincter with failure of relaxation after swallow.[64] More often the lower esophageal sphincter pressure is decreased and heart-burn is common.[61] The prognosis is poor. The neuropathy progresses relentlessly in spite of all attempted treatments. The clinical and laboratory features, based on 229 patients with primary systemic amyloid seen at the Mayo Clinic, have recently been reported. Median survival from the time of diagnosis for patients with peripheral neuropathy, carpal tunnel syndrome, orthostatic hypotension, and cardiac failure were 60, 45, 9.5, and 6.5 months, respectively.[60] Poor prognostic indices were appreciable weight loss, congestive cardiac failure, and the presence of light chains in the urine.

Multiple Myeloma-Associated Amyloid Neuropathy.   Autonomic impairment is much less common in amyloidosis associated with multiple myeloma than in sporadic systemic amyloidosis or familial amyloidotic polyneuropathy (FAP). A small fiber type neuropathy similar to FAP I has been described in three patients with multiple myeloma.[65] Amyloid infiltration of peripheral nerve is also uncommon, occurring in perhaps only 15% of cases.[66]

Familial Amyloiditic Polyneuropathy (FAP).   All forms of FAP are dominantly inherited. Prognosis for life tends to be better than for primary systemic amyloidosis. The clinical features and courses have been studied for FAP I. Age onset is younger, occurring between the ages of 20 to 40 years. Patients usually die of cardiac or renal failure or of inanition 10 to 15 years after onset. As in primary systemic amyloidosis, autonomic failure is a prominent manifestation of the neuropathy. The autonomic features of FAP I are similar to those of primary systemic amyloidosis.

The most common type of FAP is due to a point mutation in the transthyretin (prealbumin) gene, encoded on human chromosome 18.[67] Transthyretin is a single polypeptide chain of 127 amino acid residues. The most common point mutation is methionine 30, where methionine substitutes for valine and has been responsible for most cases of inherited amyloid polyneuropathy seen in the USA.[69]

DIAGNOSIS.   The pattern of dominant inheritance with onset in young adulthood, coupled with orthostatic hypotension and a dissociated pattern of sensory loss with relatively selective loss of pain and temperature perception, is suggestive of familial amyloid polyneuropathy. The electrophysiologic and autonomic features of the most common variety, FAP I, are very similar to those of primary systemic amyloidosis. Detection of the gene carrier in FAP is accomplished by isolating DNA from peripheral leukocytes and then digesting this DNA with specific restriction endonucleases that detect the various mutations, or by direct visualizations after amplification.[69,70] Rapid detection of variant transthyretin (containing the methionine-for-valine substitution at position 30) can be achieved using a radioimmunoassay based on a nonapeptide (positions 22 to 30) derived from variant transthyretin.[71]

MANAGEMENT.   There is no proven treatment of the primary process. Symptomatic treatment of autonomic failure is important.

Sensory Neuronopathy with Autonomic Failure

Sensory neuronopathy is characterized by an asymmetric sensory neuropathy which involves a disproportionate loss of proprioception and vibratory perception (large fiber type). In contrast to most neuropathies, which have a length-dependent pattern of involvement, involving the legs distally before the arms, the pattern of sensory loss in sensory neuronopathy will often begin in the upper extremity or face. These patients have a sensory ataxia with positive Rombergism and often have pseudoathetosis. The patients are areflexic and have absent sensory action potentials on nerve conduction studies. The main causes of sensory neuropathy are 1) Sjögren's syndrome, 2) pyridoxine neuropathy, 3) cisplatinum, 4) paraneoplastic, 5) monoclonal gammopathy-associated, 6) idiopathic, and 7) Vacor intoxication.

Idiopathic sensory neuronopathy[72,73] is characterized by severe sensory impairment, especially of proprioception and vibration sense (large fiber function), so that the distribution of sensory loss often involves most of the body surface. Appreciable recovery tends not to occur.

Primary Sjögren's syndrome is often associated with neuropathy. There are several neuropathic patterns. The most characteristic pattern consists of a subacute or chronic asymmetric sensory neuronopathy, with initial involvement of the upper extremity and predominant loss of vibration and position sense, Adie's pupil, trigeminal sensory loss, and combined sympathetic and parasympathetic failure.[46] However, the most common clinical pattern is probably a distal sensory or sensorimotor neuropathy. Other patterns are sensory neuronopathy, mononeuropathy multiplex, chronic inflammatory demyelinating polyradiculoneuropathy, and multiple cranial neuropathies.[46,74–76]

Laboratory confirmation of Sjögren's syndrome is essential. Keratoconjunctivitis sicca is confirmed by the Schirmer and Rose-Bengal tests. Salivation can be quantitated.[4] Labial biopsy of minor salivary glands is necessary to confirm the diagnosis, and shows perivascular round cell infiltration. Immune findings include antibodies to Ro (SSA), La (SSB), and Rheumatoid factor. There is a significant association between vasculitis and antibody to the extractable nuclear antigens (such as Ro and La[77]).

A review of 11 sural nerve biopsies at Mayo Clinic has been reported.[78] All biopsies showed perivascular inflammatory infiltrates. The histologic changes in 2/11 biopsies were considered to be diagnostic of necrotizing vasculitis, 6/11 strongly suggestive. Axonal degeneration was the predominant change. Pathologic studies on six cutaneous nerve biopsies showed perivascular round cell infiltration without necrotizing arteritis.[46] Thoracic dorsal root ganglion biopsied in three patients showed lymphocytic infiltration with degeneration of dorsal root ganglion cells.[46]

Cisplatinum chemotherapy may be associated with sensory neuronopathy and an autonomic neuropathy. Vacor poisoning may result in a sensory neuronopathy, diabetes, and autonomic failure. These two entities have been described earlier in this chapter. Pyridoxine neuropathy is associated with a sensory neuronopathy, but autonomic failure does not seem to be a prominent feature in this disorder.

Familial Dysautonomia (Riley-Day syndrome; HSAN type III)

CLINICAL FEATURES.   This recessively inherited neuropathy affects especially Ashkenazi Jews and has an onset, in infancy, of an autonomic and sensory motor neuropathy. These patients have absent fungiform papillae of the tongue and defective control of lacrimation, temperature, sweating, and blood pressure.[79] The disorder is present at birth and characteristically the infant fails to thrive, sucks poorly, and has episodes of unexplained fever. Alacrima, blotching of the skin, and corneal insensitivity are present. Hypertension and postural hypotension have been documented, as has excessive and erratic sweating. Gastrointestinal symptoms are prominent in infancy and in early childhood. There is also involvement of lower motor and sensory neurons, as suggested by hyporeflexia and kyphoscoliosis. Pain and temperature perception are more severely affected than is tactile sensation. Charcot joints resulting from insensitivity to pain have been described.

LABORATORY FINDINGS.   There is mild slowing of nerve conduction velocity. Neuropathologically there is clear-cut degeneration of all three populations of neurons with a somewhat selective involvement of small neurons (autonomic, small sensory, gamma motor neuron[6]). Homovanillic acid excretion is increased, and vanillylmandelic acid secretion is reduced. Levels of dopamine β-hydroxylase, the enzyme that converts dopamine to norepinephrine, are significantly reduced in the serum of patients with dysautonomia.[80]

COURSE AND PROGNOSIS.   Life expectancy is significantly shortened, but patients now live much longer than was originally thought.

Paroxysmal or Intermittent Dysautonomia

Dysautonomia may be paroxysmal as in certain acute peripheral autonomic storms[81] and central autonomic disorders. These paroxysmal or intermittent disorders may sometimes be acral and less dramatic, presenting as vasomotor disorders of the hands or feet. Patients with mild neuropathy may have intermittent coldness of the extremities. The disorders that are better characterized include Raynaud's phenomenon, paroxysmal hyperhidrosis, acrodynia, and erythromelalgia, characterized by prominent changes in skin color.

Erythromelalgia

Erythromelalgia refers to the acral erythema on warming, associated with an intense burning sensation. Many of these patients have a small fiber neuropathy. Some patients have a marked accentuation of the erythema and pain with warming of the feet. The mechanism of erythema and pain has, in some cases, been shown to be due to activation of neurogenic flare by a polymodal c nociceptor axon reflex, hence the term ABC syndrome (angry backfiring c nociceptor[82]). These patients often have marked relief of symptoms by cold soaks. Some patients with erythromelalgia report significant relief of symptoms with acetylsalicylic acid or ibuprofen. Some respond well to the local application of capsaicin cream.

MANAGEMENT OF THE PATIENT WITH SUSPECTED AUTONOMIC NEUROPATHY

Management needs to be individualized. The following description applies to many patients with suspected autonomic neuropathy:

Step 1 (the initial review)

This is a crucial first step. The autonomic clinician plays the decisive role in deciding if the problem is autonomic, and if it is significant enough to require a detailed evaluation. This evaluation is also important because a detailed autonomic system review should cover many autonomic areas that would not be evaluated in autonomic testing. This topic has been covered.[3]

The clinician needs to recognize the presence of an autonomic neuropathy from the symptoms and signs. It is possible to also define, in a preliminary fashion, the severity and distribution of autonomic failure or over-activity. From the temporal pattern and clinical gestalt of autonomic features, it is probable that the main differential diagnoses will have been reached. For the acute disorder, the main considerations are panautonomic neuropathy, botulism, Guillain-Barré syndrome, porphyria, and autonomic neuropathy due to drugs and toxins. The patient with chronic autonomic failure should suggest autonomic neuropathies due to diabetes, amyloidosis, immune-mediated mechanisms, inheritance, Sjögren's disease, or that of pure autonomic failure, multiple system atrophy, or the Lambert-Eaton myasthenic symptom (LEMS).

Step 2 (the initial workup)

The next step is the initial laboratory evaluation. It should comprise:

1. Autonomic reflex screen
2. Thermoregulatory sweat test

3. Routine workup
   a. Complete blood count and differential, erythrocyte sedimentation rate (ESR), chemistry group, rheumatoid factor, ANA, cholesterol
   b. Extractable nuclear antigen (ENA) group
   c. Immunoelectrophoretogram (IEPG) of blood and urine
   d. Plasma norepinephrine, supine and standing
   e. Fat aspirate for amyloid
   f. Urinary porphyrins
   g. Anti-neuronal nuclear antibody (ANNA), voltage gated calcium channel antibody
   h. EMG (fast repetitive stimulation)
   i. Cerebrospinal fluid (CSF) evaluation for protein, oligoclonal bands, CSF index.

The autonomic reflex screen is a non-invasive panel of tests that evaluates the severity and distribution of cardiovagal, postganglionic sudomotor, and adrenergic failure.[4] The thermoregulatory sweat test[83] provides a semi-quantitative evaluation of anhidrosis. The percent of anterior body surface that is anhidrotic correlates well with the severity of autonomic failure.[83] The routine workup is selected to detect evidence of collagen vascular disease (ESR, rheumatoid factor, antinuclear antibody), Sjögren's syndrome (foregoing and ENA group), amyloidosis (IEPG, and fat aspirate), porphyria (urinary porphyrins), LEMS (EMG; voltage gated calcium channel antibody), and malignant disease (ANNA).

Step 3 (additional studies)

Most cases will have been diagnosed using steps one and two. Some cases will require additional studies. These include plasma cortisol for the patient with adrenal failure. Some patients require computer-assisted sensory evaluation to better delineate the pattern of sensory loss if present. A few cases will require sural nerve biopsy. This can provide definitive evidence of amyloid infiltration, or rare causes such as Fabry's or Tangier disease. Leukocyte α-galactosidase can be measured for Fabry's disease. Lipoprotein electrophoresis can be done when Tangier disease is suspected. Conjunctival or submucosal biopsy may provide definitive diagnosis of Sjögren's disease. Genetic analysis may sort out the type of amyloid neuropathy, and reveal new types of inherited neuropathies. Finally, additional autonomic studies can be designed to study additional aspects or areas of the autonomic nervous system.

Step 4 (management strategy)

1. Treat etiology when possible; for example, porphyria, botulism, immune-mediated neuropathy, neuropathy due to drugs and poisons, the Guillain-Barré, and Lambert-Eaton myasthenic syndromes.
2. Treat manifestations of autonomic failure, including orthostatic hypotension, gastrointestinal dysmotility, erectile failure, and urinary retention or incontinence.
3. Treat dysautonomia, including the autonomic storm and pain management.

REFERENCES

1. Lambert EH, Dyck PJ. Compound action potentials of sural nerve in vitro in peripheral neuropathy. In PJ Dyck, PK Thomas, EH Lambert, R Bunge (eds), Peripheral Neuropathy, 2nd ed. Philadelphia: WB Saunders, 1984;1130–1144.
2. Low PA. Autonomic nervous system function. J Clin Neurophysiol 1993;10:14–27.
3. Low PA. Clinical evaluation of autonomic function. In PA Low (ed), Clinical Autonomic Disorders: Evaluation and Management. Boston: Little, Brown and Company, 1992;157–168.
4. Low PA. Laboratory evaluation of autonomic failure. In PA Low (ed), Clinical Autonomic Disorders: Evaluation and Management. Boston: Little, Brown and Company, 1993;169–196.
5. Low PA, McLeod JG. The autonomic neuropathies. In PA Low (ed), Clinical Autonomic Disorders: Evaluation and Management. Boston: Little, Brown and Company, 1993;395–422.
6. Low PA, Dyck PJ. Pathologic studies and the nerve biopsy in autonomic neuropathies. In PA Low (ed), Clinical Autonomic Disorders: Evaluation and Management. Boston: Little, Brown and Company, 1993;331–344.
7. Suarez G, Fealey RD, Camilleri M, Low PA. Idiopathic autonomic neuropathy: clinical, neurophysiologic, and follow-up studies on 27 patients. Neurology 1994;44:1675–1682.
8. Balm R, Zinsmeister A, Greydanus M, et al. Visceral dysautonomia in a subset of patients with idiopathic chronic intestinal pseudo-obstruction. Gastroenterology 1990;98:A324.
9. Fagius J, Wallin BG. Microneurographic evidence of excessive sympathetic outflow in the Guillain-Barre syndrome. Brain 1980;106:589–600.
10. Heafield MT, Gammage MD, Nightingale S, Williams AC. Idiopathic dysautonomia treated with intravenous gammaglobulin. Lancet 1996;347:28–29.
11. Smit AAJ, Vermeulen M, Koelman JHTM, Wieling W. Unusual recovery from acute panautonomic neuropathy after immunoglobulin therapy. Mayo Clin Proc 1997;72:333–335.
12. Pickett JB. AAEE case report #16: botulism. Muscle Nerve 1988;11:1201–1205.
13. Nix WA, Eckardt VF, Kramer G. Reversible esophageal motor dysfunction in botulism. Muscle Nerve 1985;8:791–795.
14. Critchley EM, Mitchell JD. Human botulism. Brit J Hosp Med 1990;43:290–292.
15. Vita G, Girlanda P, Puglisi RM, et al. Cadiovascular-reflex testing and single fiber electromyography in botulism, a longitudinal study. Arch Neurol 1987;44:202–206.
16. Jenzer G, Mumenthaler M, Ludin HP, Robert F. Autonomic dysfunction in botulism B: a clinical report. Neurology 1975;25:150–153.
17. Ridley A, Hierons R, Cavanagh JB. Tachycardia and the neuropathy of porphyria. Lancet 1968;2:708–710.
18. Ridley A. Porphyric Neuropathy. In PJ Dyck, PK Thomas, EH Lambert (eds), Peripheral Neuropathy. Philadelphia: WB Saunders, 1975;942–955.
19. Schirger A, Martin WJ, Goldstein NP, Huizenga KA. Orthostatic hypotension in association with acute exacerbations of porphyria. Proc Mayo Clin 1962;37:7–11.
20. Stewart PM, Hensley WJ. An acute attack of variegate porphyria complicated by severe autonomic neuropathy. Aust NZ J Med 1981;11:82–83.
21. Laiwah ACY, MacPhee GJA, Boyle P, et al. Autonomic neuropathy in acute intermittent porphyria. J Neurol Neurosurg Psychiatry 1985;48:1025–1030.
22. Rosenfeld CS, Broder LE. Cisplatin-induced autonomic neuropathy. Cancer Treat Rep 1984;68:659–660.
23. McLeod JG, Penny R. Vincristine neuropathy: an electrophysiological and histological study. J Neurol Neurosurg Psychiatry 1969;32:297–304.
24. Legha SS. Vincristine neurotoxicity. Pathophysiology and management. Med Toxicol 1986;1:421–427.
25. LeQuesne PM. Neuropathy Due to Drugs. In PJ Dyck, PK Thomas, EH Lambert, R Bunge (eds), Peripheral Neuropathy. Philadelphia: WB Saunders, 1984;2162–2179.
26. LeWitt PA. Neurotoxicity of the rat poison Vacor. A clinical study of 12 cases. N Engl J Med 1980;302:73–77.
27. Johnson D, Kubic P, Levitt C. Accidental ingestion of Vacor rodenticide: the systems and sequelae in a 25-month-old child. Am J Dis Child 1980;134:161–164.

28. Palakurthy PR, Iyer V, Meckler RJ. Unusual neurotoxicity associated with amiodarone therapy. Arch Intern Med 1987;147:881–884.

29. Martinez-Arizala A, Sobol SM, McCarty GE, et al. Amiodarone neuropathy. Neurology 1983;33:643–645.

30. Jacobs JM, Costa-Jussa FR. The pathology of amiodarone neurotoxicity. II. Peripheral neuropathy in man. Brain 1985;108:753–769.

31. Manolis AS, Tordjman T, Mack KD, Estes NA III. Atypical pulmonary and neurologic complications of amiodarone in the same patients. Report of a case and a review of the literature. Arch Intern Med 1987;147:1805–1809.

32. Bank WJ, Pleasure DE, Suzuki K, et al. Thallium poisoning. Arch Neurol 1972;26:456–464.

33. Goldstein WP, McCall JT, Dyck PJ. Metal neuropathy. In PJ Dyck, PK Thomas, EH Lambert (eds), Peripheral Neuropathy. Philadelphia: WB Saunders, 1975;1127–1162.

34. Quesne PM, McLeod JG. Peripheral neuropathy following a single exposure to arsenic. J Neurol Sci 1977;32:437–451.

35. Warkany J, Hubbard DM. Mercury in urine of children with acrodynia. Lancet 1948;1:829–830.

36. Bower DB. Pink disease: autonomic disorder and its treatment with ganglion-blocking agents. Q J Med 1954;23:215–230.

37. Altenkirch H, Mager J, Stoltenburg G, Helmbrecht J. Toxic polyneuropathies after sniffing a glue thinner. J Neurol 1977;214:137–152.

38. Steward JD, Low PA, Fealey RD. Distal small-fiber peripheral neuropathy; results of tests of sweating and autonomic cardiovascular reflexes. Muscle Nerve 1992;15:661–665.

39. Evans BA, Lussky D, Knezevic W. The peripheral autonomic surface potential in suspected small fiber peripheral neuropathy. Muscle Nerve 1988;11:982(abst).

40. Jamal GA, Hansen S, Weir AI, Ballantyne JP. The neurophysiologic investigation of small fiber neuropathies. Muscle Nerve 1987;10:537–545.

41. Low PA, Dyck PJ, Lambert EH, et al. Acute panautonomic neuropathy. Ann Neurol 1983;13:412–417.

42. Ross AT. Progressive selective sudomotor denervation–a case with co-existing Adie's syndrome. Neurology 1958;8:809–817.

43. Low PA, Fealey RD, Sheps SG, et al. Chronic idiopathic anhidrosis. Ann Neurol 1985;18:344–348.

44. Johnson RH, Spalding JMK. Disorders of the Autonomic Nervous System. Oxford: Blackwell, 1974.

45. Johnson RH, McLellan DL, Love DR. Orthostatic hypotension and the Holmes-Adie syndrome. A study of two patients with afferent baroreceptor block. J Neurol Neurosurg Psychiatry 1971;34:562–570.

46. Griffin JW, Cornblath DR, Alexander E, et al. Ataxic sensory neuropathy and dorsal root ganglionitis associated with Sjögren's syndrome. Ann Neurol 1990;27:304–315.

47. Harriman DGF, Garland HG. The pathology of Adie's syndrome. Brain 1968;91:401–418.

48. Koberle F. Chagas' disease and Chagas' syndromes. Adv Parasit 1968;6:63–116.

49. Harati Y, Low PA. Autonomic Peripheral Neuropathies: Diagnosis and Clinical Presentation. In SH Appel (ed), Current Neurology. Yearbook Med Publ, 1990;105–176.

50. Gallo Jr L, Marin-Neto JA, Manco JC, et al. Abnormal heart rate responses during exercise in patients with Chagas' disease. Cardiology 1975;60:147–162.

51. Amorim DS, Manco JC, Gallo L Jr, Martin-Neto JA. Chagas' heart disease as an experimental model for studies of cardiac autonomic function in man. Mayo Clin Proc 1982;57(Suppl):46–60.

52. Iosa D, DeQuattro V, Lee DD, et al. Plasma norepinephrine in Chagas' cardioneuromyopathy: a marker of progressive dysautonomia. Am Heart J 1989;117:882–887.

53. Manco JC, Gallo L Jr, Godoy RA, et al. Degeneration of the cardiac nerves in Chagas' disease. Circulation 1969;40:879–885.

54. Said G, Joskowicz M, Barreira AA, Eisen H. Neuropathy associated with experimental Chagas' disease. Ann Neurol 1985;18:676–683.

55. Iosa D, Massari DC, Dorsey FC. Chagas' cardioneuropathy: effect of ganglioside treatment in chronic dysautonomic patients–a randomized double-blind parallel placebo-controlled study. Am Heart J 1991;122:775–785.

56. Kirchoff LV. Trypanosomiasis. In JD Wilson, E Braunwald, KJ Isselbacher, et al. (eds), Harrison's Principles of Internal Medicine. New York: McGraw Hill, 1991;791–795.
57. Robertson D, Goldberg MR, Onrot J, et al. Isolated failure of autonomic noradrenergic neurotrnasmisison. Evidence for impaired beta-hydroxylation of dopamine. N Engl J Med 1986;314:1494–1497.
58. Mathias CJ, Bannister R, Cortelli P, et al. Clinical autonomic and therapeutic observations in two siblings with postural hypotension and sympathetic failure due to an inability to sythesize noradrenaline from dopamine because of a deficiency of dopamine beta hydroxylase. Q J Med 1990;278:617–633.
59. Dyck PJ, Lambert EH. Dissoaciated sensation in amyloidosis. Compound action potential, quantitative histologic and teased fiber, and electron microscopic studies of sural nerve biopsies. Arch Neurol 1969;20:490–507.
60. Kyle RA, Greipp PR. Amyloidosis: clinical and laboratory features in 229 cases. Mayo Clin Proc 1983;58:665–683.
61. Rubinow A, Burakoff R, Cohen AS, Harris LD. Esophageal manometry in systemic amyloidosis. a study of 30 patients. Am J Med 1983;75:951–956.
62. Sandgren O, Hofer PA. Conjunctival involvement in familial amyloiditic polyneuropathy. Acta Opthalmol 1990;68:292–296.
63. Kudo M, Griggs RC. Diagnostic usefulness of intramuscular nerve bundles. Arch Pathol Lab Med 1982;106:665–683.
64. Morita K, Yahura O, Onodera S, et al. Familial amyloidotic polyneuropathy in Hokkaido: a case report. Jpn J Med 1990;29:61–65.
65. Verghese JP, Bradley WG, Nemni R, McAdam KP. Amyloid neuropathy in multiple myeloma and other plasma cell dyscrasias. A hypothesis of the pathogenesis of amyloid neuropathies. J Neurol Sci 1983;59:237–246.
66. Vital C, Lacoste D, Deminiere C, et al. Amyloid neuropathy and multiple myeloma. Ultrastructural and immunopathological study of two cases. Eur Neurol 1983;22:106–112.
67. Wallace MR, Naylor SL, Kluve-Beckerman B, et al. Localization of the human prealbumin gene to chromosome 18. Biochem Biosphys Res Commun 1985;129:753–758.
68. Kanda Y, Goodman DS, Canfield RE, Morgan FJ. The amino acid sequence of human plasma prealbumin. J Biol Chem 1974;249:6796–6805.
69. Benson MD. Familial amyloidotic polyneuropathy. Trends Neurosci 1989;12:88–92.
70. Nichols WC, Wallace MR, Benson MD. Enzymatic amplification of prealbumin genomic sequences and potential use in diagnosis of hereditary amyloidosis. Am J Hum Genet 1987; 41:A230.
71. Nakazato M, Kurihara T, Matsukura S, et al. Diagnostic radioimmunoassay for familial amyloidotic polyneuropathy before clinical onset. J Clin Invest 1986;77:1699–1703.
72. Colan RV, Snead OC III, Oh SJ, Kashlan MB. Acute autonomic and sensory neuropathy. Ann Neurol 1980;8:441–444.
73. Okajima T, Yamamura S, Hamada K, et al. Chronic sensory and autonomic neuropathy. Neurology 1983;33:1061–1064.
74. Font J, Valls J, Cervera R, et al. Pure sensory neuropathy in patients with primary Sjögren's syndrome: clinical, immunological, and electromyographic findings. Ann Rheum Dis 1990;49:775–778.
75. Vrethem M, Lindvall B, Holmgren H, et al. Neuropathy and myopathy in primary Sjögren's syndrome: neurophysiological, immunological and muscle biopsy results. Acta Neurol Scand 1990;82:126–131.
76. Nichols WC, Wallace MR, Benson MD. Enzymatic amplification of prealbumin genomic sequences and potential use in diagnosis of hereditary amyloidosis. Am J Hum Genet 1987;41:A230.
77. Binder A, Snaith ML, Isenberg D. Sjögren's syndrome: a study of its neurological complications. Br J Rheumatol 1998;27:275–280.
78. Mellgren SI, Conn DL, Stevens JC, Dyck PJ. Peripheral neuropathy in primary Sjogren's syndrome. Neurology 1989;39:390–394.
79. Mahloudji M, Brundt PW, McKusick VA. Clinical neurological aspects of familial dysautonomia. J Neurol Sci 1970;11:383–395.

80. Weinshilboum RM, Axelrod J. Reduced plasma dopamine beta-hydroxylase activity in familial dysautonomia. N Engl J Med 1971;285:938–942.
81. Ropper AH. Acute autonomic emergencies and autonomic storm. In PA Low (ed), Clinical Autonomic Disorders: Evaluation and Management. Boston: Little, Brown and Company, 1993;747–760.
82. Ochoa J. The newly recognized painful ABC syndrome: thermographic aspects. Thermology 1986;2:65–107.
83. Fealey RD. Thermoregulatory sweat test. In PA Low (ed), Clinical Autonomic Disorders: Evaluation and Management. Boston: Little, Brown and Company, 1993;217–229.

Chapter 6
Gastrointestinal Dysfunction in Spinal Cord Disease

Ronald F. Pfeiffer

Spinal cord disease might be viewed as the "orphan" of the neurological disease spectrum. No single specialty or sub-specialty has claimed the treatment of spinal cord dysfunction as its own turf, and in everyday practice spinal cord problems are handled by a variety of medical and surgical specialists, including neurologists, neurosurgeons, orthopedic surgeons, physiatrists, and others. All too often individuals with spinal cord dysfunction are ultimately left to fend for themselves with the assistance of their primary care physicians.[1]

Individuals with spinal cord dysfunction are subject to a devastatingly diverse array of difficulties that involve motor, sensory, and autonomic malfunction. Paralysis, decubitus ulcers, and urinary dysfunction are most often the subjects of physician focus, while gastrointestinal (GI) dysfunction receives less attention. This is also evident in the medical literature, where GI dysfunction in the setting of spinal cord disease has received surprisingly little emphasis. In many respects, this chapter will reflect the relative paucity of knowledge available to aid in dealing with the GI aspects of spinal cord dysfunction.

GI dysfunction is mediated by a combination of neural, endocrine, and luminal influences.[1] Though spinal cord damage disrupts neural pathways to the gut, the enteric nervous system and endocrine mechanisms remain largely functionally intact. Because the parasympathetic and sympathetic components of the autonomic nervous system exit the central nervous system at widely different locations, there is also considerable variability in the degree of autonomic dysfunction encountered with spinal cord pathology at different levels.

Parasympathetic supply to the GI tract originates from both brainstem (vagal nuclei) and sacral locations. The parasympathetic supply to the esophagus, stomach, small intestine, and even structures as far caudal as the right (ascending) colon is derived from the vagus nerves and their nuclei in the brainstem and is completely spared in spinal cord injury (SCI), regardless of the level. Parasympathetic innervation of the left (descending) colon and anorectum is derived from the sacral parasympathetic centers in the spinal cord and is, thus, denervated in spinal cord lesions at virtually all levels. Sympathetic supply to the GI tract arises from the T_5-L_3 levels of the spinal cord and is, therefore, intact in lower lumbar cord lesions, but disrupted in cervical and upper thoracic lesions. Cord lesions at different levels may, therefore, have significantly different GI symptomology.

A variety of processes can damage or interfere with spinal cord function. Trauma is the leading cause of spinal cord damage, with 10,000 to 20,000 SCIs resulting in significant paresis occurring in the United States each year.[2] Reported incidence rates of SCI range from 11.5 to 71 injuries per million, while prevalence rates run between 721 to 906 per million population.[3–5] Traffic accidents are the most frequent source of injury, but sports and other recreation-related injuries form a significant component. Work-related injuries also certainly occur, but their frequency has actually diminished in recent years. In individuals above 65, falls constitute the most frequent mechanism of SCI.[3] Most SCIs, however, involve younger individuals between the ages of 10 to 35, with the consequence that a growing number of individuals with chronic SCIs and the various complications that accompany them confront the healthcare system today. It has been estimated that approximately 200,000 individuals with SCI are alive in the United States today.[3]

Trauma is not the only condition producing spinal cord dysfunction, however. Inflammatory, infectious, degenerative, and vascular processes also contribute to the number of individuals with spinal cord dysfunction.

SPINAL CORD INJURY

SCI results in abnormalities of both sensation and motor function as both afferent and efferent connections with cerebral centers are severed. While the disturbances of somatic sensation and voluntary muscle function following SCI are readily apparent, concomitant impairment of visceral sensation and visceral motor function are less easily discernable. The sensory abnormalities, both visceral and somatic, also magnify the difficulty in recognizing and diagnosing GI dysfunction in SCI patients.

GI dysfunction following SCI may become evident in the first days and weeks following the insult. Spinal shock is characterized by the temporary loss of reflex function in affected cord segments below the lesion immediately following the SCI, in addition to the loss of voluntary function. This results in slowing of colonic motility with consequent reflex ileus, which may develop in 8% of individuals with acute SCI, most often in those with cervical or upper thoracic cord injury.[6] Spinal shock typically persists for 3 to 4 weeks before resolving spontaneously.

During the initial days and weeks following SCI some additional acute GI emergencies can develop. In one retrospective review of 1300 cases of SCI, acute abdominal emergencies developed in seven (0.5%) individuals within the first 9 months following injury.[7] In four individuals the event occurred within 10 to 30 days of the SCI and in each instance a perforated ulcer was responsible. Other abdominal emergencies included appendicitis, peritonitis, and intestinal obstruction. Other investigators have also noted a high risk of acute abdominal emergencies in the early post-SCI patients. Life-threatening gastrointestinal hemorrhage was noted in 2.5% of SCI patients in one study,[8] sometimes within the first few days following injury, while in another large study intra-abdominal pathology developed in 4.7% of 945 cases.[9] In the latter study, the GI emergencies primarily occurred in individuals with lesions above the T5 level. In addition to GI hemorrhage, pancreatitis was noted to occur, occasionally as early as 3 days post-injury.[9] Acute acalculous cholecystitis has also been reported to follow multiple trauma with SCI.[10]

In many individuals, recognition of an acute abdominal emergency is delayed, often for 1 to 4 days, presumably because of impaired sensation secondary to the SCI.[7] Classical symptoms of acute abdominal emergency, such as abdominal tenderness, abdominal muscle rigidity, rebound tenderness, and even fever and leukocytosis are not entirely reliable indicators of acute abdominal pathology in this setting, and other symptoms and signs, such as referred shoulder tip pain, abdominal distension, and even increased spasticity in conjunction with abdominal pain, nausea, and vomiting are better predictors.[7] The most important sign of acute abdominal pathology, however, is the development of autonomic dysreflexia,[7,11] which is characterized clinically by a combination of hypertension, skin pallor, sweating, and piloerection due to massive sympathetic over-activity triggered by noxious stimuli below the level of a SCI lesion.[1] Autonomic dysreflexia presumably reflects the loss of cerebral inhibitory input on thoracolumbar outflow and, therefore, is seen in individuals with cervical and upper thoracic SCI.

Although abdominal events in the acute post-SCI period may be dramatic and life threatening, GI dysfunction in the setting of chronic SCI represents a more prevalent and pervasive challenge for both patient and physician. Chronic GI problems of sufficient severity to impair activities of daily living or require long-term management are reported in 27 to 69% of individuals with SCI.[12–16] Hospital admission for evaluation or treatment of GI dysfunction was necessary in up to 23% of SCI patients, as reported by Stone; 79% of the time admissions were for management of chronic GI problems and approximately 45% of SCI patients admitted for GI difficulties ultimately required corrective surgery.[13] There is disagreement among investigators as to whether complete cord lesions and a longer interval following injury increase the risk for developing GI dysfunction,[12,13,17,18] but all agree that problems arising at all levels of the GI tract may be seen.

Esophagus

Cervical spine trauma with cervical vertebral fractures can produce direct esophageal injury, including esophageal perforation.[19]

This may also occur as a complication of anterior spinal surgery. Symptoms may include unexplained fever, swelling of the neck, and leukocytosis, in addition to dysphagia.[20] Surgical repair is usually necessary.[19]

Symptoms of chronic esophageal dysfunction develop in a significant proportion of individuals with SCI. In a questionnaire administered to 46 consecutive new admissions with chronic SCI to a SCI service, 61% of patients reported heartburn, 52% experienced abdominal pain, 33% noted episodes of esophageal chest pain, and 30% experienced dysphagia, compared to respective frequencies of 40%, 8%, 6%, and 8% in a group of control patients.[21] When present, the frequency and severity of these symptoms were also significantly higher in the SCI group. In another study, retrospective in design and utilizing pharmacy data, an overall increase in prevalence of symptoms of gastroesophageal reflux was not documented (22% in SCI patients vs. 28% in general medical controls), but the prevalence of severe esophagitis was higher in the SCI group.[22]

Objective evidence of esophageal dysfunction is even more striking than that derived from subjective symptom reports. In 11 individuals with SCI undergoing esophagogastroduodenoscopy (EGD), histologic evidence of esophagitis was documented in 91%.[21] Esophageal motility studies demonstrated reduced contraction amplitude and contraction velocity in SCI patients, especially in the proximal esophagus.[21]

Individuals with SCI were also more likely to display an increased frequency of abnormal patterns of contraction, such as double-peaked and repetitive contractions. These abnormalities of peristaltic function with resultant esophageal dysmotility may lead to reduced esophageal acid clearance and thus to the increased incidence of esophagitis, even though the lower esophageal sphincter, which is vagally inner-vated, typically functions normally in individuals with SCI.[21] Other factors may also play a role in producing gastroesophageal reflux in persons with SCI. The increased time spent in a supine position, increased intra-abdominal pressure as a result of chronic constipation with frequent use of Valsalva maneuver, and the use of abdominal muscles for transferring may increase the likelihood of reflux.[21]

Separate from gastroesophgeal reflux disease, dysphagia is a frequent occur-rence in persons with SCI at the cervical cord level. Estimates of this problem in quadriplegic patients range from approximately 16 to 24%.[13,23] The risk of devel-oping dysphagia rises somewhat with age, but the presence of a tracheostomy and prior cervical surgery via an anterior approach are even stronger predictors of dys-phagia in cervical SCI patients.[23] Aspiration is a potentially serious complication of dysphagia and is common in those with symptomatic dysphagia. However, "silent" aspiration is also a frequent occurrence in individuals with tracheostomies on mechanical ventilation.[24]

Stomach

The effects of SCI on gastric function have been less thoroughly studied than those occurring in the lower GI tract. Gastric motility is influenced by both the sympathetic and parasympathetic systems. Because high thoracic and cervical cord lesions inter-rupt cortical inhibitory signals with consequent disinhibition of thoracic sympathetic outflow, diminished gastric motility with prolongation of gastric emptying time (GET) should occur following lesions in these locations; conversely, gastric motility should be undisturbed following spinal cord damage below a T12 level.[25] There has been some controversy, however, as to whether GET prolongation actually develops at all following SCI. While several investigators have questioned whether GET is delayed following upper cord lesions,[26,27] the preponderance of studies suggests it is.[25,28-33] In a series of studies Gondim and colleagues noted that emptying is delayed in rats following cervical cord transection and have attributed this delay to involve-ment of splanchnic pathways.[31–33] Kao and colleagues studied a group of 50 SCI patients, 24 with high-level injury above T5 and the remaining 26 with lesions below the T12 level.[25] Delayed (>124.4 minutes) gastric emptying half-time was noted in 58% of the entire group. Individuals with high cord lesions were much more likely to demonstrate impaired gastric emptying (83%) than were subjects with lower lesions (35%). A greater percentage of females than males with SCI demonstrated prolonged GET (75% vs. 47%), but this gender effect has also been noted in other studies evaluating non-SCI patients.[34] Studies provide conflicting conclusions as to whether these delays in gastric emptying diminish over time following SCI.[25,29]

The clinical significance of delayed gastric emptying in SCI patients has not been precisely delineated, but problems such as gastric distension could be a con-sequence, and delayed gastric emptying could impact on the absorption and thus the efficacy of a variety of medications.

While gastric ulcer formation has been documented in the acute post-SCI period, in the timeframe of chronic SCI, gastric ulceration is less prominent and ulcer formation in the duodenum is more typical.[6,35]

Small Intestine

Small bowel function following SCI has not been extensively evaluated. Orocecal transit time, an indirect measure of small bowel transit time, was studied by Binnie and colleagues in 10 individuals with SCI and 10 controls.[36] No difference in transit time was present between the two groups. Others have also reported intact small bowel transit following SCI.[37]

Colon

Bowel dysfunction is the best-studied and most frequently reported GI problem following SCI. An extensive array of bowel-related problems has been described in SCI patients. Abdominal bloating, constipation, fecal incontinence, and even hemorrhoid formation may occur. Most individuals note some degree of impaired bowel function following SCI.[1]

Diminished bowel movement frequency (fewer than 2 to 3 weekly) develops in up to 77% of individuals with long-standing SCI,[14] while 31 to 55% of SCI patients experience abdominal pain or distension, often as a post-prandial phenomenon.[13,38,39] Many persons with SCI also are bothered by a more vague abdominal discomfort or sensation of bloating that may be relieved by bowel care or passing flatus.[13] The reduced bowel movement frequency and abdominal bloating appear to be the consequence of delayed or slowed colonic motility. Binnie and colleagues catalogued a mean bowel movement frequency of .37 per day in 10 individuals with SCI, compared to 1.12 per day in 10 control subjects.[36] Oroanal transit time was prolonged to 187.3 hours in the individuals with SCI, compared to 68.7 hours in the controls. As noted earlier, orocecal transit time in the two groups was not significantly different, with times of 3.4 hours for SCI patients and 2.95 hours for controls, pointing to the colon as the source of the slowed transit in SCI patients.[36] Utilizing indium amberlite scintigraphy in SCI patients with thoracic lesions, Keshavarzian and colleagues calculated their velocity of colon transit to be .63 cm/hour, compared to a velocity of 2.58 cm/hour in normal controls.[40]

Whether the retardation of colonic transit involves the entire colon or just its descending and rectosigmoid portions remains a point of controversy. While scintigraphic studies seem to indicate pan-colonic delays,[39,40] investigators using other methods have noted slowing to be primarily confined to the left (descending) colon and rectosigmoid regions.[41–43] In a recent study of segmental colon transit time in SCI patients, Krogh and colleagues noted significant prolongation of transit time in the transverse and descending colon, a tendency toward significant prolongation in the ascending colon, but no prolongation of rectosigmoid transit time.[44] This stands in contrast to earlier studies, such as that of Menardo et al., where inconsistent delays in the colon transit index were documented in the right (ascending) colon and markedly slowed transit noted in the left (descending) colon and rectum.[37] The reason for these disparate results is not readily apparent and does not appear to be related to the level of SCI.

From an anatomical standpoint, more severe impairment following SCI might be expected in the descending and rectosigmoid regions, since parasympathetic supply to these structures arises from the sacral cord, while the ascending and transverse colon receive their parasympathetic supply from the posterior vagus.[45] It has, in fact, been suggested[37] that sympathetic changes are probably not critically important factors in the genesis of bowel dysfunction in the setting of SCI (or in other settings) since individuals undergoing bilateral total sympathectomy do not experience changes in bowel habits.[46]

In addition to delayed colon transit time with reduced bowel movement frequency, difficulty with the act of defecation itself develops in approximately 20% of individuals with SCI.[13,47] There is some suggestion that this is more likely to occur in persons with higher cord injuries than in those with lesions between T10 and T12[13,17] and that problems with defecatory dysfunction represent a delayed development, often taking four years or more to appear.[13] Difficulty in accomplishing defecation can compel affected individuals to spend prolonged periods of time, often 1 hour or more per day, in bowel care and may necessitate the manual evacuation of feces when more usual methods such as digital stimulation, suppositories, and enemas are not effective.[13]

The level of SCI is an important determinant of the presence and character of defecatory dysfunction. Individuals with lesions affecting the cauda equina or conus medullaris are left with flaccid external anal sphincter and puborectalis muscles, along with reduced internal anal sphinter tone.[18] This combination typically leads to fecal incontinence, which is particularly likely to occur when intra-abdominal pressure is raised. Fecal incontinence can present a problem that is of sufficient severity to warrant colostomy in a small percentage (1.5%) of individuals with conus lesions.[13]

Persons with higher cord lesions face an entirely different set of circumstances. Puborectalis and external anal sphinter muscles, as with other striated muscles below the level of the cord lesion, become disinhibited and spastic. This results in loss of conscious sphincter control and consequent anorectal dyssynergy,[18] which prevents voluntary control of defecation. Reflex pathways, however, remain intact and functional and internal anal sphincter tone is maintained[38]; some investigators have, in contrast, noted reduced anal canal pressure, even in patients with supraconal cord lesions, and have suggested that this reflects dominance of sacral parasympathetic input over lumbar sympathetic signals in the regulation of internal anal sphincter tone when control from higher centers is lost.[39] Because of these intact and autonomously functioning centers, stimulation of the rectal mucosa can be utilized to trigger the rectoanal inhibitory reflex with consequent internal anal sphincter and external anal sphincter relaxation, along with pelvic nerve-mediated peristalsis and subsequent defecation.[18,38] While occasional episodes of fecal incontinence occur in 49% or more of individuals with higher cord lesions, and then usually limited to such situations as acute illness or dietary indiscretion, recurrent episodes of fecal incontinence are unusual, being noted in one series in as few as 4%, presumably as a consequence of fecal stasis or impaction with overflow incontinence.[17]

Treatment of bowel dysfunction in persons with SCI can be a difficult and demanding process that requires dedication and determination on the part of both patient and physician. Best results can probably be achieved in a formal neurogenic bowel management program that will typically entail dietary measures, bowel training, and pharmacological approaches, including stool softeners, hyperosmolar laxatives, and suppositories.[38] Prokinetic agents such as cisapride have been recommended by some,[41] but cautioned against by others.[48] Implantable anterior sacral nerve root stimulators, typically utilized for bladder control in paraplegic patients, have also been successfully utilized to improved bowel function in SCI patients.[36]

OTHER DISEASE PROCESSES

Multiple Sclerosis

While it is quite clearly evident that GI dysfunction following SCI is the consequence of spinal cord pathology, the same conclusion cannot be so quickly drawn with multiple sclerosis (MS). By its very nature, MS is often characterized by a clinical, radiographic, and pathologic picture of multiple lesions that may involve cerebral, brainstem, and spinal cord locations simultaneously. Therefore, while individuals with MS frequently display GI symptoms, spinal cord dysfunction may not necessarily be solely to blame. Fowler and her colleagues point to the fact that 32% of patients with the clinical picture of bladder impairment and other features of spinal cord dysfunction do not experience symptoms of bowel dysfunction, and suggest that bowel dysfunction in MS may be multifactorial.[49–51] Nevertheless, it seems probable that spinal cord pathology plays a significant, though not exclusive, role in the etiology of at least some aspects of GI dysfunction in MS.

Very little has been specifically written about GI dysfunction in MS. Individuals with MS may experience dysphagia, and esophageal dysmotility has also been described, but the source of the pathology producing these symptoms is more probably in the brainstem than in the spinal cord.[52–56] Calcagno and colleagues identified dysphagia in 34% of 143 patients with MS, and noted a correlation between dysphagia and disease severity.[53] This correlation, however, has not been noted by all investigators.[54] Objective evidence of swallowing abnormalities may be present in 43 to 56% of MS patients and may include aspiration in a significant proportion of such individuals.[55]

Gastroparesis has also been noted anecdotally in the setting of MS, with typical symptoms of nausea, vomiting, and bloating.[57,58] Improvement in symptoms has been observed with prokinetic agents such as metoclopramide and cisapride.[57,58] The pathophysiological basis for gastroparesis in MS has not been addressed.

Impaired bowel function appears to be the primary manifestation of GI dysfunction in MS, and although formal studies are still few, bowel dysfunction in MS has received some specific investigative attention. Published studies suggest that some element of bowel dysfunction develops in up to 68% of MS patients.[59] Symptoms of bowel dysfunction can occur at any point in the illness, and may even precede the development of more traditional neurological symptoms.[60] Constipation is a frequent complaint of persons with MS, with reported rates of occurrence ranging from 43 to 53%.[59,61] Both decreased frequency of bowel movements and difficulty with actual defecation have been described.

Delayed colon transit time has been documented in individuals with MS and may explain the decreased bowel movement frequency.[60,62] Colon transit time was noted to be prolonged in five of seven (71%) MS patients with constipation studied by Chia and colleagues.[63] Other abnormalities of colonic function have also been described.[62] Some investigators have speculated that constipation in MS, especially when it occurs in persons with little clinical neurological deficit, might not be directly due to impaired colon transit, but rather to "some mechanism similar to that which causes fatigue in the disease."[49,50]

Difficulty with the act of defecation has also been described in individuals with MS, typically in persons with definite spinal cord dysfunction in the form of paraparesis.[49,50,64] Paradoxical contraction or failure of relaxation of the puborectalis muscle during attempted defecation may be a frequent occurrence in individuals with MS who are experiencing bowel-related difficulty.[63] In fact, Chia and colleagues noted this phenomenon in 80% of 10 such individuals they studied.[63]

Amyotrophic Lateral Sclerosis

Amyotrophic lateral sclerosis (ALS) is characterized clinically by a combination of neuromuscular features indicative of involvement of both upper and lower motor neurons. Initial clinical features are bulbar in character in 20 to 30% of individuals.[65] It has generally been considered that involvement in ALS is limited to motor pathways within the CNS and that sensation, bladder, and bowel function remain intact.[66] Some evidence, however, suggests that this may not be entirely accurate and that some element of autonomic involvement may also develop in ALS.

Dysphagia may be the initial clinical feature in persons with ALS and eventually develops in the majority of individuals. However, the dysphagia seen in ALS generally originates from bulbar structures, rather than spinal cord levels, and is the result of damage involving both corticobulbar pathways and cranial nerve motor nuclei in the brainstem itself, with consequent impairment of lingual, pharyngeal, and esophageal function.[66,67] With disease progression, the dysphagia also grows in severity and eventually forces both patient and physician to confront the issue of PEG tube placement.

Toepfer and colleagues have recently suggested that ALS may be more properly considered a multisystem disease, rather than a process limited exclusively to motor neurons.[68,69] They measured gastric emptying time in 18 patients with ALS and 14 healthy controls, using C^{13}-ontanoic acid breath testing, and demonstrated delayed gastric emptying in 15 of the 18 patients with ALS.[68] Involvement of the autonomic nervous system was proposed as an explanation for this finding.

The same group of investigators has also reported that colon transit time may be prolonged in patients with ALS, further supporting the proposition that there may be autonomic nervous system involvement in ALS.[69] In their study, colon transit time was markedly prolonged in 64% (9/14) of ALS patients studied, although prolongation did not seem to correlate with overall disease severity or duration.

The fact that fecal incontinence generally does not develop in patients with ALS has traditionally been attributed to the absence of involvement of the neurons of Onuf's nucleus in the neurodegenerative process.[70,71] However, more recent studies have, indeed, documented the presence of intracytoplasmic inclusions in the neurons on Onuf's nucleus.[72] Neuronal atrophy, though not actual cell loss, was also demonstrated. It appears, then, that while the neuronal population of Onuf's nucleus displays relative resistance to whatever is producing the neuronal degeneration in ALS, this resistance is not absolute and some involvement eventually develops. In an earlier electromyographic study, Carvalho and colleagues also demonstrated the presence of abnormalities in the external anal sphincter in at least 50% of 16 individuals with ALS who were clinically asymptomatic with regard to sphincter function.[73]

Tropical Spastic Paraparesis

HTLV-1 associated myelopathy/tropical spastic paraparesis (HAM/TSP) primarily involves the white matter of the lateral and posterior columns of the spinal cord. While bladder dysfunction, due to the loss of inhibitory influence from the pontine micturition center, is present in 75 to 100% of individuals with HAM/STP,[74] the frequency with which gastrointestinal dysfunction occurs is less fully delineated. Both constipation and fecal incontinence are described in anecdotal reports, in conjunction with other myelopathic features,[75–79] but no detailed, dedicated descriptions of GI symptoms in HAM/TSP are available. At times the constipation can become severe.

AIDS-Associated Vacuolar Myelopathy

AIDS-associated vacuolar myelopathy (VM), though often clinically asymptomatic, is present in 20 to 55% of individuals with AIDS, when determined by autopsy findings.[80,81] The symptoms of VM evolve slowly, typically emerging only in the later stages of AIDS. Formal studies that specifically address GI symptoms in VM are lacking, but constipation may be an early component of the clinical picture in affected individuals.[80]

A more rapidly evolving myelopathy can also develop in the setting of AIDS. On rare occasions this can be a primary manifestation of the AIDS itself, but more often the acute or subacute appearance of myelopathy in an individual with AIDS signals the presence of an opportunistic infection with an organism such as cytomegalovirus, herpes simplex virus type 2, varicella-zoster virus, toxoplasma, tuberculosis, or even syphilis.[80,82,83] Sphincter dysfunction may be a component of the clinical picture in each of these.

CONCLUSION

GI dysfunction, with its protean manifestations, can constitute a significant and potentially dangerous complication for a significant proportion of individuals with spinal cord dysfunction. Awareness of the potential for GI dysfunction in this population should, ideally, prompt more timely recognition of problems when they develop and lead to more expeditious and effective initiation of treatment for both acute and chronic GI abnormalities.

REFERENCES

1. Arnold EP. Spinal cord injury. In CJ Fowler (ed), Neurology of Bladder, Bowel and Sexual Dysfunction. Boston: Butterworth-Heinemann, 1999;275–288.
2. Croul SE, Flanders AE. Neuropathology of human spinal cord injury. In FJ Seil (ed), Neuronal Regeneration, Reorganization, and Repair (Advances in Neurology, Vol 72). Philadelphia: Lippincott-Raven, 1997;317–323.
3. Sekhon LHS, Fehlings MG. Epidemiology, demographics, and pathophysiology of acute spinal cord injury. Spine 2001;26:S2–S12.
4. Botterell EH, Jousee AT, Karaus AS, et al. A model for the future care of acute spinal cord injuries. Can J Neurol Sci 1975;2:361–380.

5. Kraus JF, Silberman TA, McArthur DL. Epidemiology of spinal cord injury. In EC Benzel, DW Cahill, P McCormack (eds), Principles of Spine Injury. New York: McGraw Hill, 1996;41–58.
6. Gore RM, Mintzer RA, Calenoff L. Gastrointestinal complications of spinal cord injury. Spine 1981;6:538–544.
7. Bar-On Z, Ohry A. The acute abdomen in spinal cord injury individuals. Paraplegia 1995;33:704–706.
8. Leramo OB, Tator CH, Hudson AR. Massive gastroduodenal hemorrhage and perforation in acute spinal cord injury. Surg Neurol 1982;17:186–190.
9. Berlly MH, Wilmot CB. Acute abdominal emergencies during the first four weeks after spinal cord injury. Surg Neurol 1982;17:186–190.
10. Romero Ganuza FJ, La Banda G, Montalvo R, Mazaira J. Acute acalculous cholecystitis in patients with acute traumatic spinal cord injury. Spinal Cord 1997;35:124–128.
11. Juler GL, Eltorai IM. The acute abdomen in spinal cord injury patients. Paraplegia 1985;23:118–123.
12. Han TR, Kim JH, Kwon BS. Chronic gastrointestinal problems and bowel dysfunction in patients with spinal cord injury. Spinal Cord 1998;36:485–490.
13. Stone JM, Nino-Murcia M, Wolfe VA, Perkash I. Chronic gastrointestinal problems in spinal cord injury patients: a prospective analysis. Am J Gastroenterol 1990;85:1114–1119.
14. Kannisto M, Rintala R. Bowel function in adults who have sustained spinal cord injury in childhood. Paraplegia 1995;33:701–703.
15. Levi R, Hultling C, Nash MS, Seiger A. The Stockholm spinal cord injury study: 1. Medical problems in a regional SCI population. Paraplegia 1995;33:308–315.
16. Levi R, Hultling C, Seiger A. The Stockholm spinal cord injury study: 2. Associations between clinical patient characteristics and post-acute medical problems. Parapelgia 1995;33:585–594.
17. De Looze D, Van Laere M, De Muynck M, et al. Constipation and other gastrointestinal problems in spinal cord injury patients. Spinal Cord 1998;36:63–66.
18. Lynch AC, Antony A, Dobbs BR, Frizelle FA. Bowel dysfunction following spinal cord injury. Spinal Cord 2001;39:193–203.
19. English GM, Hsu SF, Edgar R, Gibson-Eccles M. Oesophageal trauma in patients with spinal cord injury. Paraplegia 1992;30:903–912.
20. Pollock RA, Purvis JM, Apple DF Jr, Murray HH. Esophageal and hypopharyngeal injuries in patients with cervical spine trauma. Ann Otol Rhinol Laryngol 1981;90:323–327.
21. Stinneford JG, Keshavarzian A, Nemchausky BA, et al. Esophagitis and esophageal motor abnormalities in patients with chronic spinal cord injuries. Paraplegia 1993;21:384–392.
22. Singh G, Triadafilopoulos G. Gastroesophgeal reflux disease in patients with spinal cord injury. J Spinal Cord Med 2000;23:23–27.
23. Kirshblum S, Johnston MV, Brown J, et al. Predictors of dysphagia after spinal cord injury. Arch Phys Med Rehabil 1999;80:1101–1105.
24. Elpern EH, Scott MG, Petro L, Ries MH. Pulmonary aspiration in mechanically ventilated patients with tracheostomies. Chest 1994;105:563–566.
25. Kao CH, Ho YJ, Changlai SP, Ding HJ. Gastric emptying in spinal cord injury patients. Dig Dis Sci 1999;44:1512–1515.
26. Rajendrun SK, Reiser JR, Bauman W, et al. Gastrointestinal transit after spinal cord injury: effect of cisapride. Am J Gastroetnerol 1992;87:1614–1617.
27. Zhang RL, Chayes Z, Korsten MA, Bauman WA. Gastric emptying rates to liquid or solid meals appear to be unaffected by spinal cord injury. Am J Gastroenterol 1994;89:1856–1858.
28. Fealey RD, Szurszewski JH, Merritt JL, DiMagno EP. Effect of traumatic spinal cord transection on human upper gastrointestinal motility and gastric emptying. Gastroenterology 1984;87:69–75.
29. Segal JL, Milne N, Brunnemann SR, Lyons KP. Metoclopramide-induced normalization of impaired gastric emptying in spinal cord injury. Am J Gastroenterol 1987;82:1143–1148.
30. Segal JL, Milne N, Brunnemann SR. Gastric emptying is impaired in patients with spinal cord injury. Am J Gastroenterol 1995;90:466–470.
31. Gondim Fde A, da-Graca JR, de-Oliviera GR, et al. Decreased gastric emptying and gastrointestinal and intestinal transits of liquid after complete spinal cord transection in awake rats. Braz J Med Biol Res 1998;31:1605–1610.

Many MyD patients show marked weakness and atrophy of masticatory muscles, leading to prognathism and dental malocclusion.[10] Other symptoms of upper GI tract involvement include oro-pharyngeal dysphagia, nasal regurgitation, recurrent laryngeal aspirations, and heartburn. Masticatory and swallowing difficulties may contribute to the progressive weight loss, characteristic of MyD.

The great majority of MyD patients have symptoms of pharyngeal and/or esophageal involvement.[11] Rarely, dysphagia may precede other manifestations of the disease[12] or even be its only symptoms.[13] The main cause of dysphagia in MyD is associated hypomotility and abnormal coordination in the pharyngeal-esophageal area.[14] Cineradiographic, scintigraphic, and manometric studies reveal marked weakness of pharyngeal muscles, with stasis of contrast in the pyriform sinuses, regurgitation, and tracheal aspiration.[15–17] The duration of pharyngeal contraction and cricopharyngeal relaxation may be prolonged.[16] Myotonia of pharyngeal muscles has been observed,[18] though it is not easy to demonstrate it clinically.

The upper part of the esophagus, built of striated musculature, is inevitably involved in the dystrophic process of MyD, contributing to weakness of cricopharyngeal muscles and incompetence of the upper esophageal sphincter (UES).[16] Functional examinations of the esophagus show reduced motility and diffuse or segmental loss of peristalsis with subsequent esophageal distention.[15,17,19] These changes lead to delayed esophageal emptying.[20] Other esophageal findings reported in MyD patients include cricopharyngeal achalasia,[21] spasm, and antiperistaltic contractions.[22] Diminished peristaltic amplitude in the lower portion of the esophagus suggests that the smooth muscle is involved.[16] Lower esophageal sphincter function usually remains normal, although prolongation of its contraction has been observed.[23] Clinically, patients with esophageal involvement present with swallowing difficulties, initially of solid food.[20] Heartburn and acid regurgitation may also occur.[24] Many patients with instrumentally proven disturbances of esophageal motility may remain asymptomatic for several years.[22] No correlation was found between the severity of esophageal dysfunction and peripheral skeletal manifestations of MyD.[25]

The few histologic studies of the pharynx and esophagus in MyD have demonstrated typical dystrophic changes of striated muscles in the pharynx and upper esophagus, and only minimal changes in the esophageal smooth muscles.[24]

Gastric dysfunction is relatively rare in MyD,[22,26] although this may simply reflect the insensitivity of current diagnostic methods. In one study[20] of 16 patients with MyD, there were only a few who reported GI symptoms, which included mild anorexia, nausea, early satiety, and abdominal distention or pain. Scintigraphy revealed significant delay in gastric emptying, which improved after administration of metoclopramide. Another study[19] revealed the disapperance of peristaltic waves. A gastric bezoar has been described in one MyD patient, presumably due to disturbed gastric motility.[27] Another MyD patient underwent successful emergency gastrectomy because of acute gastric dilatation and pyloroantral obstruction due to gastric volvulus.[28] An autopsy of another patient, who had not suffered from GI symptoms, showed dystrophic changes with fatty infiltration of the smooth muscle of the gastric wall.[7]

Malfunction of the small intestine may contribute to GI manifestations of MyD. Diarrhea and abdominal cramps are frequent complaints in such cases,[25] but true malabsorption and steatorrhea are rare.[11] Cases of paralytic ileus and sprue-like disease[29] have also been reported, presumably due to disturbed intestinal motility. In one study,[30] x-ray examination showed dys-coordinate small bowel contractions and

dilated intestinal segments; gastroduodenal manometry revealed increased duodenal contractions in the fasting state and variability of the maximal rate of contractions. In one patient, dilatation of the duodenum, strongly resembling scleroderma,
was observed radiologically.[17] The histologic picture in the small intestine is similar to other levels of the GI tract, showing dystrophic changes in smooth muscles
with partial replacement by fat.[7]

Colonic involvement with lower abdominal cramps, chronic constipation, and
megacolon has been reported by several investigators,[8,9,12] and is sometimes associated with symptomatic esophageal impairment.[19] Radiologically, a segmental
dilatation of the colon with loss of haustrations was observed, sometimes associated with a circumscribed area of narrowed colon distal to the dilated portion,[8,17]
which was suggested to represent prolonged myotonic contraction of colonic
smooth muscles. In cases of severe megacolon, diffuse dilatation of the bowel or
its parts was evident, suggesting colonic obstruction and leading to emergency
laparotomy.[9] Pathologic findings in one patient, without clinically evident large
intestinal impairment, demonstrated typical myopathic changes in colonic smooth
muscle fibers similar to those seen in skeletal muscles.[7] In another patient who had
undergone hemicolectomy because of severe megacolon, the pathologic examination revealed normal smooth muscles and prominent degenerative changes
and neuronal loss in the myenteric plexus with decrease of the substance P- and
enkephalin-containing fibers in the muscularis externa. The authors suggested that
colonic dysfunction in MyD may be due to visceral neuropathy rather than smooth
muscle myopathy.[9]

Ano-rectal involvement in MyD patients is rarely symptomatic.[31] In most
patients without clinically evident impairment of other levels of the GI tract,
bowel habits usually remain normal. Moderate constipation is occasionally
observed. Manometric studies of MyD patients have shown significantly
decreased basal pressure, both in the external and internal anal sphincters, associated with exaggerated repetitive *rebound* contractions following rectal
distention.[32,33] Ultrasonographic measurements of anal muscle thickness have
demonstrated muscular atrophy.[32] Electromyographic findings were similar to
those found in most skeletal muscles of MyD patients, showing short polyphasic
motor unit potentials (MUP) consistent with myopathic changes and occasional
myotonic discharges. At the same time, occasional MUPs were markedly prolonged, suggesting an additional neurogenic defect. The authors suggested that
ano-rectal dysfunction represented an expression of both myopathy and neural
abnormalities.[32]

Other GI disorders occasionally associated with MyD include gallbladder
involvement with slowing of emptying, and a tendency to early gallstone formation,[34,35] alteration of bile salt metabolism,[36,37] and mild liver impairment demonstrated by elevated levels of gamma-glutamyltransferase (gamma-GT).[38]

Oculopharyngeal Muscular Dystrophy

Oculopharyngeal muscular dystrophy (OPMD) is a rare inherited muscle disease
of late onset associated with progressive ptosis of the eyelids, dysphonia, and
dysphagia. It was first described as a distinct entity in 1962 by Victor et al.[39]
The disease usually becomes evident in the fifth or sixth decade of life and has a
slowly progressive course. Other striated muscles are involved later, including

masticatory, limb girdle, and, rarely, distal limb muscles. The disease is inherited as an autosomal dominant trait, although recessive and sporadic cases have been reported.[2] Two main clusters of OPMD have been described, one among French Canadians in the province of Quebec,[40] and, the other more recently, in Jews of Bukharian (Uzbekistan) origin.[41] Several independent families with the same disease have been reported in different areas of the world. The pathogenesis of OPMD remains obscure. The gene has been recently mapped to chromosome 14q.[42]

Laboratory findings are similar to other slowly progressive muscular dystrophies with typical myopathic changes in affected muscles on EMG, and normal or slightly elevated serum creatine kinase (CK). The most striking histopathologic features of this disease are "rimmed vacuoles" seen in the sarcoplasm of affected muscle fibers, and specific characteristic filamentous inclusions, seen in about 5% of muscle nuclei. The significance of these findings remains an enigma.[2]

Involvement of the upper GI tract is an obligatory feature of OPMD and sometimes may even be the presenting symptom, preceding ptosis by several years.[43] Progressive oropharyngeal dysphagia, initially for dry solid foods and later also for liquids, leads to prolongation of the alimentation time and often to inadequate nutrition, which may result in starvation with secondary dehydration, extreme weight loss, and even death. Swallowing difficulties may increase with anxiety or after drinking cold liquids.[44] The "astrologic posture" with corrective elevation of the head due to ptosis may contribute to or aggravate dysphagia.[45] Patients with severe symptoms may be erroneously considered to suffer from esophageal cancer or psychosomatic illness.[46]

Recurrent regurgitations may result in aspiration of food and in accumulation of saliva and secretions in the nasopharynx during the night, often leading to chronic tracheo-bronchial infections. Death from pulmonary complications is not uncommon in the advanced stages of OPMD. Mild facial, temporal, and masseter muscle involvement is evident in certain patients, contributing to nutritional difficulties.[2] Weakness and atrophy of the tongue have also been reported.[47]

Cineradiographic data in OPMD confirm the involvement of pharyngeal and upper esophageal striated muscles. Weak pharyngeal contraction, delayed initiation of swallowing, and dilatation of the hypopharynx with impaired clearance of barium have been reported.[22] Reduced or absent peristalsis involving the entire esophagus indicates the involvement of both the striated and smooth esophageaal musculature.[48]

Manometric studies of the pharynx have demonstrated low pharyngeal pressure, prolongation of contraction time, and sometimes repetitive weak pharyngeal contractions.[44,49,50] In severe cases, total paralysis of the pharynx has been observed. Incomplete, prolonged, and incoordinated relaxation of the upper esophageal sphincter (UES) has been demonstrated, which contributed to difficulties in clearing the pharynx and larynx of their contents, and forced the patients to do it by repeated swallowing.[45] Resting UES pressures were low.[49]

Abnormalities of esophageal motility, although present, are generally overshadowed by involvement of the pharynx and UES. Motility studies have demonstrated weakened, nonperistaltic waves, and even lack of peristalsis in both smooth and striated muscle portions of the esophagus.[48,49,51] The function of the lower esophageal sphincter (LES) usually remains normal.[49] In a recent study, with modern solid-state manometric techniques, esophageal abnormalities were found in 10 of 11 OPMD patients, with the most common being simultaneous contractions and incomplete lower esophageal sphincter relaxation.[50]

Involvement of other levels of the gastrointestinal tract is extremely rare in OPMD. In one study, the function of the external anal sphincter was measured by EMG and rectal manometry, and subclinical involvement of the striated sphincter demonstrated.[52]

Duchenne Muscular Dystrophies

Duchenne muscular dystrophy (DMD) is usually clinically evident as early as in the third year of life, and characterized by progressive weakness and wasting of proximal lower limb muscles and pseudohypertrophic enlargement of the calves. The disease shows relentless progression, with involvement of additional muscle groups, development of fibrous contractures and secondary skeletal deformities, and, in many cases, cardiac involvement.[53] Most patients are restricted to a wheelchair by approximately 12, and die of complications during adolescence. In many cases, mild mental retardation may be observed.

Becker muscular dystrophy (BMD) represents a closely related hereditary disorder, which is operated by the same gene. The pattern of muscular system involvement is similar to DMD, but the onset occurs later and ambulation is preserved until after age 15.

Mutations in the dystrophin gene cause both DMD and BMD.[54] Dystrophin is abundant in skeletal, smooth, and cardiac muscles, tightly coupled with the cytoplasmic side of the sarcolemma, which is thought to be important in maintaining muscular membrane stability.[55] Whereas absence of dystrophin is specific for DMD, the presence of a defective form or reduced amount of dystrophin occurs in BMD. Both diseases are characterized by high levels of serum CK, a typical myopathic pattern on EMG, and severe dystrophic changes in muscle biopsy.

GI problems are not uncommon among DMD patients, and have not been reported in BMD. A case-control study of 55 children with DMD revealed a relatively high frequency of such GI complaints as dysphagia (34.4%), choking while eating (29.1%), the need to clear the throat during or after eating (23.6%), heartburn (16.3%), and vomiting during or after meals (9.1%).[56] Stomatognatic function may be impaired in DMD due to progressive weakness of masticatory muscles and macroglosia.[57,58] Poor occlusal contact with posterior crossbite or anterior open bite are typical in DMD.[59] A videotape study revealed delayed and incomplete bolus formation due to ineffective mastication.[58] The severe weight loss seen in the later stages of DMD could be due, apart from muscle wasting, also to masticatory disturbances that impair digestion.

About 60 years ago, several cases of "cardio-intestinal" syndrome were described in DMD patients, characterized by repeated attacks of vomiting, generalized abdominal tenderness, pain and diarrhea associated with tachycardia, and congestive heart failure.[60] These episodes may, in fact, have been due to acute gastric dilatation.[61,62] One patient was reported to have suffered for many years from intestinal pseudo-obstruction with recurrent episodes of nausea, vomiting, and abdominal distension. Radiologic investigations repeatedly showed significant dilatation of both small intestine and colon, and reduced motility at almost all levels of the GI tract.[63] Autopsy reports have demonstrated smooth musculature involvement of the digestive system with variation in size and shape, and fragmentation of smooth muscle fibers, as well as fatty infiltration.[62,64] The relation of these changes to dystrophin pathology still remains obscure.

In the majority of DMD patients, GI involvement may be overshadowed by the severe and debilitating peripheral manifestations of the disease. Functional studies demonstrate impairment of different levels of the GI system, even in asymptomatic patients. Manometric studies in DMD patients indicate dysfunction primarily of proximal portions of the esophagus, with significant reduction of contractions. No manometric abnormalities have been detected in the upper and lower esophageal sphincters or in the distal esophageal portion.[65] Scintigraphic studies have demonstrated a significant delay in gastric emptying,[62,65] but no changes in orocaecal transit time.[66] The constipation observed occasionally in DMD is, thus, probably not due to small intestinal impairment, but rather related to prolonged immobility and weakness of abdominal wall musculature.[66] Colonic and anal sphincter functions in DMD have not been adequately investigated.

Mitochondrial Myopathies

In recent years, a heterogeneous group of hereditary or sporadic multisystem diseases resulting from mitochondrial dysfunction have been described. Several clinically related syndromes have been identified, characterized by combinations of encephalopathy, peripheral neuropathy, myopathy, impairment of vision and hearing, as well as vascular and visceral manifestations. Different mitochondrial and nuclear DNA alterations can be associated with similar clinical phenotypes.[67] Conversely, within one kindred with a known genetic defect, different clinical manifestations may be observed, varying from progressive disease with severe disability and death, to very mild forms.[68] Involvement of the muscular system is one of the typical (but not obligatory) manifestations of these diseases. Muscle biopsy demonstrating characteristic ragged red fibers (RRF) in Gomori trichrome stain is highly suggestive of mitochondrial diseases, but more definitive diagnosis requires biochemical or genetic analysis. GI involvement may be a part of a multisystem mitochondrial disorder, or may represent its primary manifestation.

Kearns-Sayre syndrome is an adult form of predominantly ocular myopathy characterized by the triad of progressive external ophthalmoplegia, pigmentary degeneration of the retina, and myocardial conduction defects. Among associated manifestations of this condition are progressive involvement of pharyngeal and esophageal muscles with dysphagia.[69]

Mitochondrial encephalopathy with lactic acidosis and stroke-like episodes (MELAS) represents another well known phenotype of mitochondrial disease. The acronym points out its main clinical manifestations. GI involvement with disorders of gut motility, severe diarrhea, and/or constipation may be an associated feature or even a presenting manifestation of the disease.[68,70] An autopsy study of a 39-year-old patient with MELAS revealed wavy changes of the smooth fibers of the muscularis propria in the digestive system.[71]

Only one mitochondrial disease is associated with obligatory GI involvment, *mitochondrial neurogastrointestinal encephalopathy (MNGIE)*. It seems to be transmitted as an autosomal recessive trait, suggesting a nuclear DNA mutation.[72] In most reported cases, the disease became evident before age 20 with GI and/or ocular symptoms. Progressive ophthalmoplegia, sensory-motor peripheral neuropathy, and leukoencephalopathy represent other components of this multisystem disorder. The severe and often debilitating character of the disease, with resistant diarrhea and intestinal pseudoobstruction, leads to serious impairment of digestive function.[73] Functional studies have demonstrated disturbed motility of the small intestine, delayed gastric emptying, and, in certain cases, involvement of the upper gastrointestinal tract with dysmotility of the pharynx and the esophagus.[72,74] Most pathologic investigations suggest a visceral myopathic origin of GI manifestations, although evidence of neuropathic[74] and scleroderma-like changes[75] of the intestinal wall have also been reported.

Congenital myopathies (CM) encompass a heterogeneous group of rare sporadic or hereditary diseases associated with distinctive morphologic changes of muscle fibers which are evident from birth. Recent studies have permitted recognition of specific genetic abnormalities in some of these disorders.[76] Great phenotypic variability has been demonstrated in most CM, even within each affected family, ranging from generalized hypotonia and small muscle bulk, evident in early life, to mild weakness appearing in adulthood. A non-progressive course or extremely slow deterioration is typical in most cases, although examples of more rapid progression have been reported.[76] Some, but not all, CM may have GI manifestations.

Nemaline myopathy, named because of minute, rod-shaped structures (nemaline bodies) detected within muscle fibers, expresses itself by hypotonia and generalized weakness in the neonatal period. The muscles of the trunk and limbs, as well as facial, lingual, and pharyngeal muscles, are thin and hypoplastic. Infants have difficulties in sucking and swallowing, resulting in recurrent tracheo-bronchial infections, which may lead to death in the first months of life.[77] Milder forms have been described with survival for years. Adult onset may also occur. Most patients suffer from proximal myopathy with marked facial, masticatory, and pharyngeal involvement.[76]

The finding of central nuclei in muscle fibers gave the name to another kind of CM—*centronuclear myopathy*. This disease becomes evident in early life with generalized hypotonia and weakness, sometimes associated with dysmorphic features of the face.[76] Facial, masticatory, lingual, and pharyngeal muscles are weak in most cases, contributing to severe feeding and respiratory problems. Late onset cases have been recognized which are usually mild and not associated with GI symptoms.

Swallowing difficulties have also been reported in other rare forms of CM—*multicore disease,*[76] *spheroid* and *cytoplasmatic body myopathies* and *granulo-filamentous myopathy.*[78]

INFLAMMATORY MYOPATHIES

The idiopathic inflammatory myopathies (IIM) are a heterogeneous group of acquired diseases characterized by progressive muscle weakness associated with mononuclear cell infiltration in muscle.[79] They encompass three distinct disorders: polymyositis (PM), dermatomyositis (DM), and inclusion body myositis (IBM).

Differing considerably in pathogenesis and epidemiology, they share clinical features characterized by relatively slowly progressive proximal weakness, sometimes involving the pharyngeal, nuchal, respiratory, and distal limb musculature. DM can be identified clinically by a characteristic rash, which may accompany or precede muscle weakness. In PM and IBM there are no unique clinical features, and the diagnosis is established by histopathologic examination of a muscle specimen. Presumably, an autoimmune origin of PM and DM contribute to their good response to immunotherapy, whereas IBM seems to be generally resistant to all kinds of treatment.[79] Proliferation of inflammatory cells is the hallmark of all inflammatory myopathies. In DM, the inflammatory changes are predominantly perivascular and perifascicular, whereas PM and IBM are characterized by endomysial inflammation. Striking pathologic findings in IBM include typical slit-like vacuoles, containing basophilic granular material (rimmed vacuoles) and eosinophilic sarcoplasmatic inclusions.

GI manifestations of IIM consist chiefly in dysfunction of swallowing. Dysphagia is believed to be a rather common feature; its prevalence has been estimated in different studies at 10–60%.[80–83] Swallowing disturbances may also be presenting manifestations of IIM,[81] sometimes delaying diagnosis.[84] Usually the patients complain of difficulties in deglutition and/or food sticking in their throat or esophagus.[80] Heartburn and acid regurgitation have been reported.[85] Recurrent nasal regurgitations with aspiration of esophageal contents into the airways may occur, resulting in pulmonary infections.[81,86] In children, DM sometimes has a severe course, with thrombosis of smaller vessels and local infarctions in the digestive system leading to gastrointestinal hemorrhage or spontaneous perforation of the esophagus or colon.[87]

Cineradiographic and manometric studies indicate involvement of both striated and smooth esophageal muscles in most patients with IIM.[88] The typical pattern of pharyngeal and upper esophageal impairment includes prominent weakness of the hypopharynx associated with premature contractions, as well as delayed and incomplete relaxation of the crico-pharyngeal muscle.[81] Prolonged inflammation with secondary fibrosis may result in crico-pharyngeal achalasia with permanent esophageal obstruction.[86] Impairment of laryngeal elevation due to direct involvement of the suprahyoid musculature may represent an additional factor aggravating swallowing.[83] A high prevalence of functional changes in the distal portion of the esophagus has been demonstrated in several studies. Cineradiography and esophageal manometry showed reduced lower esophageal sphincter (LES) resting pressure, non-peristaltic, low amplitude, simultaneous contractions in both proximal and distal esophagus, and gastro-esophageal reflux.[80] Scintigraphic study of 13 randomly selected patients with PM and DM revealed a significant delay in both esophageal and gastric emptying, which correlated with the severity of the peripheral muscle weakness.[85] Gastric involvement usually remains asymptomatic, only occasionally resulting in clinically significant gastroparesis.[89]

Involvement of other levels of the digestive system is unusual in IIM. Facial and masticatory muscles are typically spared, with normal stomatognathic function. Besides the above mentioned intestinal complications of childhood DM, there is no evidence of significant impairment of the lower GI tract in these disorders.

METABOLIC MYOPATHIES

Thyrotoxic Myopathy

Most metabolic myopathies are only exceptionally accompanied by GI manifestations. Thyrotoxic myopathy should be mentioned here in view of its possible association with dysphagia. Progressive, but usually mild and predominantly proximal, muscle weakness has been reported to occur in the majority of thyrotoxic patients.[90] Pharyngeal and esophageal muscles may be rarely involved; this is usually associated with other signs of bulbar weakness, such as dysarthria and nasal regurgitation. Dysphagia may be a presenting symptom of hyperthyroidism[91] or may develop late in the course of the disease. Diminished esophageal peristalsis has been demonstrated radiologically in a thyrotoxic patient with dysphagia.[92]

The frequent association of hyperthyroidism with myasthenia gravis which, in turn, may result in bulbar weakness and dysphagia, represents an additional diagnostic problem.[90] The final diagnosis should be based on the results of electromyography, as well as on laboratory investigation of thyroid function and antibodies to acetylcholine receptors.

Acute thyrotoxic myopathy with extreme weakness of bulbar and limb muscles, developing within days or weeks, sometimes with fatal outcome,[93] is a rare and vague entity, the existence of which has been questioned.[94] Some cases may represent the acute onset of myasthenia gravis.[95]

MYASTHENIA GRAVIS AND MYASTHENIC SYNDROMES

Myasthenia gravis (MG) is an acquired autoimmune disorder of neuro-muscular transmission associated with alteration of the acetylcholine receptors at the neuro-muscular junction.[96] The most striking clinical feature of MG is fluctuating muscle weakness with diminished contractile power during sustained exertion, and improvement with rest. Extraocular muscles are affected initially in a majority of MG patients. Facial, masticatory, palato-pharyngeal, and tongue muscles are often involved prior to the development of more generalized weakness. Dramatic improvement of muscle weakness after administration of the short-acting anticholinesterase drug edrophonium (Tensilon) may be used as a sensitive screening test. The diagnosis should be based on the electromyographic examination demonstrating the characteristic decrement of amplitude of muscle action potential on repetitive stimulation, the pathologic results on single fiber electromyography (SFEMG), and the presence of high levels of circulating antibodies to acetylcholine receptors.

GI abnormalities in MG are usually limited to the upper levels of the digestive system. Slow mastication is common. Eating may be associated with nasal regurgitation due to velopharyngeal weakness, and recurrent choking when the glottis is incompetent.[97] It may be more difficult to eat after talking and vice versa; prolonged feeding may lead to the appearance of nasal and slurred speech.

Manometric studies of the pharynx and esophagus in MG have shown low pressures at all levels of the pharynx, decreased resting pressure of UES, and peristaltic dysfunction of the upper esophagus.[98,99] No abnormalities have been detected in LES function.[98] These impairments have correlated well with the severity of the disease and have improved after administration of anticholinesterase drugs.

Dysphagia usually develops in patients with previously diagnosed MG, but in 6 to 15% of cases it may be the initial manifestation.[1] The timely diagnosis in such cases is crucial to prevent serious complications. Moreover, the appearance of dysphagia in a myasthenic patient constitutes a neurological emergency, because it indicates the possibility of increasing bulbar paralysis, involvement of respiratory muscles, and development of myasthenic crisis. MG should, therefore, always be considered in the differential diagnosis of unexplained swallowing disorders.

Babies born to myasthenic mothers may show signs of widespread muscle weakness immediately or soon after birth, sometimes associated with prominent feeding difficulties and recurrent regurgitation, leading to secondary respiratory infections.

This *transient neonatal MG* represents a self-limited disorder resulting from the transplacental transfer of acetylcholine receptor antibodies from a myasthenic mother to the child.[92] A similar clinical picture may be observed in *congenital myasthenic syndromes*. This term encompasses a group of rare hereditary disorders characterized by different congenital pre- or postsynaptic defects of the neuromuscular junction.[100]

Botulism represents another example of a myasthenic syndrome which is typically associated with dysphagia and may be confused with MG. The disease is caused by ingestion of food contaminated with preformed neurotoxin of *Clostridium botulinum*. The toxin is spread by the bloodstream, absorbed by cholinergic nerve endings, and interferes with acetylcholine release.[101] The initial symptoms may be gastrointestinal (nausea, vomiting, abdominal cramps, diarrhea), followed by the development of a neurologic syndrome. Dysfunction of cranial nerves with diplopia, blurred vision, facial, masticatory and tongue weakness, dysphagia, and dysarthria are the most typical neurological manifestations. In the typical cases, the diagnosis is established without difficulty. In certain patients, the disease may lack symptoms of gastroenteritis and may begin with severe constipation. Electromyographic investigation showing typical incremental muscle action potential amplitude during rapid repetitive stimulation, as well as a positive mouse bioassay of serum and stool,[101] are useful in establishing the diagnosis.

CLINICAL APPROACH AND TREATMENT

In the majority of cases, GI symptoms appear relatively late in the course of the muscle diseases. The diagnosis, therefore, has usually already been established and confirmed by laboratory tests which, as a rule, include muscle biopsy. Clinical involvement of the digestive system may significantly impair the patient's clinical status and prognosis. Malnutrition may result in progressive weight loss and worsening of muscle wasting and weakness; swallowing dysfunction is often associated with recurrent aspiration and pulmonary infection. Occasionally, malabsorption is observed with secondary vitamin or microelement deficiencies. Severe constipation or diarrhea may considerably impair the quality of life. All these situations require gastroenterological evaluation.

In cases where the disease presents with GI manifestations, patients are usually referred to a general physician, gastroenterologist, or otolaryngologist, and the diagnosis may be difficult. The two main principles of the clinical approach should obviously be:

1) To distinguish between surgical, gastroenterological, and neurological diseases;
2) If the problem seems to be neurologic—to rule out treatable diseases demanding immediate therapeutic decisions.

Proper history taking and careful physical examination with special allowances for neurologic function and extramuscular manifestations often provide a clue to a proper diagnosis. The final diagnosis may require ancillary tests which are summarized in Table 7.2.

Unfortunately, for most muscle diseases there is only supportive treatment. Treatable diseases like MG, DM, PM, and thyrotoxic myopathy should be managed according to well known therapeutic guidelines presented elsewhere.[79,90,102]

Table 7.2. Ancillary Tests Useful in Diagnosis of Certain Muscle Diseases

Disease	Serum CK Level	EMG	Muscle Biopsy	Genetic Defect	Other Diagnostic Tests
MyD	Normal or moderately elevated	Myopathic pattern; myotonic discharges	Degenerative changes; ring fibers; sarcoplasmic masses	Abnormal CTG triplet repeat on chromosome 19	
OPMD	Normal or moderately elevated	Myopathic pattern	Degenerative changes; rimmed vacuoles; intranuclear inclusions	Mutation on chromosome 14q	
DMD	Markedly elevated	Myopathic pattern	Degenerative changes; necrosis; absent dystrophin	Deletion of dystrophin gene on X chromosome	
Mitochondrial myopathies	Normal or moderately elevated	Myopathic pattern	Variable	Variable	
Congenital myopathies	Normal or moderately elevated	Myopathic pattern	Variable	Variable	
PM	Elevated		Degenerative changes; necrosis; endomysial inflammation	Usually not genetic	
DM	Elevated	Myopathic pattern; abnormal electrical excitability	Degenerative changes; necrosis; perivascular inflammation; angiopathy	Usually not genetic	Skin biopsy angiopathy
IBM	Elevated		Degenerative changes; mild necrosis; endomysial inflammation; filamentous inclusions; rimmed vacuoles	Usually not genetic	
MG	Normal	Decremental response on repetitive nerve stimulation SFEMG – delayed or failed neuromuscular transmission		Usually not genetic	Elevated serum titer of acetylcholine receptor antibodies; positive Tensilon test; thymic enlargement on chest radiography

DM=dermatomyositis; DMD=Duchenne muscular dystrophy; IBM=inclusion body myositis; MG=myasthenia gravis; MyD=myotonic dystrophy; OPMD=oculopharyngeal muscular dystrophy; PM=polymyositis.

Irrespective of the etiological considerations, GI dysfunction, if present, should be treated symptomatically as soon as possible.

Impairment of mastication and weakness of the tongue may demand prescription of special soft diets. Early evaluation by an oral prosthodontist may prevent the development of malocclusion in children. Therapeutic exercise of the stomatognathic system has been reported to be effective in improving masticatory function in patients with muscular dystrophies.[103]

Oropharyngeal dysphagia is the most frequent and serious GI problem. For the majority of patients, retraining and use of various swallowing maneuvers and techniques to improve the passage of the bolus through the hypopharynx is recommended.[104] Videofluoroscopy[104] and videoendoscopy[105] have been reported to improve the results of swallowing therapy.

Cricopharyngeal myotomy represents a simple and relatively safe surgical procedure which may be helpful in certain patients with dysphagia. The procedure is widely used for a variety of swallowing disorders of different etiologies. Since its first application in motor neuron disease, it has been successfully performed in muscle diseases like OPMD[46,106] and inflammatory myopathies,[86] especially IBM.[81,83] The operation should be done only after functional evaluation of the swallowing process demonstrates failure of cricopharyngeal relaxation and opening associated with otherwise grossly intact components of swallowing. Gastroesophageal reflux (GER) represents the main contraindication for this type of surgery. Worsening of GER with pulmonary complications remains a major problem after cricopharyngeal myotomy.[104]

Oropharyngeal dysphagia, regardless of its etiology, is often associated with recurrent aspiration, resulting in acute or chronic tracheobronchial infection. There is no consensus concerning the management of this life threatening complication. In severe cases, tracheostomy affords improved pulmonary toilet, but may significantly worsen the swallowing function.[107] A variety of laryngotracheal separation procedures with relatively low morbidity, even in debilitated patients, have been advised[108] as an alternative to tracheostomy.

Adequate nutrition plays a very important role in the general management of patients with muscle diseases. In advanced cases, when oral feeding becomes insufficient, gastrostomy provides a relatively safe solution of the problem. Percutaneous endoscopic gastrostomy (PEG) is considered the method of choice,[109] although complication rates and mortality seem to be similar in PEG and in operative gastrostomy in most institutions.[110,111] Pulmonary aspiration due to GER is a contraindication to feeding gastrostomy, particularly in severely debilitated patients. Feeding jejunostomy is reported to be more appropriate in this situation.[111]

Disordered gastric and intestinal motility, although relatively rare manifestations of muscle diseases, have no clearly defined treatment approaches in the setting of neuromuscular disease. Various prokinetic agents are used, but with variable success. Cases of severe chronic intestinal pseudoobstruction are usually resistant to all kinds of treatment.[112] In such patients, dietary measures providing adequate nutrition with supplementation of multivitamins and microelements are important.

REFERENCES

1. Khan OA, Campbell WW. Myasthenia gravis presenting as dysphagia: clinical considerations. Am J Gastroenterol 1994;89:1083–1085.

2. Tomé FMS, Fardeau M. Oculopharyngeal muscular dystrophy. In AG Engel, C Franzini-Armstrong (eds), Myology, Vol. 2, 2nd ed. New York: McGraw Hill, 1994;1233–1245.
3. Graig R. The structure of the contractile filaments. In AG Engel, C Franzini-Armstrong (eds), Myology, Vol. 1, 2nd ed. New York: McGraw Hill, 1994;134–175.
4. Engel AG, Franzini-Armstrong C (eds). Myology, 2nd ed. New York: McGraw Hill, 1994.
5. Rowland LP, Dimaura S. Myopathies. In RJ Vinken, GW Bruyn, HI Klawans (eds), Handbook of Clinical Neurology. Amsterdam: Elsevier Science, 1992.
6. Sabouri LA, Mahadevan MS, Narang M, et al. Effect of the myotonic dystrophy (DM) mutation on mRNA levels of the DM gene. Nat Genet 1993;4:233–238.
7. Pruzanski W, Huvos AG. Smooth muscle involvement in primary muscle disease. I. Myotonic dystrophy. Arch Pathol 1967;83:229–233.
8. Weiner MJ. Myotonic megacolon in myotonic dystrophy. Am J Roentgenol 1978; 30:177–199.
9. Yoshida MM, Krishnamurthy S, Wattchow DA, et al. Megacolon in myotonic dystrophy caused by degenerative neuropathy of the myenteric plexus. Gastroenterology 1988;95:820–827.
10. Gazit E, Bornstein N, Lieberman M, et al. The stomatognathic system in myotonic dystrophy. Eur J Orthod 1987;160–164.
11. Chin VSW, Englert E. Gastrointestinal disturbances in myotonia dystrophica. Gastroenterology 1962;42:745–746.
12. Welsh JD, Haase GR, Bynum TE. Myotonic muscular dystrophy-systemic manifestations. Arch Intern Med 1964;76:234–236.
13. Ludman H. Dysphagia in dystrophia myotonica. J Laryngol Otol 1962;76:234–236.
14. Siciliano G, Rossi L, Fratini F, et al. Digitalized radiologic assessment of pharyngeo-esophageal function in myotonic dystrophy. Acta Cardiomyol 1990;2:45–53.
15. Hughes DTD, Swan JC, Glesson JA, Lee FI. Abnormalities in swallowing associated with dystrophia myotonica. Brain 1965;88:1037–1042.
16. Siegel CI, Thomas RH, Collins JH. The swallowing disorder in myotonia dystrophica. Gastroenterology 1966;50:541–550.
17. Krain S, Rabinowitz JG. The radiologic features of myotonic dystrophy with presentation of a new finding. Clin Radiol 1971;22:462–465.
18. Bosma JF, Brodie DR. Cineradiographic demonstration of pharyngeal area myotonia dsytrophy patients. Radiology 1969;92:104–109.
19. Goldberg HI, Sheft DJ. Esophageal and colon changes in myotonia dystrophica. Gastroenterology 1972;63:134–139.
20. Horowitz M, Maddox A, Maddern GJ, et al. Gastric and esophageal emptying in dystrophia myotonica. Effect of metoclopramide. Gastroenterology 1987;92:570–577.
21. Silbiger ML, Pikielney R, Donner MW. Neuromuscular disorders affecting the pharynx. Cineradiographic analysis. Invest Radiol 1967;2:442–448.
22. Nowak TV, Ionasescu V, Anuras S. Gastrointestinal manifestations of the muscular dystrophies. Gastroenterology 1982;82:800–810.
23. Garnett JM, DuBose TD, Jackson JE, Norman JR. Esophageal and pulmonary disturbances in myotonia dystrophica. Arch Intern Med 1969;123:26–32.
24. Eckardt VF, Nix W, Kraus W, Bohl J. Esophageal motor function in patients with muscular dystrophy. Gastroenterology 1986;90:628–635.
25. Harvey JC, Sherbourne DH, Siegel CI. Smooth muscle involvement in myotonic dystrophy. Am J Med 1965;39:89–90.
26. Schuman BM, Rinaldo JA, Darnley JD. Visceral changes in myotonic dystrophy. Ann Intern Med 1965;63:793–799.
27. Kuiper DH. Gastric bezoar in a patient with myotonic dystrophy. A review of the gastrointestinal complications of myotonic dystrophy. Am J Dig Dis 1971;16:529–534.
28. Kusunoki M, Hatada T, Ikeuchi H, et al. Gastric volvulus complicating myotonic dystrophy. Hepatogastroenterology 1992;39:586–588.
29. Woods CA, Foutch PG, Kerr DM, et al. Collagenous sprue as a cause for malabsorption in a patient with myotonic dystrophy: a new association. Am J Gastroenterol 1988;83:765–766.
30. Lewis TD, Daniel EE. Gastroduodenal motility in a case of dystrophia myotonica. Gastroenterology 1981;81:145–149.

31. Schuster MM, Tow DE, Sherbourne DH. Anal sphincter abnormalities characteristic of myotonic dystrophy. Gastroenterology 1965;49:641–648.
32. Hamel-Roy J, Devroede G, Arhan P, et al. Functional abnormalities of the anal sphincters in patients with myotonic dystrophy. Gastroenterology 1984;86:1469–1474.
33. Eckardt VF, Nix W. The anal sphincter in patients with myotonic muscular dystrophy. Gastroenterology 1991;100:424–430.
34. Schwindt ED, Bernhardt LC, Peters HA. Cholelithiasis and associated complications of myotonia dystrophica. Postgrad Med 1969;46:80–83.
35. Theodore C, Corund F, Mendez J, et al. Cholestasis and myotonic dystrophy (letter). N Engl J Med 1979;301:329–330.
36. Soderhall S, Gustafsson J, Bjorkhem I. Deoxycholic acid in myotonic dystrophy (letter). Lancet 1982;1:1068–1069.
37. Tanaka K, Takeshita K. Analysis of serum bile acids in patients with various types of muscular dystrophy (letter). Muscle Nerve 1983;6:606–607.
38. Ronnemaa T, Alaranta H, Viikari J, et al. Increased activity of serum gamma-glutamyltransferase in myotonic dystrophy. Acta Med Scand 1987;222:267–273.
39. Victor M, Hayes R, Adams RD. Oculopharyngeal muscular dystrophy. N Engl J Med 1962;267:1267–1272.
40. Barbeau A. Oculopharyngeal muscular dystrophy in french canada. In JR Brunette, A Barbeau (eds), Progress in Neuro-Ophthalmology. Amsterdam: Excerpta Medica, 1969; 3.
41. Blumen SC, Nisipeanu P, Sadeh M, et al. Clinical features of oculopharyngeal muscular dystrophy among Bukhara Jews. Neuromuscul Disord 1993;3:575–577.
42. Brais B, Xie Y-G, Sanson M, et al. The oculopharyngeal muscular dystrophy locus maps to the region of the cardiac alpha and beta myosin heavy chain genes on chromosome 14q11.2-q13. Human Mol Genet 1995;4:429–434.
43. Murphy SE, Drachman DB. The oculopharyngeal syndrome. JAMA 1968;203:1003–8.
44. Duranceau CA, Letendre J, Clermont RJ, et al. Oropharyngeal dysphagia in patients with oculopharyngeal muscular dystrophy. Can J Surg 1978;21:326–329.
45. Kilman WJ, Goyal RK. Disorders of pharyngeal and upper esophageal sphincter motor function. Arch Intern Med 1976;136:592–601.
46. Dobrowski JM, Zajtchuk JT, LaPiana FG, Hensley SD Jr. Oculopharyngeal muscular dystrophy: clinical and histopathologic correlations. Otolaryngol Head Neck Surg 1986; 95:131–142.
47. Weitzner S. Phatosis of the tongue in oculopharyngeal muscular dystrophy: report of two cases. Oral Surg Oral Med Oral Pathol 1969;28:613–617.
48. Roberts AH, Bamforth J. The pharynx and esophagus in ocular muscular dystrophy. Neurology 1968;18:645–652.
49. Bender MD. Esophageal manometry in oculopharyngeal dystrophy. Am J Gastroenterol 1976;65:215–221.
50. Castell JA, Castell DO, Durauceau CA, Topart P. Manometric characteristics of the pharynx, upper esophagus and lower esophageal sphincter in patients with oculopharyngeal muscular dystrophy. Dysphagia 1995;10:22–26.
51. Topart P, Deschamps C, Taillefer R, Duranceau A. Esophageal function in oculopharyngeal muscular dystrophy. Gullet 1992;2:149–154.
52. Teasdall RD, Schuster MM, Walsh FB. Sphincter involvement in ocular myopathy. Arch Neurol 1964;10:446–448.
53. Goldhammer G, Goldhammer E, Korczyn AD. Cardiorespiratory Involvement in Duchenne's progressive muscular dystrophy. Intern Med 1982;10:76–81.
54. Kunkel LM. Analysis of deletions in DNA from patients with Becker and Duchenne muscular dystrophy. Nature 1986;322:73–77.
55. Ahn AH, Kunkel LM. The structural and functional diversity of dystrophin. Nature Genet 1993;3:283–291.
56. Jaffe KM, McDonald CM, Ingman E, Haas J. Symptoms of upper gastrointestinal dysfunction in Duchenne muscular dystrophy: case control study. Arch Phys Med Rehabil 1990;71:742–744.
57. Ghafari J, Clark RE, Shofer FS, Berman PH. Dental and occlusal characteristics of children with neuromuscular disease. Am J Orthod Dentofacial Orthop 1988;93:126–132.

58. Marcello N, Oztaggio F, Sabadini R. The masticatory function in Duchenne muscular dystrophy patients by video-tape investigations. Acta Cardiomiol 1994;1:69–78.

59. Erturk N, Dogan S. The effect of neuromuscular diseases on the development of dental and occlusal characteristics. Quintessence Int 1991;22:317–321.

60. Berblinger W, Dunken J. Der kardio-intestinale symptomkomplex bei der progressiven muskeldystrophie. I Mitteilung: klinische und pathologisch-anatomische beobachtungen. Z Kinderheilkund 1929;47:1–26.

61. Robin GC, De Falewski G. Acute gastric dilatation in progressive muscular dystrophy. Lancet 1961;2:171–172.

62. Barohn RJ, Levien EJ, Olson JO, Mendell JR. Gastric hypomotility in Duchenne's muscular dystrophy. N Engl J Med 1988;319:15–18.

63. Leon SH, Schuffler MD, Kettler M, Rohrmann CA. Chronic intestinal pseudoobstruction as a complication of Duchenne's muscular dystrophy. Gastroenterology 1986;90:455–459.

64. Huvos AG, Pruzanski W. Smooth muscle involvement in primary muscle disease. II. Progressive muscular dystrophy. Arch Pathol 1967;83:234–240.

65. Staiano A, Del Giudice E, Romano A, et al. Upper gastrointestinal tract motility in children with progressive muscular dystrophy. J Pediatr 1992;121:720–724.

66. Korman SH, Bar-Oz B, Granot E, Meyer S. Orocaecal transit time in Duchenne muscular dystrophy. Arch Dis Child 1991;66:143–144.

67. Crimmins D, Morris JG, Walker GL, et al. Mitochondrial encephalomyopathy: variable clinical expression within a single kindred. J Neurol Neurosurg Psychiatry 1993;56:900–905.

68. Morgan-Hughes JA. Mitochrondrial diseases of muscle. Curr Opin Neurol 1994;7:457–462.

69. Shaker R, Kupla JI, Kidder TM, et al. Manometric characteristics of cervical dysphagia in a patient with the Kearns-Sayre syndrome. Gastroenterology 1992;103:1328–1331.

70. Nicoll JA, Moss TH, Love S, et al. Clinical and autopsy findings in two cases of MELAS presenting with stroke-like episodes but without clinical myopathy. Clin Neuropathol 1993;12:38–43.

71. Ban S, Mori N, Saito K, et al. An autopsy case of mitochondrial encephalomyopathy (MELAS) with special reference to extra-neuromuscular abnormalities. Acta Pathol Jpn 1992;42:818–825.

72. Hirano M, Silvestri G, Blake DM, et al. Mitochondrial neurogastrointestinal encephalomopathy (MNGIE): Clinical, biochemical, and genetic features of an autosomal recessive mitochondrial disorder. Neurology 1994;44:721–727.

73. Ionasescu V. Oculogastrointestinal muscular dystrophy. Am J Med Genet 1983;15:103–112.

74. Simon LT, Horoupian DS, Dorfman LJ, et al. Polyneuropathy, ophthalmoplegia, leukoencephalopathy, and intestinal pseudo-obstruction: POLIP syndrome. Ann Neurol 1990;28:349–360.

75. Bardosi A, Creutzfeldt W, DiMaura S, et al. Myo-, neuro-, gastrointestinal encephalopathy (MNGIE syndrome) due to partial deficiency of cytochrome-c-oxidase. A new mitochondrial multisystem disorder. Acta Neuropathol (Berl) 1987;74:248–258.

76. Faradeau M, Tomé FMS. Congenital Myopathies. In AG Engel, C Franziui-Armstrong (eds), Myology, Vol 2, 2nd ed. New York: McGraw Hill, 1994; 1487–1532.

77. Norton P, Ellison P, Sulaiman AR, Harb J. Nemaline myopathy in the neonate. Neurology 1983;33:251–256.

78. Goebel HH, Lenard HG. Congenital myopathies. In PJ Vinken, GW Bruyn, HL Klawans (eds), Handbook of Clinical Neurology, Vol 62. Amsterdam: Elsevier Science, 1992; 331–368.

79. Dalakas MC. Polymyositis, dermatomyositis and inclusion-body myositis. N Engl J Med 1991;325:1487–1498.

80. De Merieux P, Verity MA, Clements PJ, Paulus HE. Esophageal abnormalities and dysphagia in polymyositis and dermatomyositis. Arthritis Rheum 1983;26:961–968.

81. Wintzen AR, Bots GT, de Bakker HM, et al. Dysphagia in inclusion body myositis. J Neurol Neurosurg Psychiatry 1988;51:1542–1545.

82. Lotz BP, Engel AG, Nishino H, et al. Inclusion body myositis. Observations in 40 patients. Brain 1989;112:727–747.

83. Darrow DH, Hoffman HT, Barnes GJ, Wiley CA. Management of dysphagia in inclusion body myositis. Arch Otolaryngol Head Neck Surg 1992;118:313–317.

84. Thomas FB, LeBauer S, Greenberger NJ. Polymyositis masquerading as carcinoma of the cervical esophagus. Arch Intern Med 1972;129:984–986.

85. Horowitz M, McNeil JD, Maddern GJ, et al. Abnormalities of gastric and esophageal emptying in polymyositis and dermatomyositis. Gastroenterology 1986;90:434–439.

86. Kagen LJ, Hochman RB, Strong EW. Cricopharyngeal obstruction in inflammatory myopathy (polymyositis/dermatomyositis). Report of three cases and review of the literature. Arthritis Rheum 1985;28:630–636.

87. Thompson JW. Spontaneous perforation of the esophagus as a manifestation of dermatomyositis. Ann Otol Rhinol Laryngol 1984;93:464–467.

88. Jacob H, Berkowitz D, McDonald E, et al. The esophageal motility disorder of polymyositis. A prospective study. Arch Intern Med 1983;143:2262–2264.

89. Feldman F, Marshak R. Dermatomyositis with significant involvement of the gastrointestinal tract. Ann Roentgenol Radium Ther Nucl Med 1963;90:746–752.

90. Kaminski HJ, Ruff RL. Endocrine myopathpies (hyper- and hypo-function of adrenal, thyroid, pituitary, and parathyroid glands and iatrogenic corticosteroid myopathy). In AG Engel, C Franzini-Armstrong (eds), Myology, Vol 2, 2nd ed. New York: McGraw Hill, 1994;1726–1753.

91. Marks P, Anderson J, Vincent R. Thyrotoxic myopathy presenting as dysphagia. Postgrad Med J 1980;56:669–670.

92. Sweatmen MC, Chambers L. Disordered oesophageal motility in thyrotoxic myopathy. Postgrad Med J 1985;61:440–442.

93. Kammer GM, Hamilton CR Jr. Acute bulbar muscle dysfunction and hyperthyroidism. A study of four cases and review of the literature. Am J Med 1974;56:464–470.

94. Harvard CWH. Thyrotixic myopathy—a reappraisal and report of three cases. Br Med J 1962;1:440-442.

95. Laurent PE. Acute thyrotoxic bulbar palsy. Lancet 1944;1:87–88.

96. Engel AG. Acquired autoimmune myasthenia gravis. In AG Engel, C Franzini-Armstrong (eds), Myology, Vol 2, 2nd ed. New York: McGraw Hill, 1994;1769–1797.

97. Carpenter RJ 3d, McDonald TJ, Howard FM Jr. The otolaryngologic presentation of myasthenia gravis. Laryngoscope 1979;89:922–928.

98. Huang MH, King KL, Chien KY. Esophageal manometric studies in patients with myasthenia gravis. J Thorac Cardiovasc Surg 1988;95:281–285.

99. Joshita Y, Yoshida M, Yoshida Y, Kimura K. Manometric study of the pharynx and pharyngoesophageal sphincter in myasthenia gravis. Rinsho Shinkeigaku 1990;30:944–951.

100. Engel AG. Myasthenic syndromes. In AG Engel, C Franzini-Armstrong (eds), Myology, Vol 2, 2nd ed. New York: McGraw Hill, 1994;1798–1835.

101. Hughes JM. Botulism. In WM Scheld, RJ Whitley, DT Durack (eds), Infections of the Central Nervous System. New York: Raven Press, 1991.

102. Drachman DB. Myasthenia gravis. N Engl J Med 1994;330:1797–1810.

103. Kawazoe Y, Kobayashi M, Tasaka T, Tamamoto M. Effects of therapeutic exercise on masticatory function in patients with progressive muscular dystrophy. J Neurol Neurosurg Psychiatry 1982;45:343–347.

104. Logemann JA. Evaluation and treatment of swallowing disorders. Boston: College-Hill Press, 1983.

105. Bastian RW. Videoendoscopic evaluation of patients with dysphagia: an adjunct to the modified barium swallow. Otolaryngol Head Neck Surg 1991;104:339–350.

106. Montgomery WW, Lynch JP. Oculopharyngeal muscular dystrophy treated by inferior constrictor myotomy. Trans Am Acad Ophthalmol Otolaryngol 1971;75:986–993.

107. Koch WM. Swallowing disorders. Diagnosis and therapy. Med Clin North Am 1993; 77:571–582.

108. Blitzer A. Approaches to the patient with aspiration and swallowing disabilities. Dysphagia 1990;5:129–137.

109. Ponsky JL, Gauderer MW, Stellato TA. Percutaneous endoscopic gastrostomy. Review of 150 cases. Arch Surg 118:913–914.

110. Samii AM, Suguitan EA. Comparison of operative gastrostomy with percutaneous endoscopic gastrostomy. Mil Med 1990;155:534–535.

111. Stuart SP, Tiley EH 3d, Boland JP. Feeding gastrostomy: a critical review of its indications and mortality rate. South Med J 1993;86:169–172.
112. Camilleri M, Phillips SF. Acute and chronic intestinal pseudoobstruction. Adv Intern Med 1991;36:287–306.

Chapter 8

Stress, Distress, and the Gut: Physiological and Psychological Aspects

Francis Creed, Elspeth Guthrie, and David Thompson

It is well recognized in gastrointestinal practice that gut symptoms and disturbed GI function can occur without evidence of organic disease. Such problems are commonly referred to as functional disorders of the GI tract, and are known to be associated with psychological disorders, particularly anxiety.

This chapter aims to review the evidence for a functional relationship between gastrointestinal activity and the central nervous system (CNS), both at a physiological and psychological level. It is equally likely that psychological factors may contribute to gastrointestinal symptoms in patients with organic disease, including neurological disease. As little or no data exists with regard to the latter, this chapter will focus on gut function and dysfunction in functional disorders, to provide insights into interaction between the gut and the psyche, in general.

The chapter will focus attention largely on human studies both in health and in disease, but also includes experimental data from animal studies where it is felt that this information sheds new light on our understanding of stress-related pathophysiology.

BACKGROUND

Gastrointestinal Physiology and Stress

The last decade has been marked by a progressively increasing interest in the effects of experimental stress on the gastrointestinal tract both in man and in experimental animals.[1,2] While the data so far remain far from complete, there is now sufficient information for at least a broad understanding of the effects of stress, and for an approach to be made towards an understanding of the GI disturbances experienced by many patients.

Basic Concepts of Stress and the Gut

In animals, acute stressors can be demonstrated to produce major disturbances in virtually all aspects of gut function, largely working via the final common pathway of sympathetic neural activation, which acts to inhibit the intrinsic nervous system of the gut rather than by direct innervation of intestinal muscle.

In animals, stress applied either as pain or as an emotional disturbance acutely affects the stomach, inhibiting its motility and secretion, and the colon by increasing colonic activity.

An important recent discovery has been the role of corticotrophin-releasing factor (CRF) in the activation of the efferent pathways involved in these sympathetically mediated stress effects.[3,4] It now seems clear that CRF is the major neuropeptide involved in the central mechanism by which stress inhibits gastric emptying while stimulating colonic motor function. CRF, a neuropeptide, found in key areas in the brain, has been shown to influence gut function in response to stressful stimulation. In addition to initiating the endocrine and behavioral responses to stress, CRF acts in the paraventricular nucleus to trigger inhibition of gastric emptying and to stimulate colonic responses.[5,6] CRF also appears to act in the locus coeruleus to induce a selective stimulation of colonic transit without influencing gastric function.[7] These CNS effects of CRF are conveyed by sympathetic neural pathways,[8] independent of CRF stimulation of pituitary hormone secretion.[3]

A series of experimental interventions, including surgery, peritonitis, pain, or high levels of interleukin 1, are now known to initiate the release of CRF, and this may be the pathway by which such stressors induce ileus.[9] A further discovery is the interaction between cholecystokinin (CCK) and CRF within the central nervous system.[9] While traditionally regarded as a "peripheral hormone," it has now become clear that CCK functions principally as a neuromodulatory peptide, not only in the peripheral nervous system, but also within the CNS.[10-14] Within the CNS, the shorter CCK-8 molecular form predominates as a neurotransmitter.[14,15] Intracerebroventricular (ICV) injection of CRF, as well as emotional stress, induce stimulation of colonic motility in rats, an effect blocked by ICV injection of CCK-8.[16,17] This effect appears to be principally mediated via the central nucleus of the amygdala, since the effects of CCK-8 are inhibited in animals with lesions applied to the amygdala.[17]

These findings, while of considerable biological interest, are also of potential therapeutic relevance, since benzodiazepine anxiolytics act on pathways which involve CCK-8 receptor activation.

STRESS AND THE HUMAN GASTROINTESTINAL TRACT

Human studies, while necessarily limited for ethical reasons, have largely reproduced the animal data described briefly above. Gastric, small intestinal, and colonic function are disturbed by acute stresses in a similar manner.[1]

It must be recognized, however, that the stressors applicable to human studies are, of necessity, restricted in their applicability to pathophysiological states, and virtually all the information available from human studies relates to acute rather than chronic stressors.

The Esophagus

Esophageal manometry studies show that primary peristaltic amplitudes may be reduced during the application of stress and, in addition, that lower esophageal sphincter pressures are depressed.[18-21]

Stomach

The human stomach is readily disturbed by experimental stressors.[22] Antral motility is suppressed, as is secretion, and gastric emptying is delayed. Following the cessation of stress, however, it appears that a rebound increase in activity occurs, perhaps reflecting the release of the normal control mechanisms from inhibition.[2,23–28]

Small Intestine

Small intestinal function is disturbed in a number of interesting ways. Fasting motor activity is measurably disturbed by stress, with a reduction in the number of phase 3 patterns of the MMC and an inhibition of the expected number of contractions during phase 2.[29,30] After a meal, disturbance of the intestinal motor pattern is more difficult to ascertain, but intestinal transit of an ingested meal is consistently delayed, an effect independent of gastric emptying.[31] It is also known that this effect is mediated via an effect of the sympathetic neurons on intestinal smooth muscle via a beta-adrenoreceptor pathway.[27,28]

Colon

As in animals,[32,33] there is an interesting contrast between the inhibitory effects of sympathetic activation on the upper gut and an apparent increase in motor activity observed in the colon in man.[34] Various studies have shown an increase in myoelectric activity in the distal human colon in response to both cold pain and mental excitation. In the lower colorectum, an inhibition of motor activity has been demonstrated, and anal sphincter tone is inhibited. Both psychological and physical stresses inhibit external sphincter activity while increasing internal sphincter tone. The functional consequences of these changes in colonic motility appear to be an increased speed of transit of feces and increased stool frequency.[35–39]

The physiological effects of hypnotically-induced emotion on the colon have also been explored. Such a technique has a number of advantages over previously applied stressors, since it can be safely used to induce specific emotional states of considerable intensity in the same individuals. The effect on distal colonic motility of three hypnotically-induced emotions (excitement, anger, and happiness) has been studied in a group of patients with the irritable bowel syndrome. Hypnosis itself reduced colonic motility, while anger and excitement increased it.[40]

Relationships between Stress and GI Physiology in Functional Gut Diseases

In view of the relationship between the symptoms of disturbed gut function and psychological disturbances, it is not surprising that many of the studies described above have now been repeated in patients with functional disorders. While the results are of great interest, from a pathophysiological point of view, it must be admitted that, so far, they are of insufficient specificity to provide a clear guide, either to the underlying neurophysiological disturbance in patients, or to enable a relationship between stress and symptoms to be confirmed.[41,42]

Stress and Physiological Disturbances in Irritable Bowel Patients

The Small Intestine.   Because of its clearly defined pattern of fasting motility, and because of the availability of techniques to record small intestinal motor patterns over prolonged periods, it is not surprising that small intestinal manometry has been studied in detail.

The normal pattern of motility comprises a cyclical change from quiescence (phase 1), through irregular activity (phase 2), to a burst of regular activity which migrates slowly down the length of the small intestine (phase 3). The quantity of phase 2 activity and the regularity of phase 3 activity are dependent upon the level of alertness. During sleep, phase 3 becomes more regular and phase 2 virtually disappears. In patients with the irritable bowel syndrome, it appears that phase 2 activity is somewhat different, with the occurrence of periods of clustered contractions. The fact that such clustered contractions have now been reported by a series of groups suggests that this is a true finding in IBS patients, but its significance is uncertain.[43–46] The most plausible explanation would be that such activity reflects the increased alertness of an anxious individual, while an alternative explanation would be that a low grade abnormality of intrinsic neural function exists in the myenteric plexus of such patients.[42]

In IBS patients, the effects of experimental stressors are more marked than normal, with more marked inhibition of phase 3 and phase 2 activity.[29]

The Stomach.   Gastric abnormalities have also been reported in patients with the irritable bowel syndrome, even in those free of upper gut symptoms. Antral hypomotility is the abnormality most frequently reported.[42]

Stress and Colonic Motility in IBS.   It has been repeatedly reported that left-sided colonic responses to distention and to feeding are exaggerated in IBS patients. One of the intriguing findings in IBS patients is the apparent "hypersensitivity" of the colon, manifested by reduced threshold to discomfort when the gut is distended. The exact nature of this hypersensitivity and its relationship to arousal and anxiety are uncertain.[47]

Conclusions

The published data indicate that experimental stress can influence gastrointestinal function, both in normal volunteers and patients with functional GI diseases. Before firm conclusions can be drawn, the relevance, as stimuli to gut function, of acute experimental stressors to chronic environmental or emotional stress must be defined; and the relationships between observed effects of stress in health and disease and the symptoms reported by patients who are suspected of having gut dysfunction need to be established.

PSYCHOLOGICAL ASPECTS OF STRESS AND GUT FUNCTION

There has been relatively little research into the relationship between psychological status and gut function, both in healthy states and disease. Most studies of gut physiology have not included psychological measures, and most studies of psychiatric status in patients with gut symptoms have not included physiological measurements. Thus, these two important areas of research into gut symptomatology have developed independently, resulting in some instances in an unfortunate polarity: some individuals believing it is "all in the mind," while others believe it is "all in the gut."[48]

Before discussing the relationship between the gut function and psychological status, some of the difficulties and complexities involved in the measurement of psychological status will be discussed. Most gastroenterologists are unaware of these issues and may falsely believe that psychological status is easy to assess and measure.

General methodological issues concerning research involving both psychological factors and gut dysfunction will then be addressed. A brief summary of work carried out examining the effects of emotion on gut function in normal subjects will be given, followed by a more detailed review of studies on functional bowel disorders that have involved both physiological and psychological measures.

The Measurement of Psychological Status

Dimensions of Psychological Status and Behavior

Psychological functioning can be construed in many different ways. Each way is important, but provides information on only one aspect of an individual's psychological status; one piece of an elaborate jigsaw. The main aspects of psychological status that have been assessed in studies on functional abdominal disorders are: current psychological morbidity, lifetime history of psychological morbidity, personality factors, childhood experience, and treatment seeking behavior.

Current Psychological Disorder.   Current psychological disorder is the most common aspect of psychological functioning that has been studied. It can be measured either by asking the patient to complete a self-report questionnaire or by undertaking a standardized psychiatric interview. The self-report questionnaire (e.g., the SCL-90-R) usually measures symptoms like anxiety or depression, and takes a few minutes to be completed. It can be likened to a thermometer which detects a fever, but gives no indication of the cause. A standardized interview, which usually takes between 1 to 2 hours (e.g. the SCAN), is a reliable and accurate way of determining psychiatric morbidity, and could be thought of as the psychological equivalent of an endoscopy. It allows a psychiatric diagnosis (e.g., obsessional disorder or panic disorder) to be made, and rarely overestimates the prevalence of psychiatric morbidity.

Using standardized interviews, several studies in different centers have confirmed that approximately 40 to 50% of out-patients with the irritable bowel syndrome have diagnosable psychiatric morbidity.[49–51] It is important to point out that there are no studies of gut physiology that have used a standardized psychiatric interview to assess psychiatric morbidity. Those that have used self-report measures will be discussed later.

Lifetime History of Psychological Morbidity.   Current psychological status provides the researcher with a snapshot of how the patient is functioning at a particular point in time. There is increasing evidence, however, that certain groups of patients with chronic physical symptoms have a history of several episodes of psychiatric illness (sometimes preceding the onset of physical complaints), and may be psychologically different, in the context of physical symptomatology, from patients who only have one episode of psychiatric morbidity.[48] The "snapshot" approach to psychological assessment is unable to distinguish between these two groups. It is now possible to conduct a detailed assessment of past psychological ill health, but again this investigation is time consuming and has not been undertaken, so far, in any studies on gut physiology.

Personality.   Personality is a very difficult concept to define and measure. Unlike psychiatric morbidity, which should be discrete and transient, an individual's personality is stable and unchanging. It has been described in terms of characteristic patterns of emotional responses and behavior, which are present from an early age and have an enduring quality. So-called personality measures, such as Eysenck's Personality Inventory, do not actually measure personality; rather they measure a specific aspect or trait of someone's personality (e.g., anxiety traits). Detailed assessment of personality can only be carried out by a structured interview which takes several hours. To date, no studies on gut physiology have used detailed personality assessments, although a number have employed brief self-report measures to detect certain personality traits.

Childhood Experience Including Childhood Sexual Abuse.   Long before the current interest in childhood sexual abuse in relation to functional abdominal illness,[52–55] psychiatrists have been interested in the role that childhood experiences play in the development of personality and psychological and physical ill health in later life. Certain factors, such as parental illness in childhood and illness of the patient in childhood, combined with emotional neglect or trauma, have been identified as predisposing to the later development of somatic symptoms in adult life.[56]

Childhood experience is a very difficult area in which to carry out reliable or valid assessments, as independent evidence is usually unavailable. The researcher is essentially dependent upon the adult's perception of his/her childhood, not on its reality. Both are important but, at present, only the former can be studied.

Not surprisingly, there are few studies on gut physiology that have attempted to quantify differing childhood experiences in the subjects being studied.

Treatment-Seeking Behavior.   The high prevalence of psychiatric morbidity in patients with the irritable bowel syndrome has already been discussed. Individuals in the community with symptoms of gut dysfunction who do not seek medical help are psychologically normal, at least on crude testing.[57–59] This important finding has led to the suggestion that psychological factors may influence patients' concern about their symptoms and encourage treatment-seeking behavior. In extreme cases, some patients can go on seeking investigations, care, and treatment for many years despite repeated medical assurances that there is no serious underlying organic pathology. This so-called abnormal illness behavior, although striking in extremes, is difficult to measure, particularly in its more subtle forms. Several questionnaires have been developed, but none have been able to convincingly capture and accurately measure this interesting phenomenon.

Methodological Issues

There are several areas of concern regarding the methodology of studies that have attempted to combine measures of gut function and psychological status.

Definitions of Gut Symptomatology.   The problems of developing clear criteria for functional abdominal syndromes have been discussed by many authors. Most researchers now accept the importance of using explicit criteria to define symptom complexes. Although the development of the Manning[60] and the Rome[61] criteria has been a major advance in the study of functional gut disorders, other ways of categorizing patients (e.g., symptom chronicity or severity) may be as important as actual symptomatology when searching for a relationship to underlying gut physiology.

Types of Psychiatric Assessment.   In the previous section, the difference between using a psychological self-report measure and an in-depth psychiatric assessment, of either psychiatric status or personality, was highlighted. To our knowledge, no studies that have combined measures of gut physiology and psychological status have employed detailed psychiatric measuring instruments; they have all used self-report measures. It is important, therefore, to bear in mind the "crudeness" of the data that is generated by such methods, and the danger of overinterpreting the meaning of any positive findings.

Selection and Recruitment.   The importance of treatment-seeking behavior in relation to psychiatric status has already been discussed. It suggests that the way in which patients are selected and recruited to studies can have a profound influence on their results.[62] The best psychiatric studies of patients with functional abdominal pain have recruited large numbers of subjects in a consecutive manner. This ensures that the study group is, at least, representative of patients attending the particular center where the study is being carried out. The reader can then make an informed judgment as to how generalizable the results are to those of work carried out on patients from other centers or from the community.

Most studies of gut physiology have employed tiny numbers of subjects and have rarely given any information about how they have been recruited. This means that it is impossible to know whether the subjects under study are even representative of patients attending the study centers. The results cannot be generalized or meaningfully compared with other studies.

Small Numbers of Subjects: Type II Statistical Errors.   Many studies of gut motility include such small numbers that possible statistical differences between study groups are missed purely because of the small sample size. There is enough available published work in this field to be able to estimate the prevalence of psychological disorders in the study sample and controls, and to work out the minimum number of subjects necessary to carry out a meaningful experiment.

Acute Pain vs Chronic Pain.   The importance of distinguishing between acute and chronic pain has already been alluded to in the section on gut motility. Most of the physiological studies examining pain in relation to gut function focus on the effects on the gut of acute pain. Many patients with functional bowel disorder, however, describe chronic pain which physiologically may be very different from acute pain. This is important to remember when interpreting the results of physiological and psychological studies in functional bowel disorders.

Emotional Arousal and Gut Function

Emotional stress or changes in emotional arousal result in changes in bowel activity. Early pioneers in this field such as Cannon[63,64] and Grace[65] described changes in animals' and humans' gut function in relation to emotional distress.

Almy's fascinating post war experiments documented changes in rectosigmoid motility and vascular engorgement in normal subjects and patients exposed to a variety of physical and psychological stimuli.[66-69]

Welgan and colleagues studied myoelectrical and motor responses of the lower gut in IBS subjects and controls when subjected to a standardized interview designed to provoke anger. The IBS patients developed significantly greater changes in gut motility than controls.[39]

More recent work by Whorwell and colleagues demonstrated that the colonic motility index was increased in patients by the induction of certain emotions (e.g., anger) under hypnosis, and was decreased by the induction of hypnosis itself or by more pleasant emotions such as happiness.[40]

The relevance of these interesting findings to the study of gut dysfunction or psychological dysfunction is unclear. Emotions such as anger or happiness are normal, and physiological change (e.g., change in pulse, etc.) in relation to psychological change has been well documented. It is not surprising that gut function also varies in relation to normal changes in emotional arousal.

Psychological Status and Gut Motility and Sensitivity

In the last 20 years, a small number of studies of gut motility, recorded either mechanically or electrically, also employed a psychological measure, and these are summarized in Table 8.1. Recent studies looking at gut sensitivity are also included in Table 8.1, if they involved some kind of psychological assessment.

Latimer and colleagues measured myoelectrical activity in IBS patients and compared them to two control groups: normals, and psychoneurotic patients without GI symptoms. They found that IBS patients did not differ significantly from the psychoneurotic control group on any of the colonic measures, although they were significantly different from the normal subjects. They argued that the results suggested that abnormal colonic motility may be related to non-specific psychological disturbance, rather than a specific gut disorder.[70]

This study highlights some of the methodologic flaws outlined above. The numbers were small, and psychiatric disorder was over-represented in the IBS group, with a prevalence double that expected in a representative group of clinic out-patients.

It raised, however, an interesting hypothesis. Is gut dysfunction in functional abdominal disorder mediated via psychological disturbance, or is it related to some intrinsic physiological disturbance?

Table 8.1. Studies of Motility and Sensitivity that Included a Psychological Evaluation

Study	Subjects	Psychological Measure	Physiological Measure	Findings
Latimer et al, 1979	IBS	Self report	Myoelectrical activity when stressed	IBS and patients with psychological symptoms similar
Whitehead et al, 1980	IBS Normal subjects	Self report	Motility Balloon distension	IBS less tolerance than controls
Kullman and Fielding, 1981	IBS "nervous pts" Normals	Self report	Rectal distensibility	Distensibility lower in IBS than normal controls
Cook et al, 1987	IBS Crohn's Normals	Self report	Electrocutaneous pain threshold	IBS and Crohn's higher pain threshold than normals
Whitehead et al, 1990	IBS FBD LMA Normals	Self report	Rectal tolerance to balloon distension Pain threshold	IBS patients lower tolerance for balloon distension but not pain threshold
Prior et al, 1993	IBS Normals	Self report	Rectal tolerance to balloon distension	Patients with rectal sensitivity, more anxious
Zighelboim et al, 1995	IBS community Normals	Self report	Rectal tolerance to balloon distension	IBS similar to controls

FBD = functional bowel disorder; IBS = irritable bowel syndrome; LMA = lactose malabsorption.

Since Latimer's work, several interesting studies, focusing upon the role of gut visceral sensitivity, have reached findings which support the notion of intrinsic physiological disturbance. The main work in this area has been designed and conducted by Whitehead and colleagues.[71,72] In an early study, they found that IBS subjects had significantly higher scores on a psychological self-report questionnaire than normal controls, and also complained of significantly more pain when small pressure balloons were inflated in the colon.[71] Although this study appeared to support Latimer's hypothesis, a later, much more detailed study by the same team threw it into doubt. In the second study, 16 patients with classical IBS, 10 with functional bowel disorder (FBD), 25 with lactose malabsorption (LMA), and 18 normal controls were compared, psychologically and physiologically. Sensitivity to gut pain and non-gut pain (hand in ice water) was recorded. The IBS group was found to have significantly lower tolerance for balloon distention than normal controls, but the tolerance for non-gut pain was no different for IBS or FBD patients and normal controls. As expected, anxiety and depression scores were significantly elevated in patients with IBS and FBD compared with normals, but there was no significant correlation between psychological status and tolerance for gut distention.[72]

Whitehead suggested that the results pointed to a peripheral mechanism, such as altered receptor sensitivity, as being the cause of distention-induced pain in some functional bowel syndromes. He has cogently argued that his findings refute Latimer's "neurotic hypothesis."[73] Patients with IBS are more psychologically disturbed than controls, but this does not result in a generalized lowering of the pain threshold. Instead, patients with IBS have a specific lack of tolerance for gut distention. This is not the case with FBD, implying a physiological difference between IBS and FBD.[74]

It is important again to highlight some methodological concerns. The numbers in this study were small and the range of responses within each group was very large. This again raises questions about the representative nature of the patient groups. In addition, some of the other results seemed anomalous and did not fit with any hypothesis concerning gut function. For example, the LMA group had lower tolerance for ice water than normal controls.

Lower thresholds to gut pain sensitivity have since been demonstrated in IBS subjects by several different research groups.[47] The study by Mertz and colleagues[75] of patients attending a clinic in Los Angeles demonstrates that it is possible to recruit large numbers of consecutive patients (n = 100) and conduct physiological tests. This is one of the very few studies on gut physiology where the sample can be judged to be representative of IBS clinic subjects. Unfortunately, the authors do not report the use of any psychological measures! Their findings, however, are very striking. 94% of the one hundred IBS subjects showed altered rectal perception in the form of lowered thresholds for aversive sensations, increased intensity of sensations, or altered viscerosomatic referral. The authors argue that their findings suggest that altered rectal perception can be used as a biological marker for IBS.

It now seems clear that altered gut sensitivity is a common phenomenon in IBS patients, but its relationship to psychological factors and treatment-seeking behavior remains unclear.

The most careful evaluation, to date, of psychological status in relation to gut dysfunction is described in a recent study from the Mayo Clinic.[76] In contrast to the above studies, which predominantly focused upon patients, this study compared community subjects with IBS to normal community controls. In other words, the treatment-seeking element of patient behavior was removed. A variety of different psychological self-report measures were used including measures which evaluated psychological morbidity and personality traits. Stomach and rectal sensitivity were measured, as was somatic pain threshold (immersion of hand in water). As expected, the psychological measures were similar in the IBS subjects and controls, as the IBS subjects were not treatment seekers. Visceral perception was also similar in the two groups, as was the somatic pain threshold.

In other words, if IBS subjects are psychologically normal and do not show treatment-seeking behavior, then the physiological findings relating to visceral hypersensitivity will not be found. The authors suggest that visceral hypersensitivity may be related to psychological dysfunction rather than intrinsic gut processes. It is interesting, in this regard, that previous work by the Sheffield group in the UK found that anxiety was more common in those patients with IBS (i.e., treatment-seeking subjects) who demonstrated visceral sensitivity than in those who did not.[77] Galati and colleagues,[78] in another interesting study, found that IBS subjects are more sensitive to intraluminal gas distention than controls, but also reported more pain than controls in relation to sham gas. That is, they reported increased pain even when gas was not being introduced and there was no gut distention. Studies of motility and sensitivity which have included a measure of psychological disturbance[70–72,76,77,79,80] are shown in Table 8.1.

The relationship between gut dysfunction and psychological factors remains unclear. Recent studies have raised more questions than they have answered. Some of the variation in the results of the studies discussed in this section can be explained by the small numbers of subjects in most of the studies, the reliance on relatively crude psychological self-report questionnaires as opposed to detailed psychological measures, and a variety of biases in the selection and recruiting of subjects. Because of the paucity of motility studies that have included a psychological assessment, there is a danger of too much being made of the little work that has been published.

CONCLUSIONS

There is little evidence to date that supports a direct association between psychological disturbance and gut dysfunction. Psychological factors, however, appear to play an important mediating role in the relationship between gut symptoms, gut physiology, and treatment seeking behavior. It is time consuming and difficult to conduct high quality research on gut dysfunction. The inclusion of appropriate and detailed psychological measures in future physiological work, combined with improved methods of recruitment, can only enhance our understanding of this complex and confusing area. The recent application of sophisticated brain imaging techniques to this area offers promise in attempting to provide anatomical definition to gut-brain interactions.[81]

REFERENCES

1. Camilleri M, Neri M. Motility disorders and stress. Dig Dis Sci 1989;39:1777–1786.
2. Plourde V. Stress-induced changes in the gastrointestinal motor system. Canad J Gastroenterol 1999;13 (Suppl A):26A–31A.
3. Tache Y, Martinez V, Million M, Rivier J. Corticotropin-releasing factor and the brain-gut motor response to stress. Canad J Gastroenterol 1999;13 (Suppl A):18A–25A
4. Pothoulakis C, Castagliuolo I, Leeman SE. Neuroimmune mechanisms of intestinal responses to stress. Role of corticotrophin-releasing factor and neurotensin. Ann N Y Acad Sci 1998;840:635–648.
5. Martinez V, Rivier J, Wang L, Tache Y. Central injection of a new corticotropin-releasing factor (CRF) antagonist, astressin, blocks CRF- and stress-related alterations of gastric and colonic motor function. J Pharmacol Exp Ther 1997;280:754–760.
6. Martinez V, Barquist E, Rivier J, Tache Y. Central CRF inhibits gastric emptying of a nutrient solid meal in rats: the role of CRF2 receptors. Am J Physiol 1998;274:G965–G970.
7. Monnikes H, Raybould HE, Schmidt B, Tache Y. CRF in the paraventricular nucleus of the hypothalamus stimulates colonic motor activity in fasted rats. Peptides 1993;14:743–747.
8. Mancinelli R, Azzena GB, Diana M, et al. In vitro excitatory actions of corticotropin-releasing factor on rat colonic motility. J Auton Pharmacol 1998;18:319–324.
9. Coskun T, Bozkurt A, Alican I, et al. Pathways mediating CRF-induced inhibition of gastric emptying in rats. Regul Pept 1997;69:113–120.
10. Crawley JN, Corwin RL. Biological actions of cholecystokinin. Peptides 1994;15:731–755.
11. Moran TH, Schwartz GJ. Neurobiology of cholecystokinin. Crit Rev Neurobiol 1994;9:1–28.
12. Wank SA. Cholecystokinin receptors. Am J Physiol 1995;269:G628–G646.
13. Abelson JL. Cholecystokinin in psychiatric research: a time for cautious excitement. J Psych Res 1995;29:389–396.
14. Fink H, Rex A, Voits M, Voigt JP. Major biological actions of CCK—a critical evaluation of research findings. Exp Brain Res 1998;123:77–83.
15. Bueno L. Involvement of brain CCK in the adaptation of gut motility to digestive status and stress: a review. J Physiol (Paris) 1993;87:301–306.
16. Gue M, Gleizes-Escala C, Del Rio-Lacheze C, et al. Reversal of CRF- and dopamine-induced stimulation of colonic motility by CCK and igmesine (JO 1784) in the rat. Brit J Pharmacol 1994;111:930–934.

17. Gue M, Tekamp A, Tabis N, et al. Cholecystokinin blockade of emotional stress- and CRF-induced colonic motor alterations in rats: role of the amygdala. Brain Res 1994;658:232–238.
18. Anderson KO, Dalton CB, Bradley LA, Richter JE. Stress induces alteration of esophageal pressures in healthy volunteers and non-cardiac chest pain patients. Dig Dis Sci 1989; 34:83–91.
19. Soffer EE, Scalabrini P, Pope CE, Wingate DL. Effect of stress on oesophageal motor function in normal subjects and in patients with the irritable bowel syndrome. Gut 1988; 29:1591–1594.
20. Young LD, Richter JE, Anderson KO, et al. The effects of psychological and environmental stressors on peristaltic esophageal contractions in healthy volunteers. Psychophysiology 1987;24:132–141.
21. Cook IJ, Dent J, Shannon S, Collins SM. Measurement of upper esophageal sphincter pressure. Effect of acute emotional stress. Gastroenterology 1987;93:526–532.
22. Thompson DG. Central control of human gastrointestinal function. Baillieres Clin Gastroenterol 1988;2:107–122.
23. Hveem K, Hausken T, Svebak S, Berstad A. Gastric antral motility in functional dyspepsia. Effect of mental stress and cisapride. Scand J Gastroenterol 1996;31:452–457.
24. Roland J, Dobbeleir A, Vandevivere J, Ham HR. Effect of mild mental stress on solid phase gastric emptying in health subjects. Nuc Med Comm 1990;11:319–326.
25. Holtmann G, Singer MV, Kriebel R, et al. Differential effects of acute mental stress on interdigestive secretion of gastric acid, pancreatic enzymes and gastroduodenal motility. Dig Dis Sci 1989;34:1701–1707.
26. Paternico A, Stanghellini V, DeGiorgio R, et al. Effects of acute cold pressor test on vagally stimulated gastric acid secretion and circulating levels of human pancreatic polypeptide and gastrin. Digestion 1994;55:154–159.
27. Stanghellini V, Malagelada JR, Zinsmeister AR, et al. Stress-induced gastroduodenal motor disturbances in humans: possible humoral mechanisms. Gastroenterology 1983;85:83–91.
28. Stanghellini V, Malagelada JR, Zinsmeister AR, et al. Effect of opiate and adrenergic blockers on the gut motor response to centrally acting stimuli. Gastroenterology 1984; 87:1104–1113.
29. Valori RM, Kumar D, Wingate DL. Effects of different types of stress and of "prokinetic" drugs on the control of the fasting motor complex in humans. Gastroenterology 1986; 90:1890–1900.
30. Kellow JE, Langeluddecke PM, Eckersley GM, et al. Effects of acute psychologic stress on small-intestinal motility in health and the irritable bowel syndrome. Scand J Gastroenterol 1992;27:53–58.
31. Cann PA, Read NW, Brown C, et al. Irritable bowel syndrome: relationship of disorders in transit of a single solid meal to symptom patterns. Gut 1983;24:405–411.
32. Yamamoto O, Niida H, Tajima K, et al. Inhibition of stress-stimulated colonic propulsion by alpha 2-adrenoceptor antagonists in rats. Neurogastroenterol Motil 1998;10:523–532.
33. Wittmann T, Crenner F, Angel F, et al. Long-duration stress. Immediate and late effects on small and large bowel motility in rat. Dig Dis Sci 1990;35:495–500.
34. Rao SS, Hatfield RA, Suls JM. Chamberlain MJ. Psychological and physical stress induce differential effects on human colonic motility. Am J Gastroenterol 1998;93:985–990.
35. Narducci F, Snape WJ Jr, Battle WM, et al. Increased colonic motility during exposure to a stressful situation. Dig Dis Sci 1985;30:40–44.
36. Schang JC, Devroede G, Hebert M, et al. Effects of rest, stress and food on myoelectric spiking activity of left and sigmoid colon in humans. Dig Dis Sci 1988;33:614–618.
37. Sarna S, Latimer P, Campbell D, Waterfall WE. Effect of stress, meal and neostigmine on rectosigmoid electrical control activity (ECA) in normals and in irritable bowel syndrome patients. Dig Dis Sci 1982;27:582–591.
38. Welgan P, Meshkinpour H, Hoehler F. The effect of stress on colon motor and electrical activity in irritable bowel syndrome. Psychosom Med 1985;47:139–149.
39. Welgan P, Meshkinpour H, Beeler M. Effect of anger on colon motor and myoelectric activity in irritable bowel syndrome. Gastroenterology 1988;94:1150–1156.
40. Whorwell PJ, Houghton LA, Taylor EE, Maxton DG. Physiological effects of emotion: assessment via hypnosis. Lancet 1992;340:69–72.

Chapter 9
Swallowing Disorders

Peter J. Kahrilas

Swallowing disorders can result from either oropharyngeal or esophageal diseases with dysphagia being the most consistent symptom. The most severe forms of dysphagia usually affect the oropharynx.[1] Several fundamental distinctions between esophageal and oropharyngeal dysphagia should be noted. Whereas esophageal dysphagia usually results from esophageal diseases, most cases of oropharyngeal dysphagia are the result of neurological or muscular diseases, with oropharyngeal dysfunction being just one manifestation. Second, the esophagus has but one function, to serve as a conduit between the oropharynx and stomach. In this sense, it is an expendable organ. The oropharynx, on the other hand, is fundamentally involved in speech and respiration as well as swallowing, making dysfunction of greater and more obvious consequence. Finally, in most instances, esophageal dysphagia can be well treated. In contrast, this is the exception rather than the rule for oropharyngeal dyphagia.

The symptom of dysphagia must be distinguished from the continuous sensation of a lump in the throat, labeled as globus hystericus or globus sensation. Globus is prominent between swallows, whereas dysphagia occurs only during swallowing. A patient complains of dysphagia if he is aware of difficulty in the passage of food from the mouth, through the esophagus, into the stomach. In the case of oropharyngeal dysphagia, the patient's perception of the dysfunction is highly inaccurate, be it an inability to control the food within the oral cavity, inability to initiate a pharyngeal swallow response, or aspiration. The situation is different with esophageal dysphagia in which a patient's perception is of limited accuracy and the actual level of hang-up or obstruction occurs at or below the level identified by the patient.[2] Thus, dysphagia from a distal esophageal ring or achalasia will sometimes be referred to the neck. Therefore, identification of associated symptoms such as aspiration, regurgitation, nasopharyngeal regurgitation, weight loss, voice changes, drooling, chest pain, or intermittent esophageal obstruction can be of great value in localizing dysphagia.

OROPHARYNGEAL DYSPHAGIA

Oropharyngeal dysphagia can result from structural or propulsive abnormalities of either the oropharynx or the proximal esophagus.[1] Propulsive abnormalities of the oropharynx or esophagus can result from dysfunction of intrinsic musculature, peripheral nerves, or central nervous system control mechanisms. Structural abnormalities of these areas may result from trauma, surgery, tumors, caustic injury, congenital conditions, or acquired deformities. The most remedial causes of oropharyngeal dysphagia result from anatomic aberrations. A post cricoid web can effectively narrow the esophageal inlet and cause dysphagia. Similarly, a cervical osteophyte can bulge anteriorly into the hypopharynx, making the passage of a normal sized bolus difficult. Analogous situations can arise as a result of edema following the surgical stabilization of the vertebral column, the implantation of metal stabilization devices, or cervical laminectomy.

HYPOPHARYNGEAL DIVERTICULA

Hypopharyngeal diverticula can cause symptoms of dysphagia and regurgitation, especially when they are large and fixed. Hypopharyngeal diverticula can be congenital or acquired, although most are acquired. Congenital diverticula usually represent persistent pharyngeal pouches that should have disappeared during embryological development,[3] and are true diverticula in that they contain all of the structures of the full thickness of the pharyngeal wall. Acquired diverticula, on the other hand, are formed only of mucosa and submucosa, making them false diverticula. Acquired diverticula occur most commonly in men after the sixth decade of life. The most frequent site of herniation is midline between the inferior pharyngeal constrictor and the cricopharyneus muscle, corresponding to Killian's dehiscence.[4] The unifying theme of this, and less frequent locations for false diverticula formation, is that they occur through sites of potential weakness of the muscular lining of the hypopharynx. Hypopharyngeal diverticula are generally asymptomatic until they enlarge sufficiently to accommodate and store a significant amount of food or liquid. In most instances, symptoms are of post-swallow regurgitation, or even aspiration, of the material within the pharyngeal pouch.

The pathogenesis of hypopharyngeal diverticula has been the subject of much debate, having been hypothesized to result from delayed UES relaxation, failure of relaxation, and premature contraction.[5,6] However, very little data exist to support any of these hypotheses. Some clinicians have adopted the name "cricopharyngeal achalasia" to describe the findings of a cricopharyngeal bar, thereby implying an analogy to achalasia of the cardia (see below). Applying the term "cricopharyngeal achalasia" in this setting is, at best, confusing. There has been no demonstration of either motor abnormality or denervation in the pathogenesis of either cricopharyngeal bars or of hypopharyngeal diverticula.

A more plausible pathophysiologic explanation for the development of diverticula is that they form as a result of a restrictive myopathy associated with diminished compliance of the cricopharyngeus muscle. Surgical specimens of cricopharyngeus muscle strips from 14 patients with hypopharyngeal diverticula demonstrated structural changes that would decrease UES compliance and opening.[7] The cricopharyngeus biopsies from these patients had "fibro-adipose tissue replacement and fiber degeneration." The process that led to the histologic changes is unclear but, whatever the case may be, these findings support the hypothesis that fibrosis of the cricopharyngeus impairs UES opening by decreasing sphincter compliance. Thus, although the muscle relaxes normally during a swallow, it cannot distend normally, resulting in the appearance of a cricopharyngeal bar during a barium swallow.

Diminished sphincter compliance is associated with increased hypopharyngeal pressure in order to maintain trans-sphincteric flow through the smaller UES opening. Careful manometric studies have demonstrated that this restricted UES aperture results in increased intrabolus pressure in the hypopharynx during swallowing. Whereas normal individuals have compliant sphincters with upstream intrabolus pressure ranging from 6 to 18 mmHg and with swallow volumes of 2 to 30 ml, patients with cricopharyngeal bars have upstream pressures ranging from 13 to 68 mmHg for the same range of bolus volumes.[8] The same phenomena have been demonstrated in patients with Zenker's diverticula, suggesting that diverticula formation is the consequence of this increased stress on the hypopharynx.[9]

The treatment of hypopharyngeal diverticula is surgical diverticulectomy, cricopharyngeal myotomy, or both. Surgical series have reported success with diverticulectomy alone,[10] myotomy alone,[11,12] or both diverticulectomy and myotomy.[13] In all likelihood, there are instances in which a limited procedure would be adequate, but a definitive approach to the problem of pulsion diverticula should involve both diverticulectomy and myotomy. Diverticulectomy alone risks recurrence because the underlying stenosis at the level of the cricopharyngeus is not remedied. Similarly, myotomy alone risks not solving the problem of food accumulation within the diverticulum with attendant regurgitation and aspiration. Small diverticula may, however, disappear spontaneously following myotomy. A recent study examined the compliance of the cricopharyngeus following diverticulectomy with myotomy in patients with hypopharyngeal diverticula, and found that the compliance of the sphincter was restored to normal in five patients following surgery, as indicated by normal hypopharyngeal intrabolus pressure during swallowing.[9]

NEUROLOGIC DISEASES

Neurologic diseases can either selectively or uniformly affect the neural structures responsible for swallowing. Since, as far as we know, there is nothing peculiar to the neurons controlling swallowing, their involvement in disease processes is essentially random, and virtually any CNS disease can be associated with dysphagia. Neurologic involvement limited to the control of the oropharynx happens only in rare instances. More commonly, structures controlled by adjacent neuronal structures are concurrently involved.

The neuronal circuitry organizing the pharyngeal swallow is situated bilaterally beneath the nucleus of the solitary tract in the brainstem.[14] Efferent fibers from the swallow centers travel, either directly or via relay neurons, to the motoneurons controlling pharyngeal and laryngeal musculature in nucleus ambiguus. It follows from this architecture that severe dysphagia, or even complete absence of the swallow response, can occur as a result of brainstem infarcts. Bilateral involvement is more severe and less likely to show recovery than is unilateral involvement.

Dysphagia is also a potential (though less frequent) consequence of cortical strokes as opposed to brainstem strokes. However, most cortical stroke patients recover from their dysphagia within two weeks of the infarct,[15] a reflection of neuronal plasticity within the central nervous system,[16] suggesting that extensive evaluation can be delayed at least until this time. These patients do, however, merit close observation, since stroke victims with dysphagia have a higher incidence of pneumonia, dehydration, and death, compared to those who do not experience dysphagia.[17]

An old neurologic disease that has recently resurfaced is poliomyelitis. Increasing numbers of patients have been described with new symptoms traceable to their remote polio infection 30 to 40 years earlier.[18] The new, slowly progressive post-polio muscular atrophy may occur in muscles that were clinically unaffected by the acute illness. One recent investigation studied 13 patients with post-polio dysphagia and demonstrated palatal, pharyngeal, and laryngeal weakness. Over half of the patients evaluated demonstrated silent aspiration, suggesting that the clinician should maintain a low threshold for evaluating such patients with videofluoroscopy.

Other relatively common neurologic ailments in which dysphagia is often a problem are amyotrophic lateral sclerosis (ALS) and Parkinson's disease (PD). ALS is a progressive nerological disease characterized by degeneration of motoneurons in the brain, brainstem, and spinal cord. When the degenerative process involves the cranial nerve nuclei, swallowing difficulties ensue. Patients experience choking attacks, become dehydrated or malnourished, and incur aspiration pneumonia. The decline in swallowing function is progressive and predictable, invariably ending up with gastrostomy feeding. A number of patients die as a consequence of their swallowing dysfunction in conjunction with respiratory depression. Patients with PD may exhibit both oral and pharyngeal abnormalities during swallowing.[19] During the oral phase of the swallow, PD patients exhibit a typical repetitive anterior to posterior rolling pattern when attempting lingual propulsion of the bolus. This sequence of "false starts" may result from rigidity of the lingual musculature; the patient is unable to lower his tongue once it has been elevated. A recent investigation into the mechanism of oropharyngeal dysphagia in PD patients revealed impaired upper esophageal sphincter relaxation in the subset with dysphagia, resulting in diminished sphincter opening and augmented intrabolus pressure, analogous to the case with cricopharyngeal bars.[20]

MYOPATHIES

Primary muscular diseases involving the oropharynx can be associated with dysphagia. Nasality of the voice and instances of nasopharyngeal regurgitation reflect weakness or paresis of the soft palate elevators. Poor control of the bolus within the mouth results from the tongue weakness. Post swallow residua in the valeculae or hypopharynx reflect a weakened pharyngeal contraction. Aspiration suggests either weakened laryngeal elevators, with resultant impairment of laryngeal closure during swallowing, or post-swallow residua that are then aspirated after the swallow sequence is completed. As with neurologic disorders, virtually any disorder affecting skeletal muscle can result in dyphagia.[21]

The prototype myopathy causing oropharyngeal dysphagia is oculopharyngeal dystrophy, characterized by progressive dysphagia and palpebral ptosis. This disease is inherited as an autosomal dominant, with occurrences clustered in, but not limited to, families of French-Canadian descent. Oculopharyngeal dystrophy has a curious selectivity for the striated pharyngeal muscles and the levator palpebrae. The first symptom is usually ptosis, which eventually dominates the patient's facial appearance. Dysphagia may begin before or after the ptosis. Dysphagia progresses slowly but may ultimately lead to starvation, aspiration pneumonia, or asphyxia.[22] The dominant radiographic findings are a weak or absent pharyngeal contraction with hypopharyngeal stasis and occasional nasopharyngeal regurgitation.

Myasthenia gravis is a progressive autoimmune disease characterized by destruction of acetylcholine receptors at neuromuscular junctions. Musculature controlled by the cranial nerves is almost always involved, particularly the ocular muscles. Dysphagia is a prominent symptom in more than a third of myasthenia gravis cases and, in unusual instances, can be the initial manifestation of the disease.[23] In mild cases, dysphagia may not be evident until after 15 to 20 minutes of exercise. In more advanced cases, the dysphagia can be profound and associated with nasopharyngeal regurgitation and a constant nasality of the voice, even to the extent of being confused with bulbar ALS. Dysphagia, along with other manifestations of the disease, improves with therapy, but severe dysphagia is generally a poor prognostic sign signaling fulminant disease.

HEAD AND NECK CANCER

Another group of patients commonly afflicted with oropharyngeal dysphagia are head and neck cancer patients. Although the tumors themselves are sometimes associated with mild dysphagia, more commonly, problems arise as the result of surgery or radiation therapy. Radiation therapy causes diminished salivation as a result of fibrosis of the salivary glands. Afflicted individuals may complain of a viscous, mucoid saliva that is itself difficult to swallow and does not provide the normal lubrication that aids in deglutition. Other than as a consequence of radiation therapy, xerostomia can also occur as a result of drugs, autoimmune diseases, and rheumatoid arthritis. Despite its prevalence, it is unusual for xerostomia to be a patient's primary complaint; most commonly, patients report dry mouth only in response to inquiry. Symptoms associated with xerostomia are: pain, burning, and soreness of the oral mucosa, especially the tongue; difficulty in mastication, swallowing, and speech; impairment of taste; painful oral ulcers; difficulty wearing dentures; increased dental caries; and increased fluid intake. A less common cause of radiation induced dysphagia occurs a year or more after the completion of radiation therapy and is probably related to radiation induced fibrosis of the oropharyngeal musculature.

EVALUATION OF OROPHARYNGEAL DYSPHAGIA

How should oropharyngeal dysphagia be evaluated? Usually, the combination of careful history and a videofluoroscopic examination allows for evaluation of all functional elements of the swallow, assessment of the mechanism of dysfunction, and assessment of the likelihood of function being improved by compensatory therapeutic strategies. Although other diagnostic modalities such as manometry, scintigrapy, or ultrasound may corroborate the findings of videofluoroscopy, rarely, if ever, will those studies stand on their own.[1]

Critical analysis of videofluoroscopic swallowing studies suggests six main functional elements of the pharyngeal swallow: laryngeal closure, nasopharyngeal closure, UES opening, tongue loading, tongue propulsion, and pharyngeal clearance. The mechanics by which each of these events occurs has been analyzed in detail.[24–27] Laryngeal closure occurs as a result of laryngeal elevation and anterior tilting of the arytenoids, causing them to oppose the base of the epiglottis. Vocal fold closure is of secondary significance in airway protection. Nasopharyngeal closure occurs with elevation of the soft palate. UES opening is accomplished by relaxation of the sphincter, followed by traction on the anterior sphincter wall, facilitated by laryngeal elevation, and contraction of the supra and infrahyoid musculature. Bolus propulsion is facilitated mainly by tongue action, and pharyngeal residue is cleared by the longitudinal and transverse pharyngeal contractions. Dysfunction of any one of these elements of the swallow has somewhat predictable consequences. Impaired laryngeal closure results in aspiration during the swallow. Soft palate dysfunction leads to nasopharyngeal regurgitation. Impaired UES opening leads to dysphagia, post-swallow aspiration, and, in the case of cricopharyngeal bars, diverticula formation. Tongue dysfunction with attendant impaired bolus propulsion leads to a sluggish, misdirected bolus. Finally, an impaired pharyngeal contraction results in post-swallow residue in the valleculae and pyriform sinuses, with the risk of post-swallow aspiration.

Dysfunction of the swallow does not necessarily obligate an individual to non oral feeding. Depending on the severity of the impairment, level of motivation, and neurological intactness, defective elements of the swallow can be selectively compensated for.[28] Impaired laryngeal closure can be compensated for by tucking the chin during swallow and use of the "supraglottic swallow," which is done by holding the breath during swallow and coughing afterward to clear residue prior to inhaling. Impaired nasopharyngeal closure can be compensated for by using palatal elevators and by avoiding thin liquid foods. Impaired UES opening can be improved by use of a biofeedback technique using videoflouoroscopy to teach the "Mendelsohn maneuver," which is the purposeful prolongation of the anterior-superior laryngeal traction at mid swallow.[29] Finally, impaired pharyngeal clearance can be compensated for by turning the head toward the paretic side, in the case of unilateral dysfunction, or by post-swallow cough to clear residue, in the case of bilateral paresis. These maneuvers are summarized in Table 9.1.

Table 9.1. Analysis of Oropharyngeal Dysphagia According to Functional Elements of a Swallow

Swallow Element	Biomechanical Mechanism	Evidence of Dysfunction (Typical Disease)	Therapeutic Techniques
Airway protection	Laryngeal elevation, arytenoids tilt, cord closure	Aspiration during bolus transit (ALS)	Chin down, biofeedback (*supraglottic swallow*)
Nasopharyngeal closure	Soft palate elevation	Nasopharyngeal regurgitation (Myasthenia Gravis)	Avoid thin liquids (Cholinomimetics for myasthenia)
UES opening	UES relaxation, laryngeal elevation, anterior hyoid traction	Dysphagia, post-swallow residue/aspiration, diverticulum formation (Cricopharyngeal Bar, CVA, Parkinson's)	Biofeedback (*Mendelsohn maneuver*), myotomy
Bolus propulsion	Tongue contour, sensation, motor control	Sluggish, misdirected bolus (Parkinson's, surgical defects, cerebral palsy)	Avoid thin liquids
Pharyngeal clearance	Pharyngeal shortening, propagated pharyngeal contraction, epiglottic flip	Post-swallow residue/aspiration (polio, post-polio, muscular dystrophy, CVA)	Head turning (unilateral weakness), post-swallow cough

ALS = amyotrophic lateral sclerosis; CVA = cerebrovascular accident; UES = upper esophageal sphincter.

A final note is on the utility of the cricopharyngeal myotomy. As mentioned above, cricopharyngeal myotomy can be an effective mode of therapy for patients with cricopharyngeal bars or hypopharyngeal diverticula. In general, the criteria for performing a myotomy should be: 1) the presence of significant dysphagia leading to local discomfort, weight loss, or aspiration; 2) confirmation of UES dysfunction by videoradiography, preferably with intraluminal manometry; and 3) absence of clinically significant gastroesophageal reflux or gastroesophageal regurgitation. These criteria are often met in the case of hypopharyngeal diverticula, but probably not in many other clinical situations. Performing myotomies in questionable cases is not advisable because, although it is a relatively safe procedure, it can further impair diminished constrictor function, and sudden death from aspiration is a reported complication, emphasizing the need to assess lower esophageal competence preoperatively. The combination of cricopharyngeal myotomy and lower esophageal sphincter incompetence is particularly devastating, and can lead to refractory aspiration. If the myotomy is essential in this circumstance, it should be paired with an antireflux procedure.

PATTERNS OF DYSPHAGIA SUGGESTIVE OF ESOPHAGEAL DISEASE

Dysphagia is the fundamental symptom experienced by patients with esophageal disorders. However, as alluded to earlier, the differentation between oropharyngeal and esophageal lesions may be difficult on the basis of patient history. Recognizing esophageal dysphagia necessitates recognition of associated heartburn, esophagopharyngeal regurgitation, chest pain, odynophagia, or intermittent esophageal obstruction. Thus, the importance of obtaining a careful history is apparent. Interpreting the symptom of "difficulty swallowing" is heavily dependent upon the associated symptomatology, and the thoughtful diagnostic approach to the patient depends upon the array of symptoms elicited (Figure 9.1).

Of the esophageal disorders potentially resulting in swallowing difficulty, the groups most relevant to the present discussion are the motor disorders, achalasia and esophageal spastic disorders, as these are caused by dysfunction of the enteric nervous system.

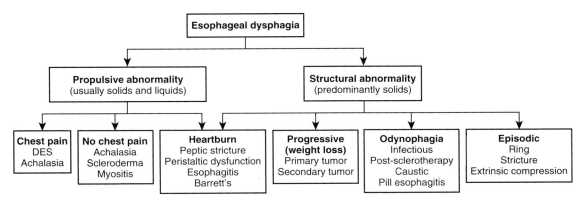

Figure 9.1. Etiologies of esophageal dysphagia.

Achalasia

Achalasia is the best defined motor disorder of the esophagus. First recognized more than 300 years ago, the disorder was initially labeled cardiospasm, reflecting the observation that it was caused by contractile dysfunction at the cardiac sphincter rather than anatomic obstruction of the esophagus, there being no obstructing lesions evident in the autopsy specimens. In 1973, Lendrum proposed that the functional esophageal obstruction resulted from incomplete relaxation of the lower esophageal sphincter, and renamed the disease achalasia ("failure to relax").[30] Achalasia is rare with an estimated incidence of about 1/100,000 population per year,[31] affecting both sexes equally and usually presenting in adult life. Although achalasia is usually idiopathic in etiology in North America, the disease can be closely mimicked by the esophageal involvement in Chagas' disease, caused by infection with the parasite *Trypanosoma cruzi*, endemic in areas of South America. A key distinction between idiopathic achalasia and that resultant from the late stages of Chagas' disease is that, whereas there is selective involvement of the esophagus with idiopathic achalasia, Chagas' disease additionally afflicts other organs, resulting in cardiomyopathy, megaureter, megaduodenum, or megacolon.[32]

Achalasia is characterized by: 1) failure of the LES to relax completely with swallowing; and 2) aperistalisis in the smooth muscle esophagus. The resting LES pressure is elevated in about 60% of achalasia cases. If there are nonperistaltic, spasm-like contractions in the esophageal body, the disease is referred to as vigorous achalasia. Achalasia is thought to result from post-ganglionic denervation of the smooth muscle esophagus, either as a result of parasitic infestation as in Chagas' disease or, more commonly, as an idiopathic entity. A recent morphologic study of 42 esophagi resected from patients with advanced achalasia revealed diminished myenteric ganglion cells and inflammation within the myenteric plexus in all cases.[33] In a further study, the same group documented myenteric inflammation and injury as the earliest lesions in early achalasia.[34] It is unclear whether the disease selectively affects excitatory or inhibitory neurons but, functionally, it is clear that the inhibitory neurons are necessarily impaired as an early manifestation of the disease. Sifrim utilized an intraesophageal balloon to demonstrate impairment of deglutitive relaxation in the esophageal body as well as the LES in early, non-dilated cases of achalasia.[35] Previously referred to as nonadrenergic, noncholinergic neurons, it is increasingly evident that the neurons responsible for deglutitive inhibition (including sphincter relaxation) utilize nitric oxide and possibly vasoactive intestinal polypeptide as neurotransmitters.[36] A working hypothesis for achalasia proposes that an initial inflammatory insult injures myenteric ganglia, and especially those involved in inhibitory neurotransmission, leading to their subsequent loss with consequent permanent loss of sphincter inhibition.[37] In support of this conclusion, patients with achalasia have been shown to lack nitric oxide synthase in the gastroesophageal junction,[36] and animal models of achalasia have been established using nitric oxide inhibitors such as L-NNA.[38]

Clinical manifestations of achalasia may include dysphagia, regurgitation, chest pain, weight loss, and aspiration pneumonia. The pattern of dysphagia in achalasics, especially in individuals with a dilated esophagus, is quite unique. They can often sense passage of material from the esophagus into the stomach and augment this by drinking a lot while eating, or applying maneuvers such as straightening the back, raising their arms over their heads, or standing to increase intraesophageal pressure.

Predictably, regurgitation can be quite problematic when large amounts of food are retained in the dilated esophagus. Classically, patients will complain of regurgitant on their bed sheets when sleeping supine, and have often elected to sleep with several pillows or upright in a chair by the time that they seek medical advice. Chest pain is a frequent complaint early in the course of the disease; its etiology is unclear. An interesting, but fortunately rare, symptom of achalasia is tracheal compression and airway compromise as a result of the dilated esophagus compressing the trachea.[39] This occurs as a result of dysfunction of the belch reflex, either because of neural degeneration or because the dilated esophagus prevents activation of stretch receptors within the esophageal wall.[40] Recent series have emphasized the variability and subtlety of symptoms at presentation[41]; many patients may begin with such atypical symptoms as heartburn, a factor which no doubt contributes to a delay in diagnosis in many cases.

The diagnosis of achalasia is made by barium swallow X-ray or esophageal manometry. The characteristic X-ray is of a dilated intrathoracic esophagus with an air-fluid level. The LES tapers to a point, giving the distal esophagus a beak-like appearance. The beak does not open with swallowing, but will open following the inhalation of amyl nitrite (a smooth muscle relaxant).[42] The radiological examination may, it must be emphasized, be normal in some cases.[41] The defining manometric features of achalasia are aperistalsis and incomplete LES relaxation. Indeed, an LES relaxation pressure ≥ 10 mmHg is highly predictive of achalasia and closely correlates with symptoms.[43] In cases of achalasia that are established by all available clinical criteria, the defining manometric features are present in >90% of patients. A recent study has clearly described the manometric features of the remaining patients. Among 58 patients with achalasia, 6 had elevated esophageal contraction amplitudes, 4 had evidence of true peristalsis in a segment of the esophagus, and single patients had either an LES relaxation pressure of less than 10 mmHg or intact transient lower esophageal sphincter relaxations (TLESRs).[44] Other manometric features provide only supportive evidence.[45] In a comparison of diagnostic modalities, one prospective study showed that achalasia was suggested by the radiologist in 21 of 33 patients who were given the diagnosis at manometry; endoscopists prospectively suggested the correct diagnosis in less than one third of the patients.[46]

Neither the radiographic nor the manometric features of achalasia are specific for idiopathic achalasia or achalasia associated with Chagas' disease; tumor-related pseudoachalasia accounts for up to 5% of cases with manometrically defined achalasia.[47] Pseudoachalasia is more likely with progressive age, abrupt onset of symptoms, and early weight loss.[48] Tumor infiltration (especially carcinoma in the gastric fundus) can completely mimic the functional impairment seen with idiopathic achalasia. It is because of this potential pitfall that a thorough anatomic examination (including endoscopy) should be done as part of the diagnostic evaluation of every new case of achalasia. A clue to the presence of pseudoachalasia on the endoscopic examination is finding more than the slightest resistance to passage of the endoscope across the gastroesophageal junction; in idiopathic achalasia, the endoscope should pop through with only gentle pressure required. If suspicion of pseudoachalasia persists, endoscopic biopsy, computerized tomography, magnetic resonance imaging, or endoscopic ultrasound may aid in further evaluation, depending upon the special circumstances.

The treatment of achalasia is to either incapacitate the LES pharmacologically or to disrupt it mechanically.[49,50] Medical treatments, on the whole, are not very effective, perhaps more indicated as temporizing maneuvers than definitive therapies. Smooth muscle relaxants such as nitrates or nifedipine,[51] administered sublingually immediately prior to eating, may offer partial relief of dysphagia. One experimental approach to the therapy of achalasia involves the use of nitric oxide agonists.[52] Another approach involves the endoscopically-delivered local injection of botulinum toxin into the sphincter muscle.[53] While initial, short-term results appeared promising,[53–55] further evaluation, with long-term follow up, has been less enthusiastic.[56,57] In most instances, therefore, definitive treatment of achalasia is still based on disruption of the LES either surgically (Heller myotomy) or by the use of a pneumatic dilator. The anticipated risk of esophageal perforation during pneumatic dilation ranges from 1 to 5%. Only one controlled trial has ever been done comparing these modalities, and it concluded that the surgical approach was somewhat superior.[58] That trial was, however, done by a surgeon.

Pneumatic dilation of the esophagus is accomplished using inflatable balloon dilators that achieve a forceful stretching of the LES to a diameter of about 3 cm. This is different from dilation done as therapy of peptic strictures and, indeed, therapy with conventional dilators (up to 56F) provides only very temporary benefit in achalasia. Pneumatic dilators are either radiographically (Rigiflex dilator) or endoscopically (Witzel dilator) positioned across the gastroesophageal junction and inflated to 6 to 9 psi for a period of 30 to 60 seconds.[59] It is neither unusual nor dangerous to repeat a pneumatic dilation 2 to 3 times in instances of an unsatisfactory result. Many practitioners routinely obtain a fluoroscopic examination of the esophagus with water soluble contrast, following pneumatic dilation, to make sure that perforation has not occurred. If any substantial perforation has occurred, surgical repair should be pursued quickly. Patients with a perforation from pneumatic dilation that is recognized and treated promptly have outcomes that are comparable to those of patients undergoing elective myotomy.[60]

The standard surgical approach to the treatment of achalasia is the Heller myotomy done via thoracotomy. Once exposed, the circular muscle layer of the esophagus is cut from the distal esophagus to the proximal stomach. Some surgeons perform an antireflux procedure concurrently with the myotomy, while others reserve this added manipulation for patients with an associated hiatal hernia.[61] Although clearly efficacious, a Heller myotomy is associated with considerable morbidity, which has led most patients to pursue pneumatic dilation as the initial intervention. However, new surgical approaches to achalasia using laparoscopic or thoracoscopic techniques may tip the balance toward employing surgery as an initial intervention, since these techniques have substantially reduced morbidity.[49,50] One recent series of 24 achalasics treated either thoracoscopically or laparoscopically had outcomes similar to those of open procedures, but a median hospitalization of only 3 days.[62]

For both of these approaches, initial results are certainly excellent (success rates = 80%); assessments of outcome performed over several years have revealed less than satisfactory outcomes in terms of either symptoms or esophageal function.[63–65]

Spastic Disorders of the Esophagus

Abnormal peristalsis can potentially cause dysphagia and chest pain. Dysphagia will typically be for both solids and liquids. The pain may mimic that of angina pectoris. An esophageal etiology of chest pain should be considered only after careful consideration of potential cardiopulmonary etiologies. However, even within the spectrum of esophageal diseases, neither chest pain nor dysphagia is specific for spastic disorders, as both symptoms are also characteristic of common esophageal disorders, including peptic or infectious esophagitis (see Figure 9.1). After these more common diagnostic possibilities have been excluded by appropriate radiographic evaluation—endoscopic evaluation and, in some instances, a therapeutic trial of antisecretory medications—spastic disorders should be considered as the etiology of the still unexplained symptoms.

Unlike the case of achalasia, the esophagus of the patient with a spastic disorder of the esophagus usually retains its ability to propagate primary peristaltic waves the majority of the time. Thus, there are no uniform radiographic, manometric, or histopathological criteria for defining esophageal spastic disorders. Partly because of this fact, the criteria for diagnosing diffuse esophageal spasm (DES) remain variable and confusing.[66] In the unequivocal case, non-peristaltic, high amplitude, prolonged contractions are seen during esophageal manometry, and these are associated with the patient experiencing chest pain. These unequivocal cases are probably associated with a defect in the neuronal architecture of deglutitive inhibition, placing them along the continuum of vigorous achalasia and achalasia.[35] The LES typically functions normally. Radiographically, DES may appear as a "corkscrew esophagus." It must be emphasized, however, that neither the tertiary contractions (non-peristaltic, simultaneous esophageal contractions) seen on X-ray, nor the simultaneous contractions seen manometrically, are pathognomonic of esophageal spasm; both may be seen in asymptomatic individuals.[47]

As alluded to above, diffuse esophageal spasm is more variably defined than is achalasia, but simultaneous contractions following ≥ 30% of swallows are not found among controls, suggesting that this finding is related to dysphagia or chest pain.[67] However, such relatively clear-cut evidence of peristaltic dysfunction is found in ≤ 5% of chest-pain patients evaluated by manometry. More commonly, the manometric findings are marginally abnormal, falling into the category of "non-specific disorders," an umbrella term encompassing manometric abnormalities insufficient to establish a diagnosis of achalasia, DES, or aperistalsis.[47] The most common manometric patterns are of exaggerated contractions in the esophageal body (increased wave amplitudes, long duration, multipeaked waves) or a hypertensive LES.[68,69] Of the group, increased wave amplitude ("nutcracker esophagus") is the most commonly detected pattern, accounting for a large portion of patients in the "non-specific disorders" category.

Similar to achalasia, the simultaneous contractions typifying diffuse esophageal spasm impair bolus transit through the esophagus, potentially explaining the associated dysphagia.[70] However, functional abnormalities associated with non-specific esophageal motor disorders are not generally recognized. Furthermore, long-term observations have shown neither a parallel in clinical course with manometric findings, nor consistency in manometric diagnosis over time.[47,71,72] Therapeutic trials with smooth muscle relaxants, tranquilizers, or bougiennage have similarly shown no parallel between modification of manometric findings and therapeutic response.[73–76] In summary, it has been difficult to determine a direct relevance of non-specific motility disturbances to either symptoms or function, making their detection of no generalizable value. More impressive has been the finding that reflux disease is often responsible for explaining symptoms of esophageal dysfunction, whether non-specific motor abnormalities are present or not. Bancewicz found that intensive anti-reflux therapy was the most useful therapy for a large group of symptomatic patients without a specific motor disorder.[77] Similarly, Achem found that antireflux therapy benefited patients with unexplained chest pain, regardless of the presence or absence of non-specific motor abnormalities.[71]

Ironically, the medical therapies of esophageal spasm are similar to those of coronary artery disease, a disease with which it can be confused. However, despite the dogma of treatment with smooth muscle relaxants, there are remarkably little controlled data on the medical treatment of esophageal spasm. Long-term outcome studies of the medical treatment of DES with smooth muscle relaxants are not available, and the entire basis for this therapy remains at an anecdotal level.[45] Likewise, there are no controlled studies of treatment of well-defined patients with DES with pneumatic dilation or myotomy. Some DES patients have been observed to evolve into achalasia, for which there are defined treatment strategies.[78] However, at this point in time, therapy of esophageal spastic disorders is typically a trial and error experience, reflecting the inhomogeneity of the patient population.

REFERENCES

1. Cook IJ, Kahrilas PJ. AGA technical review on management of oropharyngeal dysphagia. Gastroenterology 1999;116:455–478.
2. Logemann JA. Evaluation and Treatment of Swallowing Disorders. San Diego, CA: College-Hill Press, 1983.
3. Wilson CP. Diverticula of the pharynx. J Royal Coll Surg Edin 1959;4:236.
4. Zaino C, Jacobsen HG, Lepow H, Oztruk CH. The Pharyngoesophageal Sphincter. Springfield, IL: C.C. Thomas, 1970.
5. Wilson CP. Pharyngeal diverticula: their cause and treatment. J Laryngol Otol 1962;76:151–180.
6. Goyal RK. Disorders of the cricopharyngeus muscle. Otolaryngol Clin North Am 1984;17:115–130.
7. Cook IJ, Blumberos P, Cash K, et al. Structural abnormalities of the cricopharyngeus muscle in patients with pharyngeal (Zenkers's) diverticulum. J Gastroenterol Hepatol 1992; 7:556–562.
8. Dantas RO, Cook IJ, Dodds WJ, et al. Biomechanics of cricopharyngeal bars. Gastroenterology 1990;99:1269–1274.
9. Cook IJ, Gabb M, Panagopoulos V, et al. Pharyngeal (Zenker's) diverticulum is a disorder of upper esophageal sphincter opening. Gastroenterology 1992;103:1229–1235.
10. Clagett OT, Payne WS. Surgical treatment for pulsion diverticula of the hypopharynx: one stage resection in 478 cases. Dis Chest 1960;37:257–261.
11. Blakely WR, Garety EJ, Smith DE. Section of the cricopharyngeus muscle for dysphagia. Arch Surg 1968;96:745–760.
12. Van Overbeek JJ, Betlem HC. Cricopharyngeal myotomy in pharyngeal paralysis. Cineradiographic and manometric indications. Ann Otol Rhinol Laryngol 1979;88:592–602.
13. Ellis FH Jr, Schlegel JF, Lynch VP, Payne WS. Cricopharyngeal myotomy for pharyngo-esophageal diverticulum. Ann Surg 1969;170:340–349.
14. Miller AJ. The search for the central swallowing pathway: the quest for clarity. Dysphagia 1993;8:185–194.
15. Hamdy S, Aziz Q, Rothwell JC, et al. Explaining oropharyngeal dysphagia after unilateral hemispheric stroke. Lancet 1997;350:686–692.
16. Hamdy S, Aziz Q, Rothwell JC, et al. Recovery of swallowing after dysphagic stroke relates to functional reorganization in the intact motor cortex. Gastroenterology 1998; 115:1104–1112.
17. Gordon C, Hewer RL, Wade DT. Dysphagia in acute stroke. Br Med J 1987;295:411–414.
18. Dalakas M, Elder G, Hallett M, et al. A long-term follow-up study of patients with post-poliomyelitis neuromuscular symptoms. N Engl J Med 1986;314:959–963.

19. Logemann J, Blonsky E, Boshes B. Dysphagia in Parkinsonism. JAMA 1975;231:69–70.
20. Ali GN, Wallace KL, Schwartz R, et al. Mechanisms of oral-pharyngeal dysphagia in patients with Parkinson's disease. Gastroenterology 1996;110:383–392.
21. Kahrilas PJ. Disorders causing oropharyngeal dysphagia. In DO Castell (ed), The Esophagus, 2nd ed. Boston: Little Brown and Company, 1995;205–218.
22. Aarli JA. Oculopharyngeal muscular dystrophy. Acta Neurol Scand 1969;45:485–492.
23. Osserman KE. Myasthenia Gravis. New York: Grune and Stratton, 1958.
24. Jacob P, Kahrilas PJ, Logemann JA, et al. Upper esophageal sphincter opening and modulation during swallowing. Gastroenterology 1989;97:1469–1478.
25. Kahrilas PJ, Logemann JA, Lin S, Ergun GA. Pharyngeal clearance during swallowing: a combined manometric and vidoefluoroscopic study. Gastroenterology 1992;103:128–136.
26. Kahrilas PJ, Lin S, Logemann JA, et al. Deglutitive tongue action: volume accommodation and bolus propulsion. Gastroenterology 1993;104:152–162.
27. Logemann JA, Kahrilas PJ, Cheng J, et al. Closure mechanisms of the laryngeal vestibule during swallow. Am J Physiol 1992;262:G338–G344.
28. Rasley A, Logemann JA, Kahrilas PJ, et al. Prevention of barium aspiration during video fluoroscopic swallowing studies: value of change in posture. Am J Roentgenol 1993; 160:1005–1009.
29. Kahrilas PJ, Logemann JA, Krugler C, Flanagan E. Volitional augmentation of upper esophageal sphincter opening during swallowing. Am J Physiol 1991;260:G450–G456.
30. Clouse RE, Diamant NE. Esophageal motor and sensory function and disorders of the esophagus. In M Feldman, LS Friedman, MH Sleisenger (eds), Sleisenger and Fordtran's Gastrointestinal and Liver Disease: Pathophysiology, Diagnosis, Management, 7th ed. Philadelphia: WB Saunders, 2002;561–598.
31. Mayberry JF, Atkinson M. Studies of achalasia in the Nottingham area. QJ Med 1985;56:451–456.
32. Koberle F. Chagas' disease and Chagas' syndrome: the pathology of American trypanosomiasis. Adv Parasitol 1968;6:63–116.
33. Goldblum JR, Whyte RI, Orringer MB, Appelman HD. Achalasia, a morphologic study of 42 resected specimens. Am J Surg Pathol 1994;18:327–337.
34. Goldblum JR, Rice TW, Richter JE. Histopathologic features in esophagomyotomy specimens from patients with achalasia. Gastroenterology 1996;111:648–654.
35. Sifrim D, Janssens J, Vantrappen G. Failing deglutitive inhibition in primary esophageal motility disorders. Gastroenterology 1994;106:875–882.
36. Mearin F, Mourelle M, Guarner F, et al. Patients with achalasia lack nitric oxide synthase in the gastro-oesophageal junction. Eur J Clin Invest 1993;23:724–728.
37. Hirano I. Pathophysiology of achalasia. Curr Gastroenterol Rep 1999;1:198–202.
38. Helm JF, Layman RD, Eckert MD. Effect of chronic administration of Nw-Nitro-L-Arginine (LNNA) on the opossum esophagus and lower esophageal sphincter (LES) resembles achalasia. Gastroenterology 1992;103:1375.
39. Panzini L, Traube M. Stridor from tracheal obstruction in a patient with achalasia. Am J Gastroenterol 1993;88:1097–1100.
40. Massey BT, Hogan WJ, Dodds WJ, Dantas RO. Alteration of the upper esophageal sphincter belch reflex in patients with achalasia. Gastroenterology 1992;103:1574–1579.
41. Blam ME, Delfyett W, Levine MS, et al. Achalasia: a disease of varied and subtle symptoms that do not correlate with radiographic findings. Am J Gastroenterol 2002;97:1916–1923.
42. Dodds WJ, Stewart ET, Kishk SM, et al. Radiological amyl nitrite test for discriminating pseudoachalasia from idiopathic achalasia. Am J Roentgenol 1986;1:21–23.
43. Yaghoobi M, Mikaeli J, Montazarei G, et al. Correlation between clinical severity score and the lower esophageal sphincter relaxation pressure in idiopathic achalasia. Am J Gastroenterol 2003;98:278–283.
44. Hirano I, Tatum RP, Shi G, et al. Manometric heterogeneity in patients with idiopathic achalasia. Gastroenterology 2001;120:789–790.
45. McCord GS, Staiano A, Clouse RE. Achalasia, diffuse esohpageal spasm and non-specific motor disorders. Baillieres Clin Gastroenterol 1991;5:307–335.
46. Howard PJ, Maher L, Pryde A, et al. Five year prospective study of the incidence, clinical features, and diagnosis of achalasia in Edinburgh. Gut 1992;33:1011–1015.

47. Kahrilas PJ, Clouse RE, Hogan WJ. American Gastroenterological Association technical review on the clinical use of esophageal manometry. Gastroenterology 1994;107:1865–1884.

48. Kahrilas PJ, Kishk SM, Helm JF, et al. A comparison of pseudoachalasia and achalasia. Am J Med 1987;82:439–446.

49. Spiess AE, Kahrilas PJ. Treating achalasia from whalebone to laparoscope. JAMA 1998;280:638–642.

50. Vaezi MF, Richter JE. Diagnosis and management of achalasia. American College of Gastroenterology Practice Parameters Committee. Am J Gastroenterol 1999;94:3406–3412.

51. Bortolotti M, Labo G. Clinical and manometric effects of nifedipine in patients with esophageal achalasia. Gastroenterology 1981;80:39–44.

52. Marzio L, Grossi L, DeLaurentis MF, et al. Effect of cimetropium bromide on esophageal motility and transit in patients affected by primary achalasia. Dig Dis Sci 1994; 39:1389–1394.

53. Pasricha PF, Ravich WJ, Hendrix TR, et al. Treatment of achalasia with intrasphincteric injection of botulinum toxin. A pilot trial. Ann Intern Med 1994;15:121:590–591.

54. Annese V, Basciani M, Perri F, et al. Controlled trial of botulinum toxin injection versus placebo and pneumatic dilatation in achalasia. Gastroenterology 1996;111:1418–1424.

55. Cuillier C, Ducrotte P, Zerbib F, et al. Achalasia: outcome of patients treated with intrasphincteric injection of botulinum toxin. Gut 1997;41:87–92.

56. Annese V, Bassotti G, Coccia G, et al. A multicentric randomized study of intrasphincteric botulinum toxin in patients with oesophageal achalasia. Gut 2000;46:597–600.

57. Vaezi MF, Richter JE, Wilcox CM, et al. Botulinum toxin versus pneumatic dilatation in the treatment of achalasia: a randomized trial. Gut 1999;44:231–239.

58. Csendes A, Braghetto I, Henriquez A, Cortes C. Late results of a prospective randomised study comparing forceful dilation and oesophagomyotomy in patients with achalasia. Gut 1989;30:299–304.

59. Eckardt VF, Aignherr C, Bernhard G. Predictors of outcome in patients with achalasia treated by pneumatic dilation. Gastroenterology 1992;103:1732–1738.

60. Schwartz HM, Cahow CE, Traube M. Outcome after perforation sustained during pneumatic dilation for achalasia. Dig Dis Sci 1993;38:1409–1413.

61. Cushieri A. Endoscopic oesophageal myotomy for specific motility disorders and non-cardiac chest pain. Endosc Surg Allied Technol 1993;1:280–287.

62. Pellegrini CA, Leichter R, Patti M, et al. Thoracoscopic esophageal myotomy in the treatment of achalasia. Ann Thorac Surg 1993;56:680–682.

63. West RL, Hirsch DP, Bartelsman JF, et al. Long-term results of pneumatic dilation in achalasia followed for more than 5 years. Am J Gastroenterol 2002;97:1346–1351.

64. Torbey CF, Achkar E, Rice TW, et al. Long-term outcome of achalasia treatment: the need for closer follow-up. J Clin Gastronenterl 1999;28:125–130.

65. Liu HC, Huang BS, Hsu WH, et al. Surgery for achalasia: long-term results in operated achalasic patients. Ann Thorac Cardiovasc Surg 1998;4:312–320.

66. Richter JE, Castell DO. Diffuse esophageal spasm: a reappraisal. Ann Int Med 1984; 100:242–245.

67. Clouse RE, Staiano A. Manometric patterns using esophageal body and lower sphincter characteristics: findings in 1013 patients. Dig Dis Sci 1992;37:289–296.

68. Benjamin SB, Gerhardt DC, Castell DO. High amplitude, persitaltic esophageal contractions associated with chest pain and/or dysphagia. Gastroenterology 1979;77:478–483.

69. Traube M, Albibi R, McCallum RW. High-amplitude peristaltic esophageal contractions associated with chest pain. JAMA 1983;250:2655–2659.

70. Massey BT, Dodds WJ, Hogan WJ, et al. Abnormal esophageal motility. An analysis of concurrent radiographic and manometric findings. Gastroenterology 1991;101:344–354.

71. Achem SR, Crittenden J, Kolts B, Burton L. Long-term clinical and manometric follow-up of patients with nonspecific esophageal motor disorders. Am J Gatroenterol 1992; 87:825–830.

72. Swift GL, Alban-Davies H, McKirdy H, et al. A long-term clinical review of patients with oesophageal chest pain. Quart J Med 1991;81:937–944.

73. Richter JE, Dalton CB, Bradley LA, Castell DO. Oral nifedipine in the treatment of noncardiac chest pain in patients with nutcracker esophagus. Gastroenterology 1987;93:21–28.

74. Clouse RE, Lustman PJ, Eckert TC, et al. Low-dose trazodone for symptomatic patients with esophageal contraction abnormalities: a double-blind, placebo-controlled trial. Gastroenterology 1987;92:1027–1036.

75. Cattau EL, Castell DO, Johnson DA, et al. Diltiazem therapy for symptoms associated with nutcracker esophagus. Am J Gatroenterol 1991;86:272–275.

76. Winters C, Artnak EJ, Benjamin SB, Castell DO. Esophageal bougienage in symptomatic patients with the nutcracker esophagus. JAMA 1984;252:363–366.

77. Bancewicz J, Osugi H, Marples M. Clinical implications of abnormal oesophageal motility. Br J Surg 1987;74:416–419.

78. Vantrappen G, Janssen J, Henemans J, Coremans G. Achalasia, diffuse esophageal spasm and related motility disorders. Gastroenterology 1979;76:450–457.

Chapter 10
Gastroparesis

Kenneth L. Koch

The gastrointestinal tract is a neuromuscular organ system. Normal gastrointestinal motility is exemplified by highly coordinated contractions and relaxations of specific regions such as the stomach. For example, in the stomach the normal rate of peristaltic contractions that mix and empty food is three cycles per minute (cpm). Normal gastric motility is produced by the normal function of the longitudinal and circular smooth muscle, the enteric nerves and interstitial cells of Cajal within the stomach wall, the extrinsic parasympathetic and sympathetic nerves that innervate the stomach, and the brain stem nuclei and hypothalamic centers that coordinate and modulate gastric neuromuscular functions.[1-5] Cortical and emotional inputs to hypothalamic centers also influence gastric motility.

When neuromuscular function of the stomach becomes abnormal due to gastric electrical and/or contractile abnormalities, the results are disturbed gastric contractions and, ultimately, gastroparesis. The actual level of the neuromuscular lesion(s), i.e., within the stomach, extrinsic nerves, spinal cord, or central nervous system, is usually difficult to determine. In this chapter the normal neuromuscular function of the stomach will be reviewed. Abnormal gastric motility and gastroparesis will be reviewed with particular attention to neurological disorders in which gastroparesis has been found.

NORMAL GASTRIC NEUROMUSCULAR FUNCTION

Normal Gastric Electrical Activity

Gastric slow waves are spontaneous, recurrent electrical waves produced by depolarization and repolarization of the interstitial cells of Cajal.[1,3-5] These electrical waves are also termed pacesetter potentials or electrical control waves because they set the pace of gastric peristaltic contractions. Plateau and spike potentials are electrical events that occur as the circular muscle is brought to and maintains the threshold for contraction.[3] Vagal efferent activity contributes to the maintenance of slow wave rhythmicity and has a role in regulating postprandial gastric motility.[2,6] Vagal afferent nerve activity from the stomach reflects gastric tone, distention, and peristaltic activity.[7,8] Receptors are also present for temperature and a variety of nutrients.[9]

Sympathetic nerve efferent inputs from the spinal cord inhibit gastric contractions and stimulate pyloric contractions. Afferent sympathetic neurons carry nociceptive stimuli through spinal cord and brainstem pathways.[2,9] Afferent neural inputs from the parasympathetic and sympathetic nervous systems are integrated in the hypothalamus[10]; hypothalamic neurons communicate with the dorsal vagal complex and with adrenergic efferent neurons to modulate efferent parasympathetic and sympathetic nerve activity in response to ongoing afferent inputs.[11,12]

Normal Gastric Muscular Activity

Depolarizations and repolarizations of the circular muscle layer are ultimately responsible for gastric muscular activity—gastric contractions and relaxations. The coordinated relaxation and contraction of the gastric musculature results in the mixing and emptying of nutrients from the stomach (Figure 10.1).

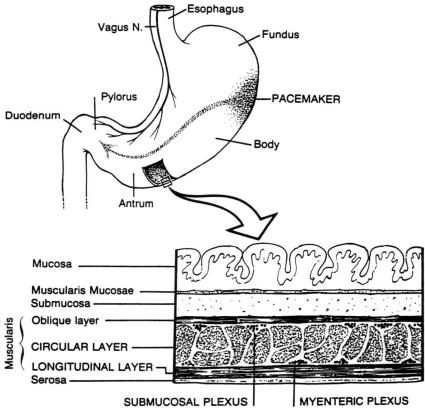

Figure 10.1. Diagram shows the major anatomical regions of the stomach including the fundus, body and antrum. As shown in the inset, the gastric wall is comprised of the mucosa and then the tunica muscularis. The muscularis has an outer longitudinal muscle layer and an inner circular muscle layer. Contractions and relaxations of these muscle layers are coordinated by the interstitial cells of Cajal and the enteric nervous system with major collections of neurons in the myenteric plexus and submucosal plexus. The vagus nerve innervates all regions of the stomach. The splanchnic nerves provide sympathetic nervous system innervation to the stomach.

In response to swallowing food, the fundus relaxes and receives the ingested solid or liquid foods. This receptive relaxation is mediated by the vagus nerve and release of nitric oxide.[2,9,13] Contractions of the corpus and antrum may be elicited by stimulating or distending the antrum, the muscular wall of the body. The gastric peristaltic waves that occur after eating are coordinated by slow waves to which the plateau or spike potentials are linked. The antral contractions mix and then empty the gastric contents from the stomach. Antro-pyloro-duodenal coordination is necessary for efficient emptying of stomach contents, as stomach contractions must coincide with pyloric and duodenal relaxation for the emptying of aliquots of nutrient suspensions into the duodenum.

ABNORMAL GASTRIC NEUROMUSCULAR FUNCTION AND GASTROPARESIS

The neuromuscular apparatus of the stomach may malfunction at many different levels after ingestion of a meal. Possible causes of neuromuscular dysfunction include enteric nervous system degeneration, smooth muscle disorders, disorders of extrinsic parasympathetic or sympathetic nervous systems, and diseases of the spinal cord and central nervous system (CNS).

Clinical gastric motility disorders are described as "gastroparesis" if gastric emptying is too slow and as "dumping" if emptying is too fast. The rate of gastric emptying is controlled by the underlying electrical and contractile activities of the stomach which were described above. Thus, gastric emptying may be delayed if the circular muscle does not contract, if gastric dysrhythmias are present, or if vagal nerve function is disordered. Disorders located in regions from the enteric nerves and interstitial cells of Cajal[14] to the central nervous system may affect gastric electrical and contractile activity and, thus, the rate of gastric emptying. Neurological diseases and disorders and their accompanying gastric disorders are reviewed below.

Symptoms of Gastroparesis

Symptoms of gastric dysrhythmias and gastroparesis include vague epigastric distress, early satiety, nausea, bloating, distention in the upper abdomen, poor appetite, and weight loss. Patients feel full very quickly after ingesting solids or liquids (early satiety); they often eat smaller portions than usual to avoid this sensation. The satiety or epigastric fullness may be reported as pain. In some patients, indeed, pain may be the presenting symptom.[15] Nausea often accompanies the sense of fullness. Nausea and fullness increase over time as the stomach fails to empty the meal normally. Thirty minutes to hours after the meal, the patient may vomit. The vomitus contains undigested food from previous meals.

Characteristics of Vomiting from Central Nervous System Disorders

Vomiting from central nervous system disorders is often abrupt in onset and precipitated by movement or changes in intracranial pressure.[16] Vomiting often occurs at the peak of headache, and is followed by improvement in headache and level of arousal. The vomitus may be projectile, and frequently does not contain undigested food. Nausea may not accompany the vomiting. Retching frequently occurs.

Tests for Gastric Neuromuscular Activity and Gastroparesis

Barium Studies

The rate of gastric emptying may be assessed quantitatively by barium studies to determine if gastric peristalses are present and to see if barium is emptied from the stomach.

Solid-Phase Gastric Emptying Tests

A quantitative and physiological test of gastric emptying is the solid-phase or liquid-phase gastric emptying study performed in nuclear medicine.[17] Typically, technetium-labeled foods, such as eggs, are ingested, and the rate of emptying is determined by measuring the isotope counts over the stomach region for two hours. Thus, time-emptying curves are developed for control subjects, and patients are compared to the control values to determine whether rapid or slow gastric emptying is present. Ultrasound may be used to determine antral cross-sectional areas over time after a liquid meal, and thus to determine gastric emptying without exposure to radiation. Delayed gastric emptying does not indicate the mechanism of the gastroparesis in terms of electrical or contractile abnormalities.

Electrogastrography

Electrogastrography is a non-invasive method for measuring the myoelectrical activity of the stomach, particularly the gastric slow wave frequency.[18] Abnormalities in gastric frequency, termed gastric dysrhythmias, are associated with nausea and vomiting[19,20] and with delayed gastric emptying.[21] Tachygastrias are abnormally fast gastric dysrhythmias ranging from 3.75 to 10.0 cpm; bradygastrias are abnormally slow rhythms ranging from flatline arrhythmias to 1 to 2.5 cpm waves.[22-24]

Intraluminal Pressure Probes

Intraluminal pressures indicate contractility of the gastric body, antrum, pylorus, or duodenum.[25] Pressure transducers mounted on flexible catheters must be passed by mouth or nose and positioned in the stomach at fluoroscopy. Poor antral contractions or poor coordination between antrum and duodenum can be defined with these tests. Contractions that do not obliterate the lumen are not detected.

Gastric Tone

Gastric tone may be measured by inflating balloons (barostats) within the proximal or distal stomach.[26,27]

ENTERIC NERVOUS SYSTEM ABNORMALITIES AFFECTING GASTRIC MOTILITY

Idiopathic, degenerative, or inflammatory disorders of myenteric plexus neurons may result in gastrointestinal dysfunction. For example, intestinal pseudoobstruction, neuropathic variety, involves the loss of myenteric neurons.[28] Disorders of function of interstitial cells of Cajal may also lead to clinical disorders, since loss of these cells in knockout mice is associated with abnormal slow waves and smooth muscle contractions.[14,29] Disorders of the extrinsic nervous system may affect myenteric neuron function, but these conditions have not been documented. Full thickness biopsies of stomach or small bowel and special silver stains are needed to detect enteric nerve abnormalities.

MUSCULAR DISORDERS OF THE GASTRIC TUNICA PROPRIA AFFECTING GASTRIC MOTILITY

Primary Muscle Disorders

Primary disorders of the gastric tunica propria are rare, and are described as intestinal pseudoobstruction, myopathic variety.[28] Histological examination shows a paucity of longitudinal muscle or circular muscle fibers or combinations of muscle wall deficits.

Secondary Muscular Disorders of the Gastric Tunica Propria

Amyloidosis

Amyloid may infiltrate the layers of gut smooth muscle and result in low-amplitude contractions.[30] Low-amplitude contractions of the stomach may lead to gastroparesis or bacterial overgrowth in the small intestine. In familial amyloidosis, a reduction in the number of neurons in the myenteric plexus has been described.[31]

Systemic Sclerosis (Scleroderma)

Motor disturbances begin with neuropathic injury to the myenteric nerves early in the course of disease; then, myopathic injury ensues due to infiltration of the muscle layers with collagenous deposits.[32] The process typically involves the esophagus and small bowel, but the stomach may also be involved.[33,34]

Dermatomyositis

Gastroparesis has been reported in patients with dermatomyositis and is proportional to skeletal muscle weakness.[35]

Myotonic Dystrophy

Abnormal smooth muscle along the entire gastrointestinal tract has been described in these patients. Gastroparesis has been described in patients with myotonic dystrophy (Figure 10.2). Metoclopramide appears to promote gastric emptying, but the precise defect(s) in muscle and/or nerve in the stomach are unknown.[36] Congenital myotonic dystrophy may also affect gut smooth muscle and result in gastroparesis.[37]

Duchenne's Muscular Dystrophy

Gastrointestinal tract involvement, including gastroparesis, has been reported in patients with variants of the muscular dystrophies.[38]

Mitochondrial Myopathy

A case report of pseudo-obstruction and gastric stasis was reported in a patient with ophthalmoplegia, hearing loss, and generalized muscle atrophy.[39]

Myasthenia Gravis

Gastroparesis has been reported in myasthenia gravis in the context of an associated auto-immune autonomic neuropathy.[40]

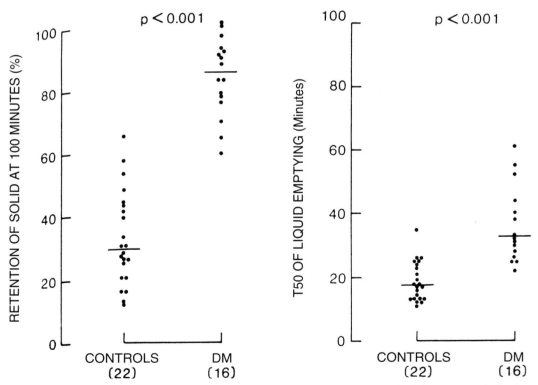

Figure 10.2. Patients with dystrophia myotonica (DM) have increased retention of solid foods in the stomach after ingestion of a standard meal and delayed gastric emptying of liquids compared with healthy control subjects. (Reproduced with permission from Horowitz M, Maddox A, Maddren GJ, et al. Gastric and esophageal emptying in dystrophia myotonica. Effect of metoclopramide. Gastroenterology 1987;92:570–577.)

EXTRINSIC NERVE DISORDERS AFFECTING GASTRIC MOTILITY

Acute Peripheral Neuropathies

Acute peripheral neuropathies from viral infections may result in nausea, vomiting, and gastroparesis. Norwalk virus has been associated with acute gastroparesis.[41] Guillain-Barré syndrome,[42] infections with herpes zoster, and Epstein-Barr viruses have been associated with gastrointestinal motility disturbances. Chronic gastroparesis following viral gastroenteritis is a clinical syndrome which may or may not resolve after many months.[43,44] Instances of gastroparesis, apparently of inflammatory origin, have also been reported.[45]

Few formal motility studies in patients with extrinsic nerve disorders have been carried out, and the level of intrinsic or extrinsic neural or muscular injury to the gastrointestinal tract is unknown.

Chronic Peripheral Neuropathies

Chronic Peripheral Neuropathy

Chronic peripheral neuropathies, resulting in gastroparesis, are most commonly seen in patients with diabetes mellitus, renal insufficiency,[46] and amyloidosis. Whether gastric dysfunction is secondary to neural damage, due to vagal nerve injury, or related to muscular degeneration/abnormal metabolism, is not clear. Symptoms attributable to gastric dysfunction are common in diabetes, though their relationship with gastric emptying rate may not always be as one would expect.[47] Decreased postprandial contractions in the antrum and duodenum of patients with diabetic gastroparesis have been recorded.[48] Other causes of diabetic gastroparesis are pylorospasm[23] and gastric dysrhythmias.[19,49] Gastric dysrhythmias predict the presence of gastroparesis in diabetic patients,[49] and correction of dysrhythmias is associated with significant improvement in symptoms, but minimal improvement in the rate of gastric emptying[19] (Figure 10.3).

Paraneoplastic Neuropathy

In one series, six of seven patients with lung cancer had gastroparesis.[24] Myenteric neurons showed degenerative changes and lymphocytic infiltrates. Cardiovagal and sympathetic dysfunction have been identified in patients with paraneoplastic syndromes and gastrointestinal neuromuscular dysfunction.[50] In some, specific anti-neuronal antibodies may be detected.[51]

Drug-Induced Neuropathy

Vincristine affects extrinsic and autonomic nerves and possibly the intrinsic nerves of the gut.[52] Nicotine,[53] morphine,[54] and levodopa[55] also decrease gastric emptying.

Neurofibromatosis

Patients with neurofibromatosis have a 10% incidence of neurofibromas in the gut, which may cause obstruction.[56] Neuropathy of the myenteric neurons, and possibly

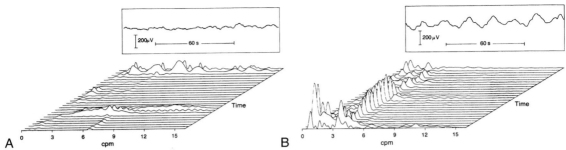

Figure 10.3. Gastric myoelectrical activity (electrogastrogram or EGG) recorded from a diabetic patient with gastroparesis. **A.** The tracing shows a "flatline" gastric dysrhythmia recorded with surface electrodes. The running spectral plot represents approximately 60 minutes of the EGG signal. No peaks are present at the normal 3 cpm gastric rhythm, but several peaks at 6 cpm (a tachygastria) are seen. **B.** Treatment with domperidone, a peripheral dopamine receptor antagonist, was associated with a restoration of normal 3 cpm EGG activity as shown in the tracing. The running spectral analysis shows many peaks at the normal 3 cpm rhythm. The patient's symptoms of nausea resolved during treatment with domperidone.

the extrinsic nerves, have been reported in patients with neurofibromatosis; not surprisingly, instances of gastroparesis have been reported.[57]

Chronic Autonomic Neuropathy with Neuronal Intranuclear Inclusions

3 to 10 micrometer intranuclear inclusions are found in the myenteric plexus and other areas of the nervous system.[58] Patients present with gut dysmotility and autonomic dysfunction of eyes, sweat glands, and heart.

Post-Vagotomy Syndromes

Vagotomy, whether deliberate or inadvertent, may be a consequence of a wide variety of surgical procedures in the upper abdomen or mediastinum, including peptic ulcer surgery, fundoplication, esophagectomy, and cardiac transplantation.[59]

AUTONOMIC NERVOUS SYSTEM DEGENERATIONS

Idiopathic Orthostatic Hypotension

Postprandial antral hypomotility has been described in a patient with idiopathic orthostatic hypotension, but the level of neural impairment is unknown.[60]

Pandysautonomias

Preganglionic or postganglionic lesions in the parasympathetic or sympathetic nervous systems may result in GI dysfunction, including gastroparesis in patients with functional dyspepsia.[61,62] Cholinergic dysfunction may be selectively present. Familial dysautonomia is associated with gastrointestinal symptoms such as dysphagia, vomiting, and constipation.[63]

Failure of Muscarinic Cholinergic Receptors

In a well reported patient with gastroparesis and small bowel pseudoobstruction, denervation hypersensitivity to cholinergic agonist and anticholinesterase drugs was found, indicating the possibility of abnormal muscarinic receptors on the gastrointestinal smooth muscle itself.[64]

SPINAL CORD DISORDERS AFFECTING GASTRIC MOTILITY

Acute Spinal Cord Injuries

Gastroparesis is usually transitory after spinal cord injuries, and responds to metoclopramide, suggesting a neuronal rather than muscular basis.[65] Refractory cases have been reported,[66] and severe gastric dilatation may occasionally occur. Ileus may be present as well; indeed, colonic and rectal motility abnormalities are more common than gastric motor dysfunction after cord injuries, due to a loss of central control of pelvic parasympathetic nerve function.

Multiple Sclerosis

Similar to spinal cord injuries, motor dysfunction of colon and rectum are more frequent than gastric dysfunction in patients with multiple sclerosis.[67] Constipation and urinary bladder problems also are frequent symptoms.

CENTRAL NERVOUS SYSTEM DISORDERS AFFECTING GASTRIC MOTILITY

Epilepsy

Nausea, bloating, and abdominal pain may be related to visceral autonomic epilepsy (with or without alteration in consciousness).[68] In one report, electroencephalographic abnormalities and neurologic symptoms were found in patients with abdominal pain, nausea, and bloating.[69] Symptoms resolved with anticonvulsants. The relationships between seizure activity and gastrointestinal neural or muscular dysfunction have not been documented. Complex partial seizures may present primarily with nausea and vomiting.

Migraines

Migraine headache and nausea and vomiting are clearly associated, but the gastric neuromuscular correlates in migraine are unknown. Cyclic vomiting syndrome is characterized by severe, intermittent nausea and vomiting with gastric dysrhythmias and a high incidence of migraine. Between episodes the patient is symptom-free.[70]

Extrapyramidal Diseases

Patients with Parkinson's disease may have delayed gastric emptying, although the anatomic level of the abnormality is unknown. Emptying delay may be exacerbated by treatment with levodopa[54]; intolerance to levodopa may relate to underlying gastroparesis.

Brainstem Lesions

Brainstem tumors, arteriovenous malformations, syringomyelia or ischemic events that affect the area postrema, tractus solitarius, or motor nucleus of the vagus may all cause abnormalities of the upper gut motility.[71]

Increased Intracranial Pressure

Increased intracranial pressure from tumors, strokes, or infections is associated with nausea and vomiting. The gastrointestinal mechanisms are unknown, but in animal experiments, increased intracranial pressure resulted in immediate suppression of antral contractions[72] (Figure 10.4).

Stress

The stress of acute vestibular stimulation results in decreased postprandial antral contractions and delays in gastric emptying.[73] These effects may be mediated in part by release of plasma norepinephrine and beta-endorphin.[74] The cold pressor test

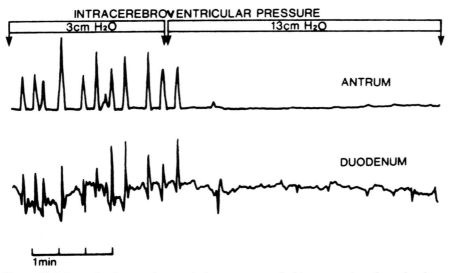

Figure 10.4. Increasing intracerebroventricular pressure resulted in suppression of antral and duodenal contractions in the conscious rabbit. (Reproduced with permission from Garrick T, Mulvihill S, Buack S, et al. Intracerebroventricular pressure inhibits gastric antral and duodenal contractility but not acid secretion in conscious rabbits. Gastroenterology 1988;95:26–31.)

increases sympathetic nervous system outflow, decreases the amplitude of 3 cpm gastric myoelectrical activity,[75] decreases the number of antral and propagated antro-duodenal pressure waves, and slows gastric emptying in healthy subjects[76] (Figure 10.5).

In patients with functional dyspepsia, stressful TENS stimulation did not unmask any autonomic nervous system dysfunction as measured by blood pressure, skin conductance, and plasma catecholamines and beta-endorphin levels.[22] Heterogeneous disorders of vagal and sympathetic nervous systems were found in other patients with functional dyspepsia, with or without abnormal gastric or small bowel motility. Thus, some patients with functional dyspepsia and normal transit studies may have disturbances in afferent nerve function.[77]

Motion Sickness

Motion can be a stressful situation in which a variety of symptoms develop: headache, sweating, nausea, and vomiting. Vection or illusory self-motion has been used to study gastric myoelectrical activity during the development of nausea. These studies have shown that the central nervous system responses to the neurosensory mismatch of vection begin with disruption of normal 3 cpm gastric myoelectrical activity, as measured with surface electrodes.[78,79] The electrogastrograms or EGGs show a shift in rhythm to tachyarrhythmias—chaotic, irregular rhythms from 3.75 to 10.0 cpm. The onset of gastric dysrhythmias occurs approximately

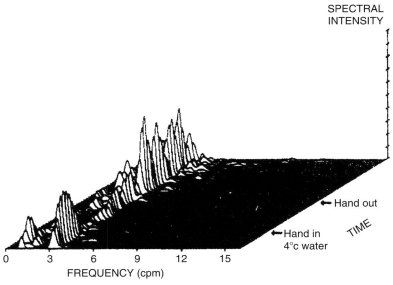

Figure 10.5. Normal 3 cpm gastric myoelectrical activity (shown by the peaks at 3 cpm) is suppressed when the subject's hand is plunged into 4°C ice water, a painful stimulus that activates the sympathetic nervous system. Normal 3 cpm peaks return when the hand is removed from the water. Spectral intensity indicates the power in the various frequencies. (Reproduced with permission from Stern RM, Hu S, Koch KL. Effects of cold stress on gastric myoelectrical activity. J Gastrointest Motil 1991;3:225–228.)

3 minutes before the subjects first report the symptom of nausea. The onset of nausea occurs during the time when plasma vasopressin levels increase significantly.[80,81] It is postulated that the gastric dysrhythmias stimulate brainstem and hypothalamic vasopressinergic neural pathways, resulting in the outpouring of plasma vasopressin (Figure 10.6).

Electroencephalographic (EEG) changes in the delta and theta bands during motion sickness resemble EEG changes seen during partial seizures.[82] Furthermore, phenytoin protects against motion sickness symptoms in the laboratory and in field studies.[83]

Emotion

The effect of emotion on gastrointestinal motility has interested many researchers over the years. The underlying neurophysiology of emotion remains unclear and undeveloped. The famous subject, Tom with the fistulated stomach, exhibited decreased gastric motility when he was fearful, and had increased gastric contractility when he was angry.[84] We observed that sham feeding usually increased the amplitude of 3 cpm EGG waves, but the subjects who reported that the thought of chewing and spitting the hot dog test meal was "disgusting" showed suppression of the normal 3 cpm EGG signal[85] (Figure 10.7). The neurohormonal physiology of emotion-gastric motility changes are fascinating but infrequently studied.

FUTURE DIRECTIONS AND IMPLICATIONS

Gastroenterologists should cultivate an increased awareness of the neurological and neuromuscular basis of normal gastrointestinal function. A better understanding of the mechanism(s) of visceral perception will help us to appreciate the origins of gastrointestinal symptoms. Loss of enteric neuron, ICC, or smooth muscle activity may cause dysfunction of the neuromuscular activity of the stomach, and stimulate afferent nerve activity that ultimately is perceived as noxious sensations or symptoms. Abnormalities in afferent neurons, spinal cord pathways, or central nervous system pathways may independently play a role in gastrointestinal symptoms. Gastric neuromuscular disorders truly require gastroenterologists to think increasingly as "neurogastroenterologists." Many poorly understood functional GI symptoms may relate more to altered neuromuscular activity and sensation, rather than structural abnormalities such as an erosion or ulcer.

Gastroenterologists also should increase their awareness of neurological disorders that present with nausea, vomiting, or gastric dysfunction in patients we see in the hospital or office. Fortunately, most of these patients have neurological signs, but subtle or variant presentations of brain tumors, arteriovenous malformations, epilepsy, Parkinson's disease, or multiple sclerosis require astute consideration of a neurological basis for symptoms of gastric neuromuscular dysfunction.

Neurologists should also cultivate an increase in awareness of gastrointestinal symptoms and an interest in the study of gastrointestinal pathophysiology in a variety of neurological disorders. Increased clinical and research interactions between neurologists and gastroenterologists will hopefully lead to a better understanding of the pathophysiology of gut-brain and brain-gut interactions, and to better therapies for GI symptoms in patients with gastric and neurological disorders.

63. Christie DL, Knauss TA. Gastrointestinal manifestations of "acquired dysautonomic" syndrome. J Pediatrics 1979;94:625–628.

64. Bannister R, Hoyes AD. Generalized smooth-muscle disease with defective muscarinic-receptor function. Br Med J 1981;282:1015–1018.

65. Segal JL, Milne N, Brunnemann SR, Lyons KP. Metoclopramide-induced normalization of impaired gastric emptying in spinal cord injury. Am J Gastroenterol 1987;82:1143–1148.

66. Clanton LJ Jr, Bender J. Refractory spinal cord injury induced gastroparesis: resolution with erythromycin lactobionate, a case report. J Spinal Cord Med 1999;22:236–238.

67. Hinds JP, Eidelman EH, Wald A. Prevalence of bowel dysfunction in multiple sclerosis. A population survey. Gastroenterology 1990;98:1538–1542.

68. Mitchell WG, Grenwood RS, Messenheimer JA. Abdominal epilepsy: cyclic vomiting as the major symptom of simple partial seizures. Arch Neurol 1983;40:251–252.

69. Peppercorn MA, Herzog AG. The spectrum of abdominal epilepsy in adults. Am J Gastroenterol 1989;84:1294–1296.

70. Fleisher DR. The cyclic vomiting system described. J Pediatr Gastroenterol Nutr 1995; 21(suppl. 1):S1–S5.

71. Wood JR, Camilleri M, Low PA, Malagelada JR. Brainstem tumor presenting as an upper gut motility disorder. Gastroenterology 1985;89:1411–1414.

72. Garrick T, Mulvihill S, Buack S, et al. Intracerebroventricular pressure inhibits gastric antral and duodenal contractility but not acid secretion in conscious rabbits. Gastroenterology 1988;95:26–31.

73. Thompson DG, Richelson E, Malagelada JR. Perturbation of gastric emptying and duodenal motility through the central nervous system. Gastroenterology 1982;83:1200–1206.

74. Stanghellini V, Malagelada JR, Zinsmeister AR, et al. Stress-induced gastroduodenal motor disturbances in humans. Possible humoral mechanisms. Gastroenterology 1983;85:83–91.

75. Stern RM, Hu S, Koch KL. Effects of cold stress on gastric myoelectrical activity. J Gastrointest Motil 1991;3:225–228.

76. Fone DR, Horowitz M, Maddox A, et al. Gastroduodenal motility during the delayed gastric emptying induced by cold stress. Gastroenterology 1990;98:1155–1161.

77. Greydanus MP, Vassallo M, Camilleri M, et al. Neurohormonal factors in functional dyspepsia: insights on pathophysiological mechanisms. Gastroenterology 1991;100:1311–1318.

78. Stern RM, Koch KL, Leibowitz HW, et al. Tachygastria and motion sickness. Aviat Space Environ Med 1985;56:1074–1077.

79. Stern RM, Koch KL, Stewart WR, Lindblad LM. Spectral analysis of tachygastria recorded during motion sickness. Gastroenterology 1987;92:92–97.

80. Koch KL, Summy-Long J, Bingaman S, et al. Vasopressin and oxytocin responses to illusory self-motion and nausea in man. J Clin Endocrinol Metab 1990;71:1269–1275.

81. Xu L, Koch KL, Summy-Long J, et al. Neurohormonal and gastric myoelectrical responses to vection in healthy Chinese subjects. Am J Physiol 1993;265:E578–E584.

82. Chelen WE, Kabrisky M, Rogers SK. Spectral analysis of the electro-encephalographic response to motion sickness. Aviat Space Environ Med 1993;64:24–29.

83. Woodard D, Knox G, Myers KJ, et al. Phenytoin as a counter measure for motion sickness in NASA maritime operations. Aviat Space Environ Med 1993;64:363–366.

84. Wolf S, Wolff HG. Human Gastric Function. New York: Oxford University Press, 1943;

85. Stern RM, Crawford HE, Stewart WR, et al. Sham feeding. Cephalic-vagal influences on gastric myoelectrical activity. J Gastrointest Motil 1991;3:225–228.

Chapter 11
Pseudo-Obstruction of the Small Bowel

G. Nicholas Verne and Charles A. Sninsky

Intestinal pseudo-obstruction is a symptom complex that is the result of abnormal intestinal motility and propulsion. Classically, it is characterized by recurrent symptoms and signs of intestinal obstruction without evidence of mechanical obstruction of the intestinal lumen.[1–8] Intestinal pseudo-obstruction may be acute or transient, or more commonly chronic and recurrent. Chronic intestinal pseudo-obstruction (CIP) is usually associated with diffuse systemic diseases such as scleroderma, myopathies, and neuropathies. More specifically, secondary causes of intestinal pseudo-obstruction can be categorized as disorders of the smooth muscle, myenteric plexus, and/or extra-intestinal nervous system. Chronic idiopathic intestinal pseudo-obstruction is the term used to describe pseudo-obstruction in which there is no obvious identifiable extra-intestinal cause. This review of intestinal pseudo-obstruction will focus on chronic or recurrent causes of pseudo-obstruction of the small bowel.

ETIOLOGY/PATHOGENESIS

Neurologic Diseases

Small bowel motility abnormalities have been described in a host of neurologic disorders (Table 11.1).[9] It is difficult to distinguish neuropathic disorders of the intrinsic (enteric) nervous system from those of the extrinsic nervous system, since most of the available diagnostic technology evaluates motor function of the intestine only.[10] Autonomic testing and careful evaluation of the extrinsic nervous system may be helpful in separating intrinsic from extrinsic nervous system disease.

Parkinson's Disease

Parkinson's disease may cause a variety of motility abnormalities as a result of a generalized extra-pyramidal motor disorder.[11–13] Constipation is perhaps the most common complaint. Gastroparesis is also commonly seen and may be further exacerbated by the effect of levodopa on inhibitory dopaminergic receptors.[14,15] The small bowel is commonly dilated in Parkinson's disease, as is the colon.[16,17]

Table 11.1. Etiology of Chronic Intestinal Pseudo-Obstruction

Neurologic diseases	Anatomical abnormalities
Parkinson's disease	Surgical changes
Postviral (herpes, varicella zoster,	Diverticulosis
Epstein-Barr)	Drugs
Brainstem strokes and neoplasms	Antiparkinsonian medications
Orthostatic hypotension syndromes	Opiates
Spinal cord trauma	Vinca alkaloids
Pandysautonomia	Isoniazid
Smooth muscle disorders	Tricyclic antidepressants
Collagen vascular diseases	Alpha$_2$ adrenergic agonists
Scleroderma	Phenothiazines
Polymyositis/dermatomyositis	Myenteric plexus disorders
Amyloidosis	Familial visceral neuropathies
Visceral myopathies	Developmental abnormalities
Muscular dystrophy	Sporadic visceral neuropathies
Diffuse lymphoid infiltration	Miscellaneous
Endocrine and metabolic disorders	Celiac sprue
Diabetes mellitus	Ceroidosis
Hypothyroidism	Radiation enteritis
Pheochromocytoma	
Hypoparathyroidism	
Acute intermittent porphyria	

The small bowel hypomotility can exacerbate constipation further in these patients. Care needs to be used in giving anticholinergic medications and dopamine agonists to patients with Parkinson's disease, as both constipation and intestinal pseudo-obstruction may be exacerbated.

Postviral (Herpes, Varicella Zoster, Epstein-Barr)

Herpes virus, Epstein-Barr virus, and varicella zoster virus have been implicated in leading to either extrinsic or intrinsic neuropathic changes in the gut.[18–20] Patients typically present with abdominal pain, bloating, and constipation that can be temporary or persist long after the acute disease has passed. Autonomic testing in patients following mononucleosis may reveal generalized involvement of sympathetic, cholinergic, and post-ganglionic parasympathetic nerves.[19,21] In herpes zoster, the inflammatory skin lesions are sometimes accompanied by intestinal motility disturbances in areas of the gut innervated by the corresponding nerve roots affecting the skin.[18] There is also a suggestion, based on both experimental animal studies and clinical observations in man, that cytomegalovirus (CMV) may also induce ileus via an effect on the enteric nervous system.[20]

Brainstem Strokes and Neoplasms

Brainstem strokes have been implicated in cases of colonic and small intestinal pseudo-obstruction.[10,22] In addition, neoplastic lesions of the brainstem can cause similar motor dysfunction in the gut.[23] A patient with a medullary glioma has been described presenting with intestinal pseudo-obstruction, manifesting as anorexia, nausea, and vomiting, without any focal neurologic findings on examination.[24] Gastrointestinal manometry revealed simultaneous activity fronts and post-prandial hypomotility. This presentation of intestinal pseudo-obstruction supports the importance of scintigraphic and manometric evaluation in patients with unexplained nausea and vomiting. A full evaluation is often warranted before the patient is considered to have idiopathic pseudo-obstruction. Anatomically, brainstem nuclei in the nucleus ambiguous, dorsal motor nucleus of the vagus, and in the medullary reticular formation may modulate upper gastrointestinal motility.[25–27]

Orthostatic Hypotension Syndromes

Neurogenic orthostatic hypotension syndromes have been described in which there is visceral denervation that results in urinary tract and gastrointestinal abnormalities. Gastrointestinal manometry may reveal a reduction of activity fronts of the migrating motor complex, lack of antral activity, uncoordinated fed and fasting antral activity, and non-propagated bursts of activity.[28] The small bowel motility abnormalities seen are secondary to the underlying autonomic dysfunction.

Spinal Cord Trauma

Spinal cord injury may cause significant effects on lower gastrointestinal motility, resulting in colonic and anorectal dysfunction.[29,30] Upper gastrointestinal motor disorders may occur; however, they are much less common. If the cervical cord is interrupted above T_5—T_{10}, sympathetic outflow to the upper gastrointestinal tract is disrupted, leading to gastroparesis and abnormal antroduodenal motility.[31] Gastroparesis and prolonged small bowel ileus following spinal cord transection have been reported to respond to metoclopramide.[32,33] Since there is no end organ dysfunction, as in diabetes mellitus, chronic sympathetic denervation of the small bowel and stomach most likely accounts for the motility abnormalities seen.[34]

Pandysautonomia

Pandysautonomia is a disorder characterized by severe parasympathetic and sympathetic dysfunction, with usually complete sparing of sensory and somatic motor function.[35] Patients may typically present with recurrent vomiting, dysphagia, diarrhea, or constipation.[36] The esophagus, stomach, and small bowel can be involved, and abnormal proximal small bowel motility and antral hypomotility have been reported.[35]

Smooth Muscle Disorders

Collagen Vascular Disease

Scleroderma.   Scleroderma is a systemic collagen vascular disease characterized by increased collagen synthesis and deposition in the skin and internal organs. Gastrointestinal involvement in scleroderma is very common, and over 50% of patients will have serious motor dysfunction.[37,38] Abnormalities of the rectum, colon, small intestine, stomach, and esophagus have been described. Small bowel involvement is very common, and patients classically present with dilated bowel, intestinal stasis, bacterial overgrowth, diarrhea, and/or steatorrhea (Figure 11.1). Small bowel manometry will typically reveal abnormal postcibal motility in addition to decreased inter-digestive motor activity.[39,40] Although the specific

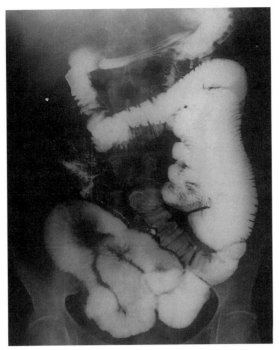

Figure 11.1. Radiological features of scleroderma. Small bowel barium x-ray demonstrating dilated small bowel loops and typical "stacked-coin" appearance of the duodenal and jejunal folds.

pathogenetic mechanism is unknown, it is believed that, early in the course of the disease, a neuropathy occurs, followed later by myopathy as the smooth muscles are infiltrated with fibrous tissue.[40] Cohen and colleagues have shown that a primary neurogenic defect occurs in the lower esophageal sphincter in scleroderma, since an intact response is present after testing with edrophonium, gastrin, and methacholine.[41] Intrinsic cholinergic pathways may also be impaired.[42] An antimyenteric neuronal antibody has been described in the sera of some patients with scleroderma that may be instrumental in neuropathic-based dysmotility in scleroderma.[43]

Polymyositis/Dermatomyositis.   Polymyositis and dermatomyositis may involve the entire gastrointestinal tract. Patients may typically present with abdominal pain, dysphagia, and constipation.[44] In addition to delayed gastric emptying, these patients may also have small bowel motility abnormalities reflected as megaduodenum and prolonged small bowel transit time.[44,45] The esophagus is most commonly involved, and many patients may develop dysphagia secondary to a delay in esophageal transit.[45,46] A thorough gastrointestinal tract examination is warranted in all patients, as approximately one-third will be found to have a gastrointestinal tumor.[47]

Amyloidosis

The gastrointestinal tract is frequently involved in systemic amyloidosis, resulting in altered gastrointestinal motility.[48] The amyloid deposits may lead to malabsorption, mucosal lesions, intestinal ischemia, perforation, and hemorrhage. Intestinal pseudo-obstruction can occur in amyloidosis, leading to massively dilated small bowel that leads to obstructive symptoms.[49] Patients with systemic amyloidosis may present with a picture similar to scleroderma, in which initially they may have mild symptoms that progress as the disease advances and more extensive infiltration of muscle layers occurs. It is still not fully clear whether the motility dysfunction is secondary to the effects of amyloid on the autonomic nervous system or on the smooth muscle.[48] Gastrointestinal motility abnormalities have also been described in mitochondrial neurogastrointestinal encephalomyopathy.[50]

Visceral Myopathy

Visceral myopathies are relatively rare disorders of the intestinal smooth muscle that may occur sporadically, congenitally, or may be familial. All three types of visceral myopathies are characterized by vacuolar degeneration and fibrosis of the muscularis propria.[51–54] Smooth muscle of the bladder, ureters, iris, and uterus may also be affected.[51–53,55,56] This is in contrast to other smooth muscle disorders that do not cause vacuolar degeneration, but are characterized by progressive fibrosis and muscle atrophy, such as scleroderma.[57,58] The disease severity and extent of involvement varies. Some patients may present initially with recurrent urinary tract infections reflective of bladder dysfunction well before gastrointestinal symptoms develop.

Muscular Dystrophy

Progressive muscular dystrophy may be complicated by intestinal pseudo-obstruction with dilated loops of small bowel and recurrent attacks of nausea, vomiting, and abdominal distention.[59] Smooth muscle fibrosis is observed along the entire gastrointestinal tract that is very similar to that observed in scleroderma. Motility abnormalities have been described throughout the gastrointestinal tract from the anus to the pharynx.[60–65]

Diffuse Lymphoid Infiltration

Diffuse lymphoid infiltration is a rare cause of intestinal pseudo-obstruction in which a widespread lymphoid infiltrate in the myenteric plexus, lamina propria, and muscularis propria occurs.[66] Small bowel peroral and full-thickness biopsies reveal sparse crypts and flat intestinal mucosa.[67] The lymphoid proliferation is polyclonal and is similar to the pattern of benign lymphoplasmacytic intestinal infiltrate seen in association with diarrhea and malabsorption, and reported in third world countries and Europe.[66]

Endocrine and Metabolic Disorders

Diabetes Mellitus

Diabetic autonomic neuropathy involving the gastrointestinal tract is very common and up to 75% of diabetics may experience one or more gastrointestinal symptoms, including constipation, abdominal pain, nausea, vomiting, dysphagia, diarrhea, and fecal incontinence.[68–71] Even though constipation is the most frequent gastrointestinal symptom in diabetics, gastroparesis has received more attention. Patients with diabetic gastroparesis have markedly reduced Phase II and Phase III activity in the stomach.[72] The small bowel is also frequently involved in diabetic gastroparesis, and abnormal gastrointestinal motility has been reported with reduced or non-propagated bursts of pressure activity.[73] Pyloric dysfunction ("pylorospasm") has also been implicated in patients with diabetes mellitus and may further contribute to recurrent nausea and vomiting[74]; others have failed to confirm this finding.[71]

Hypothyroidism

Hypothyroidism is a relatively rare cause of intestinal pseudo-obstruction that should be considered when no other cause is apparent.[75] If myxedema is severe, paralytic ileus may develop and surgical intervention would not be warranted.[76] The importance of recognizing hypothyroidism lies in the fact that myxedema ileus can be completely reversed with thyroid hormone administration.[77]

Pheochromocytoma

Intestinal pseudo-obstruction is a rare manifestation of pheochromocytoma.[78,79] The etiology is most likely related to high levels of catecholamines that cause relaxation of intestinal smooth muscle.[80] Other rare causes of intestinal pseudo-obstruction include hypoparathyroidism and acute intermittent porphyria.[81,82]

Anatomical Abnormalities

Surgical Changes

Surgery of the gastrointestinal tract is a common cause of altered intestinal motility. Bezoar formation is frequently seen in patients who have undergone various small bowel and gastric resections. Abdominal pain, nausea, and vomiting may be seen in the Roux-en-Y syndrome where the Roux limb acts as a functional obstruction.[83]

Diverticulosis

Intestinal pseudo-obstruction may be a manifestation of jejunal diverticulosis that can be associated with abnormalities of the myenteric plexus or smooth muscle.[84] Jejunal diverticulosis may also present as an early manifestation of scleroderma. These patients may have limited progressive systemic sclerosis of the gastrointestinal tract, producing localized areas of weakness in the muscle with protrusion of the entire wall, or uncoordinated spastic motility resulting in protrusion of the submucosa and mucosa through gaps in the muscular wall created by the entry of blood vessels along the mesenteric wall.[84] It is the abnormal motility that produces symptoms, not the diverticula themselves. The diverticula may, however, lead to intestinal stasis and bacterial overgrowth that may contribute to abdominal distention and pain.

Drugs

There are several pharmacological agents that may promote the development of intestinal pseudo-obstruction.

Anti-parkinsonian Medications

Anti-parkinsonian medications are perhaps the most well known pharmacologic cause. Care is needed when administering dopamine agonists and anticholinergic medications to Parkinson's patients.[14,15]

Opiates

The "narcotic bowel syndrome" has been described in some patients who take large doses of opiates for pain relief.[85] These patients typically present with increasing abdominal pain, nausea, intermittent vomiting, and weight loss. There is radiographic evidence of ileus and large amounts of stool in the colon.

Vinca Alkaloids

The vinca alkaloids are another group of pharmacological agents that may affect the autonomic and peripheral nervous systems, leading to intestinal pseudo-obstruction. Vincristine is the most well known of these medications, and our laboratory has reported the effects of vincristine on myoelectric recordings in the rat.[86]

Isoniazid

Isoniazid is another drug which can lead to intestinal pseudo-obstruction by damaging the myenteric plexus.[87]

Other Drugs

Other drugs that have been implicated in producing intestinal pseudo-obstruction include tricyclic anti-depressants, alpha-adrenergic agonists, and phenothiazines.

Myenteric Plexus Disorders

Myenteric plexus disorders that may lead to intestinal pseudo-obstruction include the familial visceral neuropathies, developmental abnormalities, and the sporadic visceral neuropathies.

Familial Visceral Neuropathies

Familial visceral neuropathy is one subset of myenteric plexus abnormalities that include a number of different gastrointestinal disorders.[88–91] The most common of these is neuronal intranuclear inclusion disease, in which neurons have intranuclear inclusions both in the submucosa and myenteric plexus.[92–94]

Developmental Abnormalities

Developmental abnormalities of the myenteric plexus may also occur, usually in early childhood or infancy, and include neuronal intestinal dysplasia, aganglionosis, and maturational arrest.[95] Neuronal intestinal dysplasia is characterized by disorganization of the myenteric plexus. Structural changes include increased acetylcholinesterase activity, formation of giant ganglia, and hyperplasia of the myenteric plexus.[96] The disease may occur as a clinical entity in itself, and frequently gives rise to signs and symptoms similar to that of Hirschsprung's disease. It may also occur in a disseminated form and involve the entire gastrointestinal tract.[96] Neurofibromas or ganglionomas within the enteric nervous system may also be seen in neuronal intestinal dysplasia.[97] Patients with maturational arrest may have mental developmental delays or mental retardation, and the myenteric plexus contains a deficient number of neurons.[98,99] The most severe developmental abnormality of the myenteric plexus that usually affects the colon and most of the small bowel is aganglionosis.[100] This condition is most frequently manifest as Hirschsprung's disease, in which the defective formation of ganglion cells is limited to the colon.

Sporadic Visceral Neuropathies

The sporadic visceral neuropathies encompass a number of degenerative disorders of the myenteric plexus and submucosal plexus, such as paraneoplastic visceral neuropathy, inflammatory visceral neuropathy, and inflammatory axonopathy. Sporadic visceral neuropathies are best visualized with silver staining, and one may see degeneration in neurons, dendrites, and axons that may be associated with inflammatory changes.[7,67] Glial scar formation may actually replace neurons if the inflammation and destruction is severe enough. Paraneoplastic visceral neuropathy is characterized by inflammatory changes in the myenteric plexus, and is usually secondary to small cell carcinoma of the lung,[101–105] possibly due to hormones or antibodies produced by the tumor that affect or damage the myenteric plexus.[103,104] This syndrome may feature loss of interstitial cells of Cajal within the gut wall.[106] Symptoms of constipation, gastroparesis, intestinal pseudo-obstruction, and central nervous system dysfunction can actually precede the diagnosis or presentation of lung cancer. Therefore, patients with idiopathic intestinal pseudo-obstruction and significant weight loss and wasting, without an obvious cause, should be carefully evaluated to rule out any evidence of an underlying lung cancer or other malignancy.[101] To complicate matters further, a similar syndrome, including the presence of circulating autoantibodies directed against enteric neurons, has been described in the absence of neoplasia.[107]

Inflammatory visceral neuropathies may be caused by several different types of infections. Chagas' disease may cause an inflammatory neuropathy due to a destruction of ganglion cells, either through a toxic effect of the parasite, the immune response, destruction of Schwann cells, or inflammation.[108,109] Cytomegalovirus has also been reported to cause intestinal pseudo-obstruction as a result of viral inclusions within the neurons.[110] An idiopathic inflammatory axonopathy, formerly regarded as a rare cause of visceral neuropathy, features damage limited to the axons[111]; more recent reports suggest that inflammation in relation to myenteric ganglia (ganglionitis) may be a relatively common cause of CIP in adults.[112]

With the recognition of the key roles of interstitial cells of Cajal (ICC) in pacemaking and neurotransmission in the gut, and with the development of specific morphological markers for these cells, it should come as no surprise that there have been several reports of loss of ICC in relation to a variety of manifestations of CIP.[106,113,114] Of interest, a similar loss of ICCs has been reported in relation to an intensely inflammatory condition of the bowel—Crohn's disease.[115] Whether the loss of ICCs, in CIP, is the primary event or occurs secondary to inflammation, is unclear.

Miscellaneous

Other rare causes of intestinal pseudo-obstruction include ceroidosis, celiac sprue, and radiation enteritis.[116]

DIAGNOSIS

General Aspects

The successful diagnosis of chronic intestinal pseudo-obstruction requires a thorough and comprehensive approach to the patient. A detailed history is imperative. Many patients present with a prolonged history of dysphagia, nausea, vomiting, abdominal pain, bloating, early satiety, weight loss, or constipation. There may be months to years of symptoms that suggest intermittent pseudo-obstruction. Presenting symptoms may reflect involvement of the colon, stomach, and esophagus, as well as the small bowel. Patients will often give a history of previous exploratory laparotomies for a possible obstructing lesion. In approximately 30% of patients, a family history may be elicited.[5,6]

   A detailed physical examination is also important in the initial evaluation of these patients. Many will have evidence of abdominal distention, sucussion splash, evidence of malnutrition, a distended bladder, or signs of systemic disease (e.g., scleroderma). Orthostatic hypotension or other neurologic signs may be present that indicate disease of the peripheral, central, or autonomic nervous system.[28] Since a brain stem stroke or malignancy may cause intestinal pseudo-obstruction, a computerized tomography or magnetic resonance imaging (MRI) of the brain and brainstem are important, especially if focal neurologic findings are present.[22,24] In addition to the routine neurologic examination, autonomic nervous system testing should be done in patients who have evidence of orthostatic hypotension, distended bladder, or anhydrosis.[10] Suspicion of peripheral neuropathy may best be evaluated by nerve conduction studies. Finally, systemic muscle diseases should be excluded by electromyography.

   Laboratory tests should be performed on these patients to evaluate for electrolyte abnormalities and to assess for the degree of malnutrition. Thyroid function studies are important to exclude hypothyroidism. Antinuclear antibodies should be done to rule out evidence of a systemic collagen vascular disease, such as scleroderma. Since bacterial overgrowth is very common in this group of patients, a ^{14}C D-Xylose breath test or hydrogen breath test should be done to evaluate for bacterial overgrowth. A serum creatinine phosphokinase (CPK) to look for evidence of dermatomyositis or polymyositis should be obtained, as should porphyrinogens to exclude acute intermittent porphyria. Serologic examination for Chagas' disease should be obtained if the patient has been in an endemic area.

Radiological and Scintigraphic Studies

A thorough radiologic examination of the entire gastrointestinal tract is extremely important in these patients, since involvement of other areas of the bowel would further support a diagnosis of intestinal pseudo-obstruction if no obvious underlying etiology is present (Figure 11.2). In addition to plain films of the abdomen, an upper

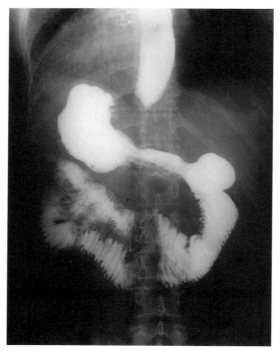

Figure 11.2. Upper GI barium study in a patient with myopathic pseudo-obstruction. Note dilated proximal duodenum (megaduodenum) and dilated esophagus with appearance suggestive of achalasia.

gastrointestinal series and small bowel follow-through to look for evidence of small bowel dilatation or obstruction is important. In general, enteroclysis is usually preferred, as this is more sensitive in evaluating for mechanical small bowel obstruction,[117] and may also provide evidence of dysmotility.[118] If mechanical obstruction cannot be ruled out by enteroclysis and the abnormalities are limited to the small intestine, then small bowel manometry and/or exploratory laparotomy or laparoscopy should be considered to rule out mechanical obstruction. With the advent of laparoscopy for gastrointestinal surgery, biopsies may be obtained from the small intestine, and both silver staining and light microscopy can be performed on the specimens.[20] Urologic imaging with intravenous pyelogram or retrograde cystogram should be considered if the patient has urinary symptoms. Dilated ureters or bladder suggest a diffuse smooth muscle disorder as may be seen in visceral myopathy.[54]

Radionucleotide gastric emptying studies should also be considered in these patients, in addition to barium studies, since delayed gastric emptying is quite common in intestinal pseudo-obstruction and may contribute significantly to the patient's symptoms. Scintigraphic transit studies of the colon and small intestine may also give important information regarding the severity and location of the motility abnormalities present.[119] Finally, since lung cancer may present with a paraneoplastic syndrome resulting in intestinal pseudo-obstruction, a chest x-ray and CT scan of the chest should also be considered, especially if the patient has no underlying etiology for the pseudo-obstruction and has considerable weight loss and wasting.[104]

Antroduodenal and Small Intestinal Manometry

Antroduodenal manometry may play an important role in both the diagnostic evaluation and determination of specific pharmacological therapy in patients with intestinal pseudo-obstruction.[120] Gastrointestinal manometry has become more widely available, but remains largely confined to referral centers. There are several proposed indications for small bowel manometry: distinguishing functional from organic intestinal disorders, gastroparesis refractory to prokinetic agents, refractory/recurrent bacterial overgrowth, and to evaluate postoperative motility.[121–123] Despite the increased availability of small bowel manometry, there are still many limitations to its use, which include the specificity of abnormal patterns and technical difficulties related to the study itself.[124,125] With the exception of the radiolabelled amberlite technique,[119] which is very limited in availability, there are few less invasive alternatives available to manometry for the patient in whom pseudo-obstruction is suspected, but has not been confirmed or excluded by other means. In the small bowel, the widely available transit studies are insufficiently sensitive and specific, and are subject to considerable problems in interpretation.

In general, small bowel manometry has been used to classify altered motility into either neuropathic or myopathic disorders/patterns. A neuropathic process characteristically will exhibit a normal amplitude of motor activity; however, this will be uncoordinated. A myopathic pattern, on the other hand, is classically characterized by either low or no pressure wave activity with little response in the fed state. One must be careful, however, in classifying abnormal intestinal motility into neuropathic versus myopathic disease processes based on motility patterns alone. There is still considerable controversy regarding this classification, and there is some preliminary evidence to suggest that there may be no difference in the patterns of motor activity between neuropathic and myopathic varieties of chronic intestinal pseudo-obstruction.[126]

Four basic manometric abnormalities have been described, in chronic intestinal pseudo-obstruction[127] (Figure 11.3). First, one may see aberrant propagation or configuration of the migrating motor complex (MMC), the dominant motor pattern of

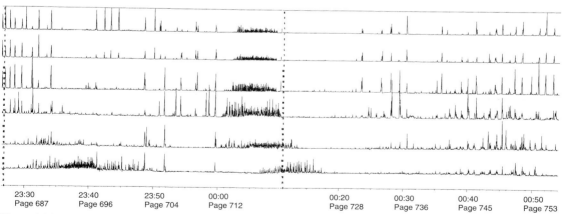

Figure 11.3. Fasting small bowel motility recording from a patient with diabetic neuropathic pseudo-obstruction demonstrating a simultaneous activity front that does not propagate normally during the fasting state *(center of trace)*, an isolated and sustained phase 3-type pressure wave activity *(lowest channel on left)*, and recurrent brief bursts of pressure wave activity *(all channels on right)*.

the fasted gut. Phase III of the MMC may fail to propagate in its usual aboral manner and may, instead, appear retrograde or simultaneous. In addition, marked tonic rises of the baseline (>30 mmHg of amplitude, > 3 minutes duration) may be observed. Another major abnormality that may be seen consists of bursts of non-propagated pressure wave activity in both the fasting and fed states that last at least two minutes, with an amplitude of greater than 20 mmHg and that occur at a frequency of 10 to 12 cycles per min (Figure 11.3). These bursts are not propagated in a normal fashion and are not followed by a normal quiescent period. Another pattern observed is sustained (> 30 min) and intense pressure wave activity that occurs in only one segment of the small intestine, while simultaneously there is either reduced or normal activity in other areas of the small intestine (Figure 11.3). The above patterns are all classically seen in the fasting state. In the fed state, one may see the inability of a meal to induce the normal fed pattern. Postcibal hypomotility in both the antrum and proximal small bowel is often observed in patients with scleroderma[40] (Figure 11.4). In addition to delineating these abnormalities of motility pattern, small bowel manometry may also be useful in differentiating mechanical obstruction from pseudo-obstruction.[128,129] In diabetes mellitus, uncoordinated antral and small bowel pressure wave activity may occur and lead to increased gastric outlet resistance and delayed gastric emptying.[73,130]

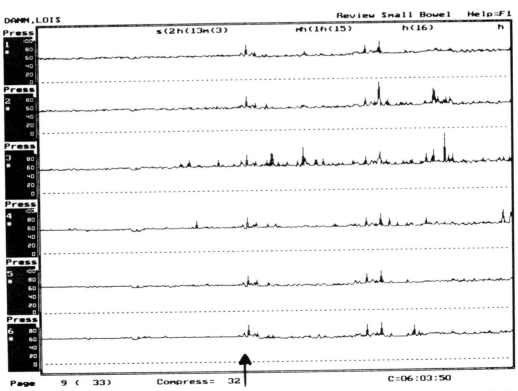

Figure 11.4. Small bowel motility recording from a patient with progressive systemic sclerosis, after a standardized meal *(indicated by arrow)*. Note the postcibal hypomotility in both the antrum (top 3 traces) and proximal small bowel *(lower 3 traces)*.

Perhaps one of the most important uses of small bowel manometry is to predict individual patient responses to specific prokinetic agents. In order to perform such a task, small bowel manometry needs to be extended from the classically-devised 5-hour study (3 hours fasting, 2 hours post prandial) to a 24-hour study. After a sufficient baseline of approximately 8 hours, prokinetic agents may be given. Our laboratory uses metoclopramide, erythromycin and, more recently, octreotide to determine individual patient response. It is important to note that varying doses of these prokinetic agents may be needed, since not all patients will respond similarly.[131]

Other Investigations

Biopsies obtained during upper gastrointestinal endoscopy in patients with chronic intestinal pseudo-obstruction may occasionally provide diagnostic information, by revealing amyloid infiltration or the histological features of celiac sprue, for example. Diseases that involve the submucosal plexus, such as amyloidosis, neuronal intestinal dysplasia, neuronal intranuclear inclusion disease, and inflammatory neuropathies, may be diagnosed with rectal biopsies.[94,95] Rarely, will full-thickness rectal biopsies add additional information, with the possible exception of the instance of visceral myopathy reported in a patient who was initially felt to have Hirschsprung's disease.[132]

TREATMENT

One of the most important considerations in the treatment of patients with chronic intestinal pseudo-obstruction is that therapy needs to be individualized to the patient. It is important to define the specific regions of the bowel affected, the severity of the symptoms, and the underlying pathophysiology of the altered motility. Unfortunately, there are few treatments which are curative, and most therapy is specifically aimed at improving the patient's symptoms and quality of life. The two major goals in these patients are, first, to restore small bowel motility and, secondly, to correct any underlying malnutrition that may be present. In patients with mild disease without evidence of malnutrition, control of symptoms and provision of reassurance are of primary importance.

Prokinetic Agents

Prokinetic agents that have been used in chronic intestinal pseudo-obstruction include metoclopramide, erythromycin, octreotide, and cisapride. In both medium and long-term treatment, cisapride appeared to be the most favorable prokinetic agent for treatment of pseudo-obstruction.[133] Cisapride acts through the release of acetylcholine from postganglionic neurons in myenteric plexus, and also appears to have 5-HT4 agonist activity and 5-HT3 antagonist activity.[134] In several placebo-controlled studies, cisapride has been shown to hasten gastric emptying in addition to accelerating small bowel transit.[135,136] Despite this improvement in small bowel transit, a 6-week trial of cisapride failed to improve symptoms significantly more than placebo.[136] Several studies have recently attempted to find criteria that may predict which patients with intestinal pseudo-obstruction will respond favorably to cisapride.[137,138] Those patients who have intestinal pseudo-obstruction and associated abdominal vagal dysfunction are less likely to have a significant response to cisapride.[138] In addition, patients who appear to have myopathic disease and have absent migrating motor complexes in the fasting state, during small bowel manometry, or who have a biopsy proven visceral myopathy, also tend not to have a significant response to cisapride.[137] Patients who have an enlarged bowel diameter typically respond poorly to cisapride. Another subset of patients who do not improve with prokinetic agents, such as cisapride, may actually have altered afferent visceral sensation as a cause of their symptoms.[139] Cisapride has been associated with rare, though potentially significant, cardiac toxicity, which is especially likely to occur in those who are on other medications which affect cisapride metabolism, or affect cardiac conduction.[140] This has led to the withdrawal of the drug from many countries, or to the imposition of severe restrictions on its prescription, and has presented both patients and physicians, alike, with a significant therapeutic dilemma: when to consider the drug in the patient with a refractory motility disorder?[141]

Among available prokinetics, few possess evidence of efficacy in CIP. Metoclopramide, for example, has been used for years to treat gastroparesis and as an anti-emetic; it appears, however, with the possible exception of a report of improvement of prolonged ileus after acute spinal cord injury,[32,142] to be ineffective in stimulating small bowel motility. We have also observed, in our laboratory, that patients with intestinal pseudo-obstruction will exhibit antral activity, but no small bowel activity, when intravenous metoclopramide is given during antroduodenal manometry.

Domperidone, available in many countries apart from the USA, has shown some promise in the treatment of gastroesophageal reflux disease and gastroparesis; its effects on small bowel motility do not appear to be significant.[143] There is, however, one case report of a patient with chronic intestinal pseudo-obstruction, secondary to neuronal dysplasia, who did respond well to domperidone 60 mg a day.[144] Erythromycin, a macrolide antibiotic, which possesses prokinetic properties by virtue of its stimulation of motilin receptors on intestinal smooth muscle, is a potent stimulant of antral motility and gastric emptying[145-147] but, again, has little effect on small intestinal propulsion.

Octreotide, a long-acting somatostatin analogue, has recently emerged as a potential prokinetic agent. An initial study of five patients with scleroderma, who had bacterial overgrowth and chronic symptoms of intestinal pseudo-obstruction, showed that octreotide in a dose of 100 micrograms given subcutaneously at night improved not only bacterial overgrowth, but also the other chronic symptoms.[148] In addition, octreotide was shown to increase the frequency of the interdigestive migrating motor complexes in the small bowel in all five patients with scleroderma. We have also shown that octreotide increases the frequency of the migrating motor complex in patients with scleroderma-associated pseudo-obstruction, but not idiopathic pseudo-obstruction.[131] It is important to note that, in our study, patients with a myopathic pattern at baseline, in the fasting state, did respond to octreotide. This is in contrast to other reports which suggest that patients with myopathic type patterns do not respond to prokinetic agents. We also found that many patients responded to lower doses of octreotide (25 to 50 micrograms) at night and that larger doses, such as 100 micrograms, tended to suppress small bowel activity. Thus, it may be important that octreotide is given only at night since our study and others have shown that antral activity is suppressed by octreotide.[131,148]

Tegaserod (Zelnorm) is currently the only available 5-HT$_4$ (serotonin) receptor agonist available for use. Tegaserod accelerates gastric emptying, increases both small bowel and colonic transit, increases the peristaltic reflex, and reduces visceral hypersensitivity.[149-151] It has received a Grade A recommendation from the American College of Gastroenterology for the treatment (6 mg po bid) of women with constipation predominant IBS.[152] Tegaserod should prove to be beneficial in patients with chronic intestinal pseudo-obstruction.[149-151]

Other Measures

In addition to augmentation of small bowel motility in chronic intestinal pseudo-obstruction, treatment of bacterial overgrowth with antibiotics is very important and may alleviate some of the symptoms such as abdominal bloating, abdominal pain, and diarrhea. Bacterial overgrowth, as a consequence of intestinal stasis, is quite common in patients with intestinal pseudo-obstruction. It has also been suggested that the abnormal bacterial flora and bacterial overgrowth may, in fact, further alter motility and cause worsening of symptoms and distention.[153] Antibiotics that may be useful include metronidazole, tetracycline, and amoxicillin, and should be given for a full 10 to 14-day course. Some patients with irreversible structural changes leading to intestinal pseudo-obstruction may actually need rotating courses of antibiotics one week out of every month, in order to keep bacterial counts suppressed.

In advanced disease, where patients have severe nutritional deficiencies, supplementation with vitamins, low fiber and low fat diet, in addition to liquid meals during periods of exacerbations, may be helpful. However, some patients may have such severe disease that even liquids are not well tolerated. These patients need to be considered for total parenteral nutrition.[154-156] Patients who require long-term total parenteral nutrition may require supplementation of trace elements in addition to vitamins.[157] Long-term parenteral nutrition may have significant morbidity and mortality associated with it, such as large vessel thrombosis and line sepsis, even though nutritional deficiencies may be improved.

The last therapeutic resort for patients with chronic intestinal pseudo-obstruction is surgery.[158] Surgery should be limited to patients who are refractory to medical therapy and have unrelenting symptoms. A focused approach to the patient's primary symptoms is needed, and a variety of surgical procedures have been used, including venting enterostomy, side-to-side duodenojejunostomy for megaduodenum, and colectomy for isolated colonic pseudo-obstruction. Small bowel transplantation[159] and the use of intestinal pacemakers are still in the experimental stages, but may play a future role in the treatment of patients who are refractory to medical therapy.[160-161]

SUMMARY

Chronic intestinal pseudo-obstruction is a symptom complex that is caused by ineffective intestinal propulsion and may be caused by a variety of different diseases, including several neurological diseases. It can present at any age, and the symptoms may include constipation, abdominal pain, abdominal distention, nausea, or diarrhea. The workup includes a comprehensive search for an underlying etiology, in addition to functional studies of the stomach, small bowel, and colon. Treatment is primarily aimed at maintaining or improving nutrition, and limiting symptoms secondary to small intestinal stasis and resulting bacterial overgrowth. Currently, there are few options available with respect to prokinetic agents. Total parenteral nutrition and surgery should be reserved for those patients who are refractory to all types of medical therapy.

REFERENCES

1. Faulk DL, Anuras S, Christensen J. Chronic intestinal pseudo-obstruction. Gastroenterology 1978;4:922–931.
2. Camilleri M, Phillips SF. Disorders of small intestinal motility. Gastroenterol Clin N Amer 1989;18:405–424.
3. Christensen J, Dent J, Malagelada JR, Wingate DL. Pseudo-obstruction. Gastroenterol Int 1990;3:107–119.
4. Colemont LJ, Camilleri M. Chronic intestinal pseudo-obstruction: diagnosis and treatment. Mayo Clin Proc 1989;64:60–70.
5. Coulie B, Camilleri M. Intestinal pseudo-obstruction. Ann Rev Med 1999;50:37–55.
6. Quigley EMM. Intestinal pseudo-obstruction. In MC Champion, WC Orr (eds), Evolving Concepts in Gastrointestinal Motility. Oxford: Blackwell Science, 1996;171–199.
7. Schuffler MD, Janak Z. Chronic idiopathic intestinal pseudo-obstruction caused by a degenerative disorder of the myenteric plexus: the use of Smith's method to define the neuropathy. Gastroenterology 1982;82:476–486.
8. Mann SD, Debinski HS, Kamm MA. Clinical characteristics of chronic intestinal pseudo-obstruction in adults. Gut 1997;41:675–681.
9. Quigley EMM. Gastrointestinal dysfunction in neurological disease. The Neurologist 1999;5:101–110.
10. Camilleri M. Disorders of gastrointestinal motility in neurologic disorders. Mayo Clin Proc 1990;65:825–846.
11. Pallis CA. Parkinsonism: natural history and clinical features. Br Med J 1971;3:683–690.
12. Quigley EMM. Gastrointestinal dysfunction in Parkinson's disease. Semin Neurol 1996; 16:245–250.
13. Edwards LL, Quigley EMM, Pfeiffer RF. Gastrointestinal dysfunction in Parkinson's disease: frequency and pathophysiology. Neurology 1992;42:726–732.
14. Berkowitz DM, McCallum RW. Interaction of levodopa and metoclopramide on gastric emptying. Clin Pharmacol Ther 1980;27:414–420.
15. Evans MA, Broe GA, Triggs EJ, et al. Gastric emptying rate and the systemic availability of levodopa in the elderly Parkinsonian patient. Neurology 1981;31:1288–1294.
16. Berenyi MR, Schwartz GS. Megasigmoid syndrome in diabetes and neurological disease: review of 13 cases. Am J Gastroenterol 1967;47:311–320.
17. Lewitan A, Nathanson LM, Slade WP Jr. Megacolon and dilatation of the small bowel in Parkinsonism. Gastroenterology 1951;17:367–374.
18. Wyburn-Mason MA. Visceral lesions in herpes zoster. Br Med J 1957;1:678–681.
19. Vassallo M, Camilleri M, Caron BL, Low PA. Gastrointestinal motor dysfunction in acquired selective cholinergic dysautonomia associated with infectious mononucleosis. Gastroenterology 1991;100:252–258.
20. Quigley EMM. Enteric neuropathology—recent advances and implications for clinical practice. The Gastroenterologist 1997;5:233–241.
21. Schuffler MD, Rohrmann CA, Chaffer RG, et al. Gastrointestinal motor dysfunction in acquired selective cholinergic dysautonomia associated with infectious mononucleosis. Gastroenterology 1991;100:252–258.
22. Reynolds BJ, Eliasson SG. Colonic pseudo-obstruction in patients with stroke. Ann Neurol 1977;1:305.
23. Quigley EMM. Gastric and small intestinal motility disorders. In LR Schiller (ed), Small Intestine; Vol. 7, M Feldman (ed), Gastroenterology and Hepatology. The Comprehensive Visual Reference. Philadelphia: Churchill Livingstone, 1997;6.2–6.20.

24. Wood JR, Camilleri M, Low PA, Malagelada JR. Brainstem tumor presenting as an upper gut motility disorder. Gastroenterology 1985;89:1411–1414.
25. Eliasion S. Activation of gastric motility from the brain stem of the cat. Acta Physiol Scand 1954;30:199–214.
26. Kalia M, Mesulam MM. Brainstem projections of sensory and motor components of the vagus complex in the cat. II. Laryngeal, tracheobronchial, pulmonary, cardiac, and gastrointestinal branches. J Comp Neurology 1980;193:467–508.
27. Pagani FD, Norman WP, Kasbekar DK, Gillis RA. Effects of stimulation of nucleus ambiguous complex on gastroduodenal function. Am J Physiol 1984;246:G253–G262.
28. Camilleri M, Malagelada JR, Stanghellini V, et al. Gastrointestinal motility disturbances in patients with orthostatic hypotension. Gastroenterology 1985;88:1852–1859.
29. Fajardo NR, Pasiliao RV, Modeste-Duncan R, et al. Decreased colonic motility in persons with chronic spinal cord injury. Am J Gastroenterol 2003;98:128–134.
30. Krogh K, Olsen N, Christensen P, et al. Colorectal transport during defecation in patients with lesions of the spinal cord. Neurogastroenterol Motil 2003;15:25–32.
31. Fealey RD, Szurzewski JA, Merritt JL, DiMagno EP. Effect of traumatic spinal cord transection on human upper gastrointestinal motility and gastric emptying. Gastroenterology 1984; 87:69–75.
32. Miller F, Fenzl TC. Prolonged ileus with acute spinal cord injury responding to metoclopramide. Paraplegia 1981;19:43–45.
33. Sagel JL, Milne V, Brunnemann SR, Lyons KP. Metoclopramide-induced normalization of impaired gastric emptying in spinal cord injury. Am J Gastroenterol 1987;82:1143–1148.
34. Fox S, Behar J. Pathogenesis of diabetic gastroparesis: a pharmacological study. Gastroenterology 1980;78:757–763.
35. Low PA, Dyck PJ, Lambert EH, et al. Acute panautonomic neuropathy. Ann Neurol 1983; 13:412–417.
36. Christie DL, Knauss TA. Gastrointestinal manifestations of "acquired dysautonomic" syndrome. J Pediatrics 1979;94:625–628.
37. Cohen S, Laufer I, Snape WJ Jr, et al. The gastrointestinal manifestations of scleroderma: Pathogenesis and management. Gastroenterology 1980;79:155–166.
38. Weston S, Thumshirn M, Wiste J, Camilleri M. Clinical and upper gastrointestinal motility features in systemic sclerosis and related disorders. Am J Gastroenterol 1998; 93:1085–1089.
39. Rees WD, Christofides ND, Bloom SR, Turnberg LA. Interdigestive motor activity in patients with systemic sclerosis. Gastroenterology 1982;83:575–580.
40. Greydanus MP, Camilleri M. Abnormal postcibal antral and small bowel motility due to neuropathy or myopathy in systemic sclerosis. Gastroenterology 1989;96:110–115.
41. Cohen S, Fisher R, Lipshultz W, et al. The pathogenesis of esophageal dysfunction in scleroderma and Raynaud's disease. J Clin Invest 1972;51:2663–2668.
42. DiMarino AJ, Carlson G, Myers A, et al. Duodenal myoelectric activity in scleroderma: abnormal responses to mechanical and hormonal stimuli. N Engl J Med 1972;289: 1220–1223.
43. Howe S, Eaker EY, Sallustio JE, et al. Antimyenteric neuronal antibodies in scleroderma. J Clin Invest 1994;94:761–770.
44. Kleckner FS. Dermatomyositis and its manifestations in the gastrointestinal tract. Am J Gastroenterol 1970;53:141–146.
45. Horowitz M, McNeil JD, Maddern GJ, et al. Abnormalities of gastric and esophageal emptying in polymyositis and dermatomyositis. Gastroenterology 1986;90:434–439.
46. DeMerieux P, Verity MA, Clements PJ, Paulus HE. Esophageal abnormalities and dysphagia in polymyositis and dermatomyositis. Arthritis Rheum 1983;26:961–968.
47. Malkinson FD, Rothman S. Changes in the gastrointestinal tract in scleroderma and after diffuse connective tissue disease. Am J Gastroenterol 1956;26:414–432.
48. Battle WM, Rubin MR, Cohen S, Snape WJ Jr. Gastrointestinal motility dysfunction in amyloidosis. N Engl J Med 1979;301:24–25.
49. Lesse DA, Wollaeger EE, Carlson HC. Intestinal pseudo-obstruction in systemic amyloidosis. Gut 1970;11:764–767.

50. Mueller LA, Camilleri M, Emslie-Smith AM. Mitochondrial neurogastrointestinal encephalomyopathy: manometric and diagnostic features. Gastroenterology 1999; 116:959–963.

51. Schuffler MD, Pope CE II. Studies of idiopathic intestinal pseudo-obstruction. Hereditary hollow visceral myopathy: family studies. Gastroenterology 1977;73:339–344.

52. Anuras S, Mitros FA, Nowak TV, et al. A familial visceral myopathy with external ophthal-moplegia and autosomal recessive transmission. Gastroenterology 1983;84:46–53.

53. Anuras S, Mitros FA, Milano A, et al. A familial visceral myopathy with dilation of the entire gastrointestinal tract. Gastroenterology 1986;90:385–390.

54. Schuffler MD, Pagon RA, Schwartz R, Bill AH. Visceral myopathy of the gastrointestinal and genito-urinary tracts in infants. Gastroenterology 1988;84:982–988.

55. Schuffler MD, Lowe MC, Bill AH. Studies of idiopathic intestinal pseudo-obstruction. I. Hereditary hollow visceral myopathy: clinical and pathological studies. Gastroenterology 1977;73:327–328.

56. Faulk DL, Anuras S, Gardner GD, et al. A familial visceral myopathy. Ann Int Med 1978;89:600–606.

57. Schuffler MD, Beegle RG. Progressive systemic sclerosis of the gastrointestinal tract and hereditary hollow visceral myopathy: two distinguishable disorders of intestinal smooth mus-cle. Gastroenterology 1979;77:664–671.

58. Jayachander J, Frank JL, Jonas MM. Isolated intestinal myopathy resembling progressive systemic sclerosis in a child. Gastroenterology 1988;95:1114–1118.

59. Leon SH, Schuffler MD, Keffler M, Rohrman CA. Chronic intestinal pseudo-obstruction as a complication of Duchenne's muscular dystrophy. Gastroenterology 1986;90:455–459.

60. Goldberg HI, Sheft DJ. Esophageal and colon changes in myotonic dystrophia myotonica. Gastroenterology 1972;63:134–139.

61. Lewis TD, Daniel EE. Gastroduodenal motility in a case of dystrophia myotonica. Gastroenterology 1981;81:145–149.

62. Swick HM, Werlin SC, Dodds WJ, Hogan WJ. Pharyngo-esophageal motor function in patients with myotonic dystrophy. Ann Neurol 1981;10:454–457.

63. Nowak TV, Anuras S, Brown BP, et al. Small intestinal motility in myotonic dystrophy patients. Gastroenterology 1984;86:808–813.

64. Hemel-Roy J, Devroede G, Arhan P, et al. Functional abnormalities of the anal sphincter in patients with myotonic dystrophy. Gastroenterology 1984;86:1469–1474.

65. Horowitz M, Maddox A, Maddern GJ, et al. Gastric and esophageal emptying in dystrophia myotonica. Gastroenterology 1987;92:570–577.

66. McDonald GB, Schuffler MD, Kudin ME, Tytgat GN. Intestinal pseudo-obstruction caused by diffuse lymphoid infiltration of the small intestine. Gastroenterology 1984;89:882–889.

67. Krishnamurthy S, Schuffler MD. Pathology of neuromuscular disorders of the small intestine and colon. Gastroenterology 1987;93:610–639.

68. Feldman M, Schiller LR. Disorders of gastrointestinal motility associated with diabetes mellitus. Ann Int Med 1983;98:378–384.

69. Camilleri M. Gastrointestinal problems in diabetes. Endocrinol Metabolism Clin N Amer 1996;25:361–378.

70. Quigley EMM. The pathophysiology of diabetic gastroenteropathy: more vague than vagal? Gastroenterology 1997;113:1790–1794.

71. Quigley EMM. Diabetic gastric and intestinal motility disorders. Resident and Staff Physicians 1999;45:9–16.

72. Malagelada JR, Rees WD, Mazzete LJ, Go VL. Gastric motor abnormalities in diabetic and post-vagotomy gastroparesis: effect of metoclopramide and bethanechol. Gastroenterology 1980;78:286–293.

73. Camilleri M, Malagelada JR. Abnormal intestinal motility in diabetics with the gastroparesis syndrome. Eur J Clin Invest 1984;14:420–427.

74. Mearin F, Camilleri M, Malagelada JR. Pyloric dysfunction in diabetics with recurrent nausea and vomiting. Gastroenterology 1986;90:1919–1925.

75. Wells I, Smith B, Hinton M. Acute ileus in myxedema. Br Med J 1977;1:211–212.

76. Hohl RD, Nixon RK. Myxedema ileus. Arch Intern Med 1965;115:145–150.

77. Abbasi AA, Douglass RC, Bissell GW, Chen Y. Myxedema ileus: A form of intestinal pseudo-obstruction. JAMA 1975;2324:181–183.

78. Turner CE. Gastrointestinal pseudo-obstruction due to pheochromocytoma. Am J Gastroenterol 1983;78:214–217.

79. Mullen JP, Cartwright RC, Tisherman SE, et al. Case report: pathogenesis and pharmacologic management of pseudo-obstruction of the bowel in pheochromocytoma. Am J Med Sci 1985;290:155–158.

80. Interlandi JW, Hundley RF, Kusselberg AG, et al.Hypercortisolism, diarrhea with steatorrhea, and massive proteinuria due to pheochromocytoma. South Med J 1985;78:879–883.

81. Clarkson B, Knowlassar OD, Horwith M, Sleisenger MH. Clinical and metabolic study of a patient with malabsorption and hypoparathyroidism. Metabolism 1960;9:1093–1106.

82. Stein JA, Tschudy DP. Acute intermittent porphyria: a clinical and biochemical study of 46 patients. Medicine 1970;49:1–16.

83. Mathias JR, Fernandez A, Sninsky C, et al. Nausea, vomiting, and abdominal pain after roux-en-Y anastomosis: motility of the jejunal limb. Gastroenterology 1985;88:101–107.

84. Krishnamurthy S, Kelly MM, Rohrmann CA, Schuffler MD. Jejunal diverticulosis: a heterogeneous disorder caused by a variety of abnormalities of smooth muscle or myenteric plexus. Gastroenterology 1983;85:538–547.

85. Rogers M, Cardu JJ. Editorial: The narcotic bowel syndrome. J Clin Gastroenterol 1987;11:132–135.

86. Sninsky CA. Vincristine alters myoelectric activity and transit of the small intestine in rats. Gastroenterology 1987;92:472–478.

87. Smith B. The myenteric plexus in drug-induced neuropathy. J Neurol Neurosurg Psychiat 1967;30:506–510.

88. Siman LT, Haroupin DS, Dorfman LJ, Marks M. Polyneuropathy, ophthalmoplegia, leukoencephalopathy, and intestinal pseudo-obstruction polyp syndrome. Ann Neurol 1960;28:349–360.

89. Cockel R, Hill EE, Rushton DI, et al. Familial steatorrhea with calcification of the basal ganglia and mental retardation. Q J Med 1973;42:771–783.

90. Mayer EA, Schuffler MD, Retter JI, et al. A familial visceral neuropathy with autosomal dominant transmission. Gastroenterology 1986;91:1528–1535.

91. Faber J, Fich A, Steinberg A, et al. Familial intestinal pseudo-obstruction dominated by a progressive neurologic disease at a young age. Gastroenterology 1987;92:786–790.

92. Schuffler MD, Bird TD, Sumi SM, Cook A. A familial neuronal disease presenting as intestinal pseudo-obstruction. Gastroenterology 1978;75:889–898.

93. Patel H, Norman MG, Perry TL, Barry KE. Multiple system atrophy with neuronal intranuclear inclusions. Report of a case and review of the literature. J Neurol Sci 1985;67:57–65.

94. Barnett JL, McDonnell WM, Appelman HD, Dobbins WO. Familial visceral neuropathy with neuronal intranuclear inclusions: diagnosis by rectal biopsy. Gastroenterology 1992;102:684–691.

95. Achem SR, Owyang C, Schuffler MD, Dobbins WO. Neuronal dysplasia and chronic intestinal pseudo-obstruction: rectal biopsy as a possible aid to diagnosis. Gastroenterology 1987;92:805–809.

96. Scharl AF, Meier-Ruge W. Localized and disseminated forms of neuronal intestinal dysplasia mimicking Hirschsprung's disease. J Pediatr Surg 1981;16:164–170.

97. Feinstat T, Tesluk H, Schuffler MD, et al. Megacolon and neurofibromatosis: A neuronal intestinal dysplasia. Gastroenterology 1984;86:1573–1579.

98. Tanner MS, Smith B, Lloyd JK. Functional intestinal obstruction due to deficiency of argyrophilic neurons in the myenteric plexus. Familial syndrome presenting with short small bowel, malrotation, and pyloric hypertrophy. Arch Dis Child 1976;51:837–841.

99. Navarro J, Sonsino E, Boige N, et al. Visceral neuropathies responsible for chronic intestinal pseudo-obstruction syndrome in pediatric practice: analysis of 26 cases. J Pediatr Gastroenterol Nutr 1990;11:179–195.

100. Boggs JD, Kidd JM. Congenital abnormalities of intestinal innervation. Absence of innervation of jejunum, ileum, and colon in siblings. Pediatrics 1958;21:261–265.

101. Schuffler MD, Baird HW, Fleming CE, et al. Intestinal pseudo-obstruction as the presenting manifestation of small-cell carcinoma of the lung: a paraneoplastic neuropathy of the gastrointestinal tract. Ann Intern Med 1983;98:129–134.

102. Chinn JS, Schuffler MD. Paraneoplastic visceral neuropathy as a cause of severe gastrointestinal motor dysfunction. Gastroenterology 1988;95:1279–1286.

103. Lennon VA, Sas DF, Buck MF, et al. Enteric neuronal antibodies in pseudo-obstruction with small-cell lung carcinoma. Gastroenterology 1991;100:137–142.

104. DiBaise JK, Quigley EMM. Tumor-related dysmotility. Dig Dis Sci 1998;43:1369–1401.

105. Lee HR, Lennon VA, Camilleri M, Prather CM. Paraneoplastic gastrointestinal motor dysfunction: clinical and laboratory characteristics. Am J Gastroenterol 2001; 96:373–379.

106. Pardi DS, Miller SM, Miller DL, et al. Paraneoplastic dysmotility: loss of interstitial cells of Cajal. Am J Gastroenterol 2002;97:1828–1833.

107. Smith VV, Gregson N, Foggenstiner L, et al. Acquired intestinal aganglionosis and circulating autoantibodies without neoplasia or other neural involvement. Gastroenterology 1997; 112:1366–1371.

108. Earlam RJ. Gastrointestinal aspects of Chagas' disease. Am J Dig Dis 1972;17:559–571.

109. Brandt de Oliveira R, Troncon LE, Dantas RO, Meneghelli UC. Gastrointestinal manifestations of Chagas' disease. Am J Gastroenterol 1998;93:884–889.

110. Sonsino E, Mouy R, Foucard P, et al. Intestinal pseudo-obstruction related to cytomegalovirus infection of myenteric plexus. N Engl J Med 1984;31:196–197.

111. Krishnamurthy S, Schuffler MD, Belic L, Schweid AJ. An inflammatory axonopathy of the myenteric plexus producing a rapidly progressive intestinal pseudo-obstruction. Gastroenterology 1986;90:754–758.

112. De Giorgio R, Barbara G, Stanghellini V, et al. Clinical and morphofunctional features of idiopathic myenteric ganglionitis underlying severe intestinal motor dysfunction: a study of three cases. Am J Gastroenterol 2002;97:2454–2459.

113. Jain D, Moussa K, Tandon M, et al. Role of interstitial cells of Cajal in motility disorders of the bowel. Am J Gastroenterol 2003;98:618–625.

114. Boeckxstaens GE, Rumessen JJ, de Wit L, et al. Abnormal distribution of the interstitial cells of Cajal in an adult patient with pseudo-obstruction and megaduodenum. Am J Gastroenterol 2002;97:2120–2126.

115. Porcher C, Baldo M, Henry M, et al. Deficiency of interstitial cells of Cajal in the small intestine of patients with Crohn's disease. Am J Gastroenterol 2002;97:118–126.

116. Husebye E, Skar V, Hoverstad T, et al. Abnormal intestinal motor patterns explain enteric colonization with gram-negative bacilli in late radiation enteropathy. Gastroenterology 1995;109:1078–1089.

117. Shrake PD, Rex DK, Lappas JC, Maglinte DD. Radiographic evaluation of suspected small bowel obstruction. Am J Gastroenterol 1991;86:175–178.

118. Fidler JL, Coleman KL, Quigley EMM. Small bowel motility disturbances: a comparison of small-bowel series and antroduodenal manometry. Acad Radiol 1999;6:570–574.

119. Camilleri M, Zinsmeister AR, Greydanus MP, et al. Towards a less costly but accurate test of gastric emptying and small bowel transit. Dig Dis Sci 1991;36:609–615.

120. Camilleri M, Hasler WL, Parkman HP, et al. Measurement of gastrointestinal motility in the GI laboratory. Gastroenterology 1998;115:747–762.

121. Camilleri M. Study of human gastroduodenojejunal motility. Applied physiology in clinical practice. Dig Dis Sci 1993;38:785–794.

122. Quigley EMM. Intestinal manometry in man: a historical and clinical perspective. Dig Dis Sci 1994;12:199–209.

123. Quigley EMM, Deprez P, Hellstrom P, et al. Ambulatory intestinal manometry: a consensus report on its clinical role. Dig Dis Sci 1997;92:2395–2400.

124. Quigley EMM. Intestinal manometry—technical advances, clinical limitations. Dig Dis Sci 1992;37:10–13.

125. Quigley EMM, Donovan JP, Lane MJ, Gallagher TF. Antroduodenal manometry. Usefulness and limitations as an outpatient study. Dig Dis Sci 1992;37:20–28.

126. Lindberg G, Tornblom H, Iwarzon M, et al. Manometry cannot predict pathology in patients with chronic intestinal pseudo-obstruction. Gastroenterology 2000;118:A153.

127. Stanghellini V, Camilleri M, Malagelada JR. Chronic intestinal pseudo-obstruction: clinical and intestinal manometric findings. Gut 1987;28:5–12.

128. Camilleri M. Jejunal manometry in distal subacute mechanical obstruction: significance of prolonged simultaneous contractions. Gut 1989;30:468–475.

129. Frank JW, Sarr MG, Camilleri M. Use of gastroduodenal manometry to differentiate mechanical and functional intestinal obstruction: an analysis of clinical outcome. Am J Gastroenterol 1994;89:339–344.

130. Camilleri M, Brown ML, Malagelada JR. Relationship between impaired gastric emptying and abnormal gastrointestinal motility. Gastroenterology 1986;91:94–99.

131. Verne GN, Eaker EY, Hardy E, Sninsky CA. Effect of octreotide and erythromycin on idiopathic and scleroderma-associated intestinal pseudo-obstruction. Dig Dis Sci 1995; 40:1892–1901.

132. Leon SH, Schuffler MD. Visceral myopathy of the colon mimicking Hirschsprung's disease. Diagnosis by deep rectal biopsy. Dig Dis Sci 1986;31:1381–1386.

133. Camilleri M. Appraisal of medium and long-term treatment of gastroparesis and chronic intestinal dysmotility. Am J Gastroenterol 1994;89:1769–1774.

134. McCallum RW. Cisapride: a new class of prokinetic agent. Am J Gastroenterol 1991; 86:135–149.

135. Camilleri M, Brown ML, Malagelada JR. Impaired transit of chyme in chronic intestinal pseudo-obstruction: correction by cisapride. Gastroenterology 1986;91:619–626.

136. Camilleri M, Malagelada JR, Abell TL, et al. Effect of six weeks of treatment with cisapride in gastroparesis and intestinal pseudo-obstruction. Gastroenterology 1989;96:704–712.

137. Hyman PE, DiLorenzo D, McAdams L, et al. Predicting the clinical response to cisapride in children with chronic intestinal pseudo-obstruction. Am J Gastroenterol 1993;88:832–836.

138. Camilleri M, Balm RK, Zinsmeister AR. Determinants of response to prokinetic agent in neuropathic chronic intestinal motility disorder. Gastroenterology 1994;106:916–923.

139. Mearin F, Cucala M, Azpiroz F, Malagelada JR. The origin of symptoms on the brain-gut axis in functional dyspepsia. Gastroenterology 1991;101:999–1006.

140. Quigley EMM. Chronic intestinal pseudo-obstruction. Curr Treat Options Gastroenterol 1999;2:239–250.

141. Jones MP. Access options for withdrawn motility-modifying drugs. Am J Gastroenterol 2002;97:2184–2188.

142. Lipton AB, Knauer CM. Pseudo-obstruction of the bowel. Therapeutic trial of metoclopramide. Am J Dig Dis 1977;22:263–265.

143. Davis RH, Clench MH, Mathias JR. Effects of domperidone in patients with chronic unexplained upper gastrointestinal symptoms. A double-blind, placebo-controlled study. Dig Dis Sci 1988;33:1505–1511.

144. Turgeon DK. Domperidone in chronic intestinal pseudo-obstruction. Gastroenterology 1990;99:1194.

145. Richards RD, Davenport K, McCallum RW. The treatment of idiopathic and diabetic gastroparesis with acute intravenous and chronic oral erythromycin. Am J Gastroenterol 1993; 88:203–207.

146. Ramirez B, Eaker EY, Drane WE, et al. Erythromycin enhances gastric emptying in patients with gastroparesis after vagotomy and antrectomy. Dig Dis Sci 1994;39:2295–2300.

147. Maganti K, Onyemere K, Jones MP. Oral erythromycin and symptomatic relief of gastropareis: a systematic review. Am J Gastroenterol 2003;98:259–263.

148. Soudah HC, Hasler WL, Owyang C. Effect of octreotide on intestinal motility and bacterial overgrowth in scleroderma. N Engl J Med 1991;325:1461–1467.

149. Camilleri M. Review article: Tegaserod. Aliment Pharmacol Ther 2001;15:777–789.

150. Prather CM, Camilleri M, Zinsmeister AR, et al. Tegaserod accelerates orocecal transit in patients with constipation-predominant irritable bowel syndrome. Gastroenterology 2000; 118:463–468.

151. Degen L, Matzinger D, Mertz M, et al. Tegaserod, a 5-HT$_4$ receptor partial agonist, accelerates gastric emptying and gastrointestinal transit in healthy male subjects. Aliment Pharmacol Ther 2001;15:1655–1666.

152. Brandt LJ, Locke GR, Olden K, et al. An evidence-based approach to the management of irritable bowel syndrome in North America. Am J Gastroenterol 2002;97:S20–S22.

153. Justus PG, Fernandez A, Martin JL, et al. Altered myoelectric activity in the experimental blind loop syndrome. J Clin Invest 1983;72:1064–1071.

154. Warner E, Jeejeebhoy KN. Successful management of chronic intestinal pseudo-obstruction with home parenteral nutrition. J Parenter Enteral Nutr 1985;9:173–178.

155. Pitt HA, Mann LL, Berquist WE, et al. Chronic intestinal pseudo-obstruction. Management with total parenteral nutrition and a venting enterostomy. Arch Surg 1985;120:614–618.

156. Mughal MM, Irving MH. Treatment of end stage chronic intestinal pseudo-obstruction by subtotal enterectomy and home parenteral nutrition. Gut 1988;29:613–617.

157. Kadowaki H, Ouchi M, Kaga M, et al. Problems of trace elements and vitamins during long-term total parenteral nutrition. A case report of idiopathic intestinal pseudo-obstruction. JPEN 1987;11:322–325.

158. Murr MM, Sarr MG, Camilleri M. The surgeon's role in the treatment of chronic intestinal pseudo-obstruction. Am J Gastroenterol 1995;90:2147–2151.

159. Quigley EMM. Small intestinal transplantation – Reflections on an evolving approach to intestinal failure. Gastroenterology 1996;110:2009–2012.

160. Tougas G, Huizinga JD. Gastric pacing as a treatment of intractable gastroparesis: shocking news? Gastroenterology 1998;114:598–601.

161. Bortolotti M. The "electrical way" to cure gastroparesis. Am J Gastroenterol 2002; 97:1874–1883.

Chapter 12
Malabsorption and Neurological Disease

Joseph A. Murray and Mark A. Ross

INTRODUCTION

The major function of the gastrointestinal system is the digestion and absorption of nutrients. Digestion is the breakdown and hydrolysis of food macromolecules in the lumen of the gastrointestinal tract and absorption is the assimilation of the nutrients across the gut wall. These two functions are inextricably linked and disorders of these processes frequently co-exist. Digestion commences as soon as the food enters the oral cavity. The food is initially mechanically broken down by mastication and admixed with the lipase and other enzymes present in the saliva. Once in the stomach, the food is churned and mixed with hydrochloric acid and pepsin. At this point, most of the macromolecules remain intact. The solid food particles are usually reduced to a size less than 3 mm in diameter before exiting the stomach. The stomach empties its contents into the small intestine in a controlled fashion, which allows the small intestine to perform its vital role in digestion and absorption efficiently. Overly rapid emptying of the stomach can overcome the capacity of the small intestine to cope with the nutrients delivered.

The majority of the digestive and absorptive processes occur in the small intestine. This 20 to 26 foot long organ is uniquely adapted for this purpose. Not only is the lining pleated into many folds but these are covered with many finger-like projections called villi. It is at this interface between the lumen and the mucosal surface that most digestion and absorption occur. The gastric chyme is mixed with pancreatic enzymes and intestinal secretions to achieve breakdown of proteins and carbohydrates into amino acids and sugars. Bile salts serve to emulsify the fats and allow packaging of lipids into micelles for ease of absorption. The fats undergo digestion primarily by pancreatic lipase. The small intestine has a remarkable reserve capacity. Individuals have survived without the need for parenteral nutrition with as little as 10%, or even less, of small bowel remaining. The small intestine is remarkably similar in structure throughout its length, however some significant regional specialization of functions exists. For example, iron and folate are absorbed in the proximal small intestine, while bile acids and vitamin B12 are absorbed in the distal small bowel. Diseases that specifically affect these areas are most likely to give rise to corresponding combinations of nutrient deficiencies. Loss of the distal ileum and the ileocecal valve can give rise to significant diarrhea due to the

203

irritating effects of the lost bile acids in the colon. The interruption of the entero-hepatic circulation of bile can lead to its gradual depletion and consequent fat maldigestion and malabsorption.

Maldigestion

Disorders of digestion not associated with malabsorption may be common, but usually do not have consequences for the nervous system. An example is primary lactase deficiency, in which the small intestine lacks the enzymatic ability to digest lactose, milk sugar. This and other isolated maldigestive disorders have little, if any, impact on the nervous system. Digestive problems may indicate the presence of an underlying malabsorptive disease. Maldigestion of nutrients frequently co-exists with malabsorption, and these are dealt with together.

Malabsorption

There are many causes of malabsorption. The most common of these are listed in Table 12.1. While many of these entities are rarely seen in clinical practice, collectively they constitute a significant cause of neurologic dysfunction. Malabsorptive disorders can be classified according to whether or not there is mucosal disease. The classic mucosal malabsorptive disease is celiac disease, also known as gluten sensitive enteropathy, in which the mucosa is diffusely affected. Other diseases may affect the gross anatomy of the small intestine, such as short bowel syndrome or jejunal diverticulosis. The diverticuli serve as reservoirs for bacterial overgrowth and consequent malabsorption. The intervening mucosa is often normal. These entities are usually easily differentiated on the basis of mucosal biopsies, and the latter is usually diagnosed with small bowel contrast x-rays (Figure 12.1). The small intestine is completely normal in the malabsorption of pancreatic insufficiency. This entity is suspected by the presence of large amounts of fat in the stools and normal small bowel mucosal and gross anatomy.

General Clinical Features of Malabsorption and Maldigestion

The clinical manifestations of malabsorption are protean. Gastrointestinal symptoms classically include steatorrhea. Patients or their families complain of very malodorous, bulky stools that float and may be difficult to flush. They may remark on a light or gray color. Weight loss is common; however, the patients may be able to compensate by eating tremendous quantities of foods. Post prandial bloating and flatulence are often due to the accompanying disaccharide maldigestion. The undigested disaccharide is acted upon by the colonic microflora to produce gas. Remaining sugars are osmotically active and result in diarrhea. Fasting usually stops the diarrhea due to maldigestion/malabsorption. Abdominal pain may be due to the distension of the intestine by gas or fluid, or it may result from the inflammatory nature of the disease. Excessive fatigue is almost universal and reflects nutritional deficiency or a chronic inflammatory process. Many patients with a malabsorptive disease have minimal or no gastrointestinal symptoms and their only manifestations are extra-gastrointestinal (Table 12.2). If the malabsorption was

Table 12.1. Causes of Malabsorption

Disorder	Pathogenic Mechanisms	Investigation	Intestinal Biopsy	Treatment
Diffuse mucosal disease				
Celiac disease	Gluten intolerance	Endomysial and tissue transglutaminase antibodies, serum carotene	Villous atrophy, ↑IEL's, plasma cell infiltrate, crypt hyperplasia	Gluten-free diet
Tropical sprue	Multiple bacterial infections	Travel history	Villous blunting, milder than CD	Antibiotics and folic acid
HIV enteropathy	HIV, opportunistic infections (MAI, CMV, isospora, cryptosporidia, microsporidia, cyclospora)	HIV test, stool tests, EM on biopsy	Variable, organisms, viral inclusions, inflamed lamina propria	Nutritional support, treat specific infection
Graft-versus-host disease	Graft immune attack on intestine	History (30–180 days post transplant, apoptosis in biopsy, clinical features)	Partial villous atrophy, apoptosis	Steroids, immunosuppressives
Giardiasis	Parasite, giardia lamblia, more frequent in selective IgA deficiency and common variable hypogammaglobulinemia	Stool for giardia antigen, jejunal aspirate	Giardia, mild patchy villous blunting and inflammation.	Metronidazole, quinacrine
Radiation enteritis	Radiotherapy to cervix, lymphoma, bladder or other viscera	Intestinal strictures on contrast x-rays, mucosal telangiectasias on endoscopic examination	Normal to total villous atrophy fibrosis, atypical fibroblasts in submucosa	Steroids, Azulfidine
Whipple's disease	Bacterium (*Tropheryma whippelii*)	PCR on blood (investigational)	PAS stain on biopsy, EM, molecular probe	Long-term antibiotics
Lymphangiectasia	Lymphatic obstruction, lymphoma, filariasis, idiopathic, Hekkeman's syndrome, radiation, Whipple's disease	Hypoalbuminemia, hypogammaglobulinemia, raised alpha-1 antitrypsin in stool	Dilated lymph channels	Very low fat diet, medium chain triglyceride oil supplement
Amyloidosis	Unknown; proliferative disorders associated with deposition of amyloid protein	Immunofixation electrophoresis	Congo red stain of biopsy	

Table continued on following page

Table 12.1. Causes of Malabsorption—*Continued*

Disorder	Pathogenic Mechanisms	Investigation	Intestinal Biopsy	Treatment
Systemic endocrine disorders	Impaired fat digestion/ absorption, mild GI disease. Hyperthyroidism leads to hyperphagia and rapid transit; hypothyroidism may cause decreased pancreatic function	Check thyroid function, search for hypoadrenalism, diabetes, systemic sclerosis		
Abetalipo-proteinemia	Recessive hereditary absence of lipoprotein B, cholesterol malabsorption	No VLDL, LDL or chylomicrons on lipoprotein electrophoresis	Yellow duodenal mucosa, fat droplet laden surface enterocytes	
Alpha heavy chain disease, IPSID	Neoplastic disease, poor nutrition, plasma cell proliferation of IgA secreting cells, may progress into a lymphoma. Occurs in the Near East	Broad band on serum electrophoresis, immuno-fixation electrophoresis, identify incomplete IgA chains (heavy chains) in the serum/intestinal secretions; demonstrate lack of light chains	Plasma cell proliferation on biopsy	Early with antibiotics, treat parasites, nutritional support, later treat lymphoma
Vascular hyalinosis	Familial abnormality of small vessels, gray hair, poikiloderma, cerebrovascular calcifications	Alpha-1 antitrypsin in stool	Hyalinosis of basement membrane of intestinal capillaries	
Tangier disease	Recessive inherited congenital degradation of apoprotein A leading to cholesterol ester accumulation, yellow tonsils hepatospleno-megaly, peripheral neuropathy	Lipoprotein electrophoresis		
T-cell lymphoma	Enteropathy associated lymphoma, celiac disease, HTLV-1.	CT scan, enteroclysis, laparotomy/scopy, enteroscopy	Mixed large cell, small cell lymphoma with T-cell markers, non-lymphomatous mucosa resembles celiac disease	
Diseases associated with normal mucosa				

Table continued on opposite page

include effects on the musculoskeletal system (myopathy and osteomalacia), reproductive system, skin, growth, and development in children. Disorders of absorption specifically may affect the integrity and function of the nervous system. Deficiencies of individual micronutrients may result in a variety of neurological disorders, which are described in the first part of this review. Neurological disease seen in association with diseases of malabsorption may not be due to the deficiency of a specific nutrient. For example, Whipple's disease leads to malabsorption and neurological dysfunction by direct infection of each organ system. Similarly, amyloidosis can lead to both malabsorption and peripheral neuropathy by direct involvement of both tissues (Figure 12.3). Pernicious anemia, though not considered by many to be a malabsorptive state, causes the very specific deficiency of vitamin B12. Other diseases that result in malabsorption may also be associated with neurological syndromes, though the neurological defect is not caused by the deficiency state.

SPECIFIC NUTRITIONAL DEFICIENCY STATES

The gastrointestinal tract not only provides the body with macronutrients (protein, carbohydrates, and fat), but also many micronutrients essential for numerous enzymatic functions. Deficiencies of many of these micronutrients may result in neurological dysfunction (Table 12.5). Many micronutrient deficiencies do not result from malabsorption, but rather from starvation or chronic dietary deficiency of specific vitamins or minerals. Several micronutrient deficiencies may be associated with diseases of the small intestine. For example, fat malabsorption may cause

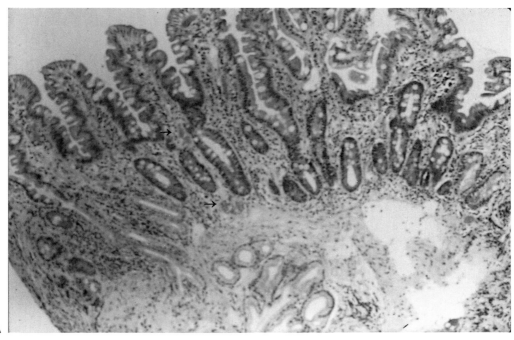

A

Figure 12.3. A. Small intestinal amyloid deposition *(arrow)* in the small bowel of a patient whose underlying condition was multiple myeloma with monoclonal gammopathy.   *Figure continued on following page*

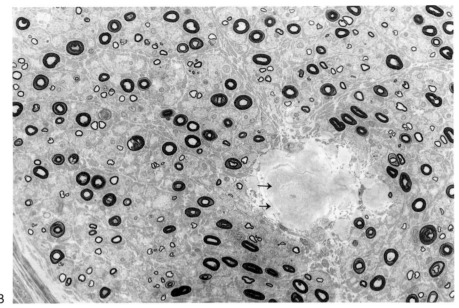

Figure 12.3 *Continued.* **B.** Amyloid deposits in the peripheral nerve of the same patient (pictures courtesy of F. Mitros and S. Moore).

deficiency of the fat soluble vitamins A, D, E, and K. Isolated deficiency of the micronutrient vitamin B12 may present as a major neurological syndrome.

Cobalamin (Vitamin B12) Deficiency

Biology

Vitamin B12, or cobalamin, is a water soluble vitamin that is a required co-factor in several enzymatic reactions. Its essential structure is a corrin ring surrounding a cobalt atom. Attached at the upper pole of the molecule is a variable ligand that differentiates the various forms of the molecule. At least three forms occur naturally in animals: hydroxyl-, adenosyl-, and methyl-cobalamin. Cyanocobalamin, the

Table 12.5. Micronutrient Deficiencies That Lead to Neurologic Dysfunction

Vitamin B12[*]
Vitamin D[*]
Vitamin A
Vitamin E[*]
Pyridoxine[*]
Niacin
Vitamin C
Choline
Thiamine

[*]Commonly associated with malabsorption.

common pharmaceutical form, is a synthetic compound that does not occur in nature. The corrin ring of cobalamin is synthesized by some microorganisms, and the resulting cobalamin compounds are concentrated in animal tissue. Cobalamin cannot be manufactured by man or absorbed from the colonic flora. Plants are poor sources of cobalamin, hence the occasional occurrence of cobalamin deficiency in strict vegetarians.

The process of assimilation of cobalamin is a complex sequence of events requiring structural and functional integrity of the gastrointestinal system (Figure 12.4). Dietary cobalamins are cleaved from the proteins, primarily by the action of pepsin and other proteases in the stomach. The transport of cobalamin through the intestine to its primary storage site in the liver, and hence to its site of biologic action in the cell, requires many different transport factors and receptor molecules.[2] First, the

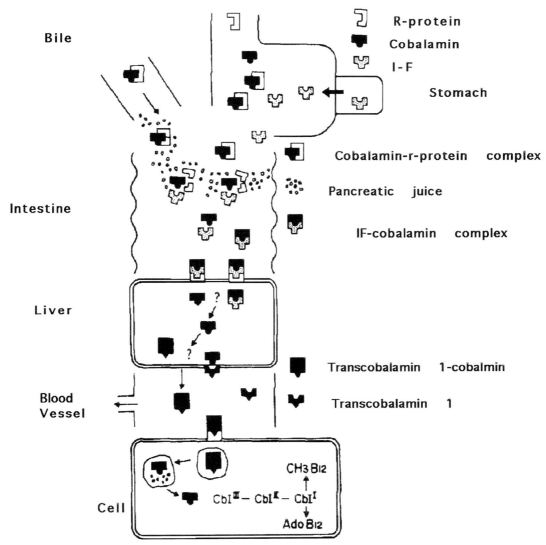

Figure 12.4. Diagram of the GI tract featuring the mechanism of cobalamin, absorption. (Reproduced with permission from Cano N. Disorders of cobalamin metabolism. Crit Rev Oncol Hematol 1995;3:1–34.)

liberated cobalamin is bound to r-proteins in the stomach. The r-proteins originate in the salivary glands. The r-protein-cobalamin complex passes into the proximal small intestine, where the r-protein is cleaved from the cobalamin and replaced by intrinsic factor (IF). Intrinsic factor is produced by the parietal cells of the gastric body and fundus. The IF-cobalamin complex passes through the small intestine to the distal ileum where it binds to receptors for IF that allow the efficient absorption of cobalamin. Very little free cobalamin is absorbed without these factors and receptors. In the enterocyte, cobalamin is attached to another r-protein, transcobalamin II. This complex is bound by specific receptors on the cell surfaces and taken up by endocytosis. The complex is cleaved by proteases and the free cobalamin is converted into the active forms, primarily methylcobalamin and adenosylcobalamin. Why man has developed this circuitous mechanism for absorption of cobalamin is not known. It is speculated that the r-proteins (which are actually glycoproteins) serve to prevent cobalamin from being utilized by bacteria.

Large quantities of cobalamin are stored in the liver, usually as adenosylcobalamin and hydroxycobalamin. Total body stores may exceed 2000 μg, while daily requirements are on the order of 2 to 5 μg. Cobalamin bound to r-proteins is also secreted into the bile. Much of this is reabsorbed in the intestine, following cleavage and attachment to intrinsic factor. This large hepatic store of B12 and the efficient enterohepatic circulation lead to a long delay before clinical deficiency becomes evident.

Functions

Cobalamin acts as a co-enzyme for three enzymes in animals: 5-methyl homocysteine methyl transferase, methylmalonyl CoA mutase, and leucine 2,3 aminomutase (Figure 12.5). Methyl-cobalamin, in which the cobalt is in the 2+ oxidation state, is

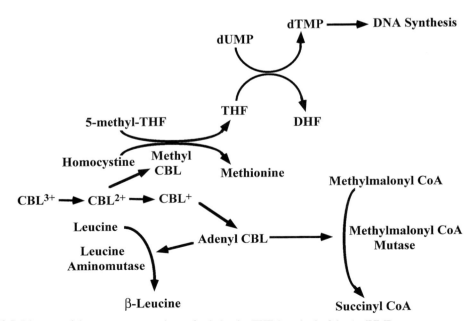

Figure 12.5. Diagram of the coenzyme reactions of cobalamin. THF (tetrahydrofolate); dUMP (d uranyl monophosphate).

essential for the formation of methionine from homocysteine, and the simultaneous formation of tetrahydrofolate from 5-methyl tetrahydrofolate. Cobalamin deficiency can result in accumulation of folic acid as the unusable form of N-methyl tetrahydrofolate. Tetrahydrofolate is necessary for the formation of thymidine from uracil and subsequent DNA synthesis. Interference with DNA synthesis explains the development of megaloblastic anemia in cobalamin deficiency. Indeed, in some cases, megaloblastic anemia can be overcome by giving very large doses of folic acid.

The adenosyl-cobalamin is necessary for the conversion of methylmalonyl-CoA to succinyl CoA. Failure of this conversion leads to impaired fatty acid metabolism and accumulation of methylmalonyl-CoA. The neurologic sequelae of cobalamin deficiency are believed to result from accumulation of methylmalonyl-CoA, which competes with the malonyl CoA in myelin sheath formation. Methylmalonyl-CoA mutase is also important in the metabolism of branch chain fatty acids. Accumulation and substitution of these fatty acids for malonyl CoA could also interfere with myelin sheath formation.

The third enzymatic pathway that requires cobalamin is leucine 2,3 aminomutase, which is involved in the interconversion of alpha-leucine and beta-leucine. This reaction may be involved in leucine synthesis, but its importance in cobalamin deficiency is not known.[3] The aminomutase may not even be present in humans.[4]

Cobalamin Deficiency

The recognized clinical features of cobalamin (vitamin B12) deficiency have changed since the classic descriptions of the classic features of pernicious anemia. The classic syndrome is the result of an autoimmune gastropathy targeting the parietal cells which produce intrinsic factor. The parietal cell is also the acid secreting cell of the stomach. Hence, loss of parietal cells results in both loss of intrinsic factors and gastric acid secretion.

Etiology of Cobalamin Deficiency.   The complex absorption of cobalamin presents many opportunities for defects to occur (Table 12.6). Dietary deficiency is limited to strict vegetarians or totally breast fed infants of mothers with cobalamin deficiency. While B12 deficiency can affect all races, the underlying etiology may vary among ethnic groups. For instance, pernicious anemia is more common among Caucasians, while tropical sprue predominates in those patients from developing nations. A history of ingestion of raw fish raises the possibility of fish tapeworm infestation (diphyllobothrium latum) which, while it is more common in countries and cultures where the consumption of raw fish is common, can occur elsewhere. The tapeworm is a fresh water parasite whose larvae, when ingested by fish, are deposited in the flesh. If the fish is then not properly cooked, the larvae can develop in the small intestine, where they consume B12. Most infestations are asymptomatic, with diarrhea or abdominal pain occurring rarely. Eosinophilia may prompt suspicion of the condition. It is diagnosed by the identification of the eggs in the stool. Treatment is with praziquantil or niclosamide orally.

Acute neurological features of vitamin B12 deficiency may occur following repeated nitrous oxide gas exposure with recreational use. Rarely, in individuals who have marginally low B12 levels, symptoms may develop acutely with a single exposure.[5] Nitrous oxide inactivates methylcobalamin by oxidation of the cobalt ion. This causes neuropathic features similar to vitamin B12 deficiency.[6] Serum B12 levels may be normal. Elderly patients with marginal B12 stores may present

Table 12.6. Causes of Cobalamin Deficiency

Dietary deficiency
    Vegetarian diet
    Breast fed infants of mothers with cobalamin deficiency
Intrinsic factor deficiency
  Associated with hypochlorhydria
    Autoimmune gastritis (pernicious anemia)
    Intrinsic factor blocking antibody
    Gastrectomy
    Helicobacter-associated atrophic gastritis
  Not associated with hypochlorhydria
    Congenital IF deficiency
Inhibition of binding of cobalamin to IF
    Pancreatic insufficiency
    Zollinger Ellison syndrome
    Bacterial overgrowth/Blind loop syndrome
Consumption of cobalamin
    Bacterial overgrowth
    Diphyllobothrium latum infestation
    Drug-induced destruction
Malabsorption
    Intestinal diseases
      Crohn's disease
      Celiac disease
      Tropical sprue
      Diffuse small bowel malignancy
      HIV infection[187]
    Intestinal resection
    Imerslund-Grasbeck's disease (congenital)
Congenital defects in transport proteins
Inactivation of cobalamin with nitrous oxide gas

---

with a neurologic syndrome post-operatively, due to nitrous oxide scavenging of B12. Hypochlorhydria may lead to failure to cleave the protein bound B12 in food. B12 deficiency has been seen in this scenario in cases of gastric resection or vagotomy. Drug induced acid suppression can impair B12 absorption; however, clinical B12 deficiency has not been identified in patients taking omeprazole continuously for 4 years.[7-10]

Clinical Features of Cobalamin Deficiency.   The syndrome of anemia, neurologic abnormalities, and achlorhydria of the stomach was recognized in the late 19th century. Severe B12 deficiency can result in impaired cell differentiation in the mucosa of the gastrointestinal tract. This may cause a secondary malabsorption that resolves with B12 repletion. Glossitis may be identified by what is called a strawberry tongue. This is occasionally seen in some individuals with pernicious anemia. In the past, treatment of this syndrome with liver extract produced a prompt improvement, usually in the anemia and also in the neurologic sequelae. In the 1940s, B12 was identified as the active therapeutic modality in liver extract.

Megaloblastic Anemia.   Erythropoiesis is impaired in cobalamin deficiency, resulting in decreased production of mature red cells, accumulation of megaloblastic red cells in the bone marrow, and increased numbers of circulating immature red cells. There is usually a prompt response to cobalamin administration.

Neurologic Syndromes Associated with Cobalamin Deficiency. Cobalamin deficiency may cause damage or dysfunction of the peripheral nerves, the spinal cord, and more rarely, the brain.[11] Isolated abnormalities, such as optic neuropathy or other cranial nerve disorders, are quite rare. A common clinical presentation is the complaint of distal paraesthesias without objective neurologic signs. The neurologic syndromes are outlined in Table 12.7.

While B12 deficiency causes both megaloblastic anemia and neurologic disorders, these two conditions do not always co-exist. In fact, roughly 25% of patients with neurologic disorders associated with B12 deficiency have an entirely normal blood count.[12] Frequently, neurologic symptoms precede anemia. The single most common neurologic symptom is distal symmetrical paresthesia, occurring in more than 70% of patients. This usually involves the feet and occasionally the hands. This may also be associated with impaired proprioception or other sensory deficits. Less commonly, paresthesias exclusively involve the hands. Other symptoms include numbness, gait disturbance, lower limb weakness, and cognitive or psychiatric disturbances. The single most common abnormality apparent on physical examination is impaired or absent vibration sense, particularly in the lower limbs. Other objective abnormalities seen in descending order of frequency include ataxia, mental impairment, paraparesis, and quadriparesis, with these rarely being seen as a sole manifestation. Abnormalities of the autonomic nervous system are quite rare and usually accompany other findings. Dementia or psychosis is a common form of neurologic presentation of cobalamin deficiency, and also may occur in the absence of hematological abnormalities.[13] The cerebral dysfunction is most commonly a global dementia or occasionally a specific memory loss. Psychotic features may be superimposed. Cerebral dysfunction is rarely an isolated finding, and is usually seen in association with motor or sensory deficits. There appears to be a correlation between low cognitive ability and low vitamin B12 levels.[14] Psychiatric disturbances may take the form of dementia, depression, behavioral disturbances, personality changes, and hallucinations.[15,16] Quite rarely, patients may experience orthostatic hypotension and anosmia, or visual disturbances.

It has been suggested that B12 deficiency may increase the likelihood of chronic tinnitus and noise induced hearing loss, some of which is reversible with B12 replacement.[17] Severe clumsiness of the upper limbs was identified in a single

Table 12.7. Neurologic Syndromes Associated with Cobalamin Deficiency

Peripheral neuropathy	Distal symmetric sensory deficit with absent ankle reflexes, may have distal weakness and atrophy, no upper motor neuron signs
Myelopathy	Spasticity, extensor plantar responses, hyperreflexia, weakness, large fiber sensory deficit (impaired vibration and position sense, ataxia)
Cerebral dysfunction	Defects in cognitive function, neuropsychiatric disturbances, dementia
Miscellaneous	Optic neuropathy, noise induced deafness and chronic tinnitus

Note: Subacute combined degeneration refers to pyramidal tract involvement and posterior column involvement. When myelopathy is present, as evidenced by upper motor neuron (pyramidal) findings, it is impossible to differentiate large fiber sensory abnormalities due to posterior column from peripheral nerve involvement.

individual. This was, however, seen in association with paresthesias of the hands and feet and ataxia.[18] Optic neuropathy has occasionally been identified in patients with B12 deficiency, and rarely can be the sole manifestation, with symmetric optic neuropathies resulting in bilateral centrocecal scotomas.[19] Interestingly, tobacco-alcohol amblyopia, which also produces centrocecal scotomas, may occasionally be improved by the administration of cyanocobalamin. A chiasmal visual defect has also been identified, producing a bitemporal hemianopia.[20]

Diagnosis.   Suspicion of the diagnosis might be raised by the presence of macrocytic anemia. However, a significant number of patients may not be anemic. The most common blood index abnormality is a raised MCV, which is often marked with an MCV of greater than 110. Blood smear evaluation may reveal hypersegmented neutrophils. A bone marrow aspirate will always reveal a megaloblastic picture. In approximately 20% of all patients with neurologic abnormalities, there is no apparent abnormality in hematopoiesis. In particular, the hemoglobin, hematocrit, and MCV may be normal. It is interesting that folic acid supplementation may correct the blood abnormalities, while the neurologic abnormalities progress or appear de novo.

The serum cobalamin level is the single best screening test, and is abnormal in the vast majority of B12 deficient patients. There are three types of assays for plasma B12 levels: chemiluminescent, bacterial, and radioimmune. It is important to note that normal ranges vary by the technique used. The chemiluminescent is the most widely used test due to its simplicity. Bacterial assays utilize bacteria that require cobalamin for growth, such as lactobacillus leishmannii. This is a reliable and specific test; however, it is not very practical. It has been replaced by sensitive radioimmunoassays utilizing pure intrinsic factor as a detector. The radioimmunoassay is reasonably sensitive, but occasionally detects cobalamin analogues that have no biologic activity. There may be elevated serum levels with cellular deficiency, especially in hematopoietic diseases. Chemiluminescent levels have found widespread acceptance due to ease of use.

Cobalamin deficiency can occur when the B12 levels are in the low normal range. Homocysteine and methylmalonic acid accumulate in B12 deficiency. Measurements of these may be helpful when suspicion for B12 deficiency is high and the levels are in the low normal range. Homocysteine levels may also be elevated in B6 deficiency and in renal impairment. These levels usually respond quite rapidly to repletion with the appropriate vitamin.

B12 levels do not correlate with the severity of the neurological disorders. Indeed, some patients with a low but normal B12 level and an associated neurologic disorder have responded to B12 supplementation. The severity of neurologic syndromes correlates with the duration of symptoms and absence of hematological abnormalities. Severity may also be greater in Caucasian patients than in other ethnic groups. This may be a reflection of the increased frequency of pernicious anemia that causes just B12 deficiency. This is in contrast to the B12 deficiency that occurs in association with generalized malabsorption, leading to earlier presentation affecting other nutrients.

The confirmation of B12 deficiency is only the first step in diagnosis. When B12 deficiency is confirmed, the cause should be determined. Positive intrinsic factor blocking antibody (IFBA), parietal cell antibody, or a high fasting gastrin would support the diagnosis of pernicious anemia, and there is little need to proceed to further investigation.

Tests of Cobalamin Absorption.* The presence of IF antibody in the untreated patient confirms essentially the diagnosis of pernicious anemia, however it is only 50% to 60% sensitive. False positive IFBA can occur shortly after parenteral B12 administration. Parietal cell antibodies are positive in 90% of patients with pernicious anemia, but are much less specific for pernicious anemia, particularly for individuals over the age of 70.

Obvious factors in the history, such as prior gastric resection or small bowel surgery, suggest a specific cause and should allow truncating the usual diagnostic strategies. Other tests may help identify pernicious anemia, and these can include elevated fasting gastrin levels. Gastrin produced by the antrum of the stomach is increased in the setting of achlorhydria and can reach levels of over 1000 ng/ml in pernicious anemia. While upper endoscopy with biopsies of the gastric body may reveal mucosal atrophy, this is seldom necessary if the other tests indicate pernicious anemia. Helicobacter pylori infection of the stomach may be associated with mucosal atrophy and decreased acid production. This hypochlorhydria results in failure of splitting the bound cobalamin away from food proteins.[27] In this situation, the Schilling test is usually normal because there is adequate IF production, but the lack of acid interferes with the separation of cobalamin from the food protein and decrease in absorption.[28] This shortcoming can be overcome by the use of the egg yolk-cobalamin absorption test (EYCAT).[29]

If there are significant upper gastrointestinal symptoms, then endoscopy should be carried out, not only to detect chronic gastritis related to the Helicobacter infection, but also the rare occurrence of gastric carcinoma or carcinoid, conditions that are more frequent in pernicious anemia.

---

*The original Schilling test measures the absorption of vitamin B12 using radio labeled cobalamin compounds. It is performed in two stages. The first stage Schilling test consists usually of the oral administration of a radiolabeled unbound cobalamin. An injection of unlabeled cobalamin is given after the radiolabeled dose to displace the absorbed labeled cobalamin into the urine. The subsequent collection of urine is assayed for the excreted radiolabeled compound.[21] Excretion of less than 8% of the oral dose is indicative of defective absorption. If the Stage I test is abnormal, then the test is repeated with addition of intrinsic factor (Stage 2). The correction of the excretion with the addition of intrinsic factor indicates atrophic gastritis or some other cause of IF deficiency. Failure to correct indicates a small intestinal disease. Attempts at one-step Schilling tests utilizing a combination of differentially labeled Cr57 cobalamin and Cr58–IF-cobalamin have been developed.[22] The ratio of Cr57 to Cr58 in the urine is supposed to indicate the relative absorption of the two compounds; however, exchange of Cr58 cobalamin for Cr57-cobalamin bound to IF in vivo renders the test unreliable.[23] The standard crystalline B12 used in the Schilling test may not detect protein bound B12 malabsorption.[24] This may be overcome by the use of a protein bound radiolabeled B12.[25] A non-radioactive version of the Schilling test has been proposed, but has not gained widespread use, possibly due to the pretest restrictions for the patients.[26] It must be pointed out that the cost of the Schilling test may exceed the cost of lifetime replacement of vitamin B12, by injection. The cost and inconvenience of the various forms of the Schilling test limits its clinical utility.

If the preliminary tests are negative, then a Stage 2 Schilling test should be carried out using IF-cobalamin. An abnormal test suggests that there is small intestinal malabsorption or rarely consumption of B12. Other tests, such as gastrointestinal contrast x-rays, may reveal an anatomic abnormality, such as jejunal diverticulosis or Crohn's disease.

In terms of neurological investigations, nerve conduction studies and somatosensory evoked potentials often demonstrate abnormalities suggestive of an axonopathy involving both sensory and motor fibers. Visually evoked potentials may also be delayed due to central involvement.

Therapy.   As most causes of B12 deficiency, with the exception of vegan diets and diphyllobotrium latum infestation, are essentially irreversible, repletion and maintenance doses of cyanocobalamin administered parenterally are required. Even in those patients with reversible causes of B12 depletion, such as parasitic infestation of the small intestine, celiac disease, tropical sprue, or bacterial overgrowth of the intestine, parenteral B12 therapy should usually be provided to replete the stores of cobalamin.

The usual pharmacological form of cobalamin is cyanocobalamin. A typical repletion schedule is 1000 μg i.m. weekly of cobalamin over the initial 4 to 6 weeks. Maintenance strategies have varied quite a bit, but aim to provide 100 μg monthly. There are some other forms of cobalamin that have been developed, including a depot form of cyanocobalamin that would only need to be given once every three months.[30] Oral, nasal, or sublingual replacement therapy with 1000 micrograms daily has become popular in Europe, and usually is sufficient, even in the absence of intrinsic factor. The 1 to 2% of the ingested B12 that is absorbed is adequate for repletion of B12 stores.[31–34] Hydroxycobalamin has been used in some countries and is more effectively absorbed and converted into utilizable forms.[35] The response of hematological abnormalities is usually dramatic, with a rapid rise in reticulocyte counts within 48 hours and correction of the anemia in 4 to 8 weeks. The majority of patients with neurologic abnormalities will show some improvement, but it is often a more gradual response than the hematological response. Nearly half of the patients with neurologic syndromes will have complete recovery. Patients with psychosis may have a dramatic and often complete resolution of symptoms within days or weeks of the institution of the therapy.[36] The remaining patients have a partial recovery of their neurologic abnormalities. Usually, the first symptoms to respond are the distal paresthesias; however, other symptoms, such as paraparesis or cerebral dysfunction, may take weeks or occasionally months to show improvement. While maximal response is usually seen within the first months, on occasion, maximal recovery may not be complete for 2 to 3 years following initiation of cobalamin therapy. A poor response to therapy is predicted by longer duration of symptoms prior to diagnosis and with the pretreatment severity. Relapse of neurologic abnormalities may occur when patients have inadvertently stopped their cobalamin supplementation.

Folic Acid Deficiency

Biology

Folic acid (pteroylglutamate) is primarily derived from plants. It exists for the most part as a polymer that must be hydrolyzed by a brush border enzyme present only in the jejunum. It can then be absorbed via a carrier exchange mechanism that extrudes hydroxyl ion into the lumen. This process is dependent on a slightly acidic luminal pH. Folic acid is predominantly protein bound in the serum. Folic acid is usually reduced and methylated in the liver to the active form, tetrahydrofolate. Some is secreted in the bile, only to be reabsorbed in the intestine, with the majority being distributed to the sites of action.

Function

Folic acid and its metabolites are essential cofactors for DNA synthesis. Its availability is vital in rapidly dividing cells, such as the bone marrow. Folic acid also seems critical for neural tube development.[37] Indeed the USA and some other countries require the addition of folic acid to most grain products, with the expectation of reducing the incidence of neural tube defects.

Clinical Features of Folic Acid Deficiency

The most common effect of folic acid deficiency is megaloblastic anemia. Common causes of folic acid deficiency include gastric resection and diffuse disorders that damage the jejunum, such as celiac disease, tropical sprue, bacterial overgrowth syndrome, and giardiasis. Loss of gastric acid results in alkalinization of the jejunal lumen, with consequent reduction in hydrolysis of the folic acid by the brush border enzyme. While many drugs can interfere with folic acid absorption, only a few give rise to clinical folic acid deficiency states. Diphenylhydantoin, in particular, interferes with hydrolysis of folic acid and occasionally causes megaloblastic anemia.[38,39] Antiepileptic-induced folic acid deficiency in the mother may be responsible for the increased risk of fetal abnormalities.[40] Both supplemental folic acid, 4 mg/day started preconceptually, and minimizing the dose of antiepileptic are prudent considerations in women of reproductive capacity.[41] Methotrexate, a commonly used chemotherapeutic and immunosuppressive agent, inhibits the conversion of folic acid to its active metabolite, folinic acid. If methotrexate is given repeatedly by the intrathecal route, an acute severe encephalopathy may occur that corrects with folinic acid.

Clinicians are generally aware that folic acid treatment alone may correct the hematological abnormalities, but worsen or even precipitate the neurological complications of B12 deficiency.[42] It is not as well recognized that folic acid deficiency alone may cause some cases of subacute combined system degeneration in which vitamin B12 levels are normal.[43] In such cases, the neurological abnormalities respond to repletion of folic acid alone.[44] The most common symptoms in these patients were leg weakness, ataxia, and incontinence. Physical exam revealed paraparesis, impaired vibration sense, up-going plantar responses, and absent muscle stretch reflexes.[45] The etiology most frequently identified for the folic acid deficiency was alcoholism. Dementia has also been associated with low levels of folic acid, although a causal relationship has not been established.[46] Folic acid deficiency may be the cause of the syndrome of epilepsy and intracranial calcifications seen in celiac disease,[47] and may also mimic the Sturge-Weber syndrome.[48]

Diagnosis

Most patients with a folic acid deficiency have a megaloblastic anemia. Serum folic acid levels can be measured with normal values ranging from 6 to 20 ng/mL. The red blood cell folic acid level more accurately reflects the folic acid availability at the tissue level, and this value is not as easily affected by recent intake as the serum level is. Cerebrospinal fluid folic acid levels have also been measured.

Treatment

Treatment of folic acid deficiency requires simultaneous recognition of the patient's B12 status, to avoid precipitating neurologic manifestations of B12 deficiency. However, if the serum B12 is >300 pg/mL, then it seems reasonable to treat folic acid deficiency with folic acid alone. A daily intake of 0.4 mg of folic acid is enough to avoid deficiency if demands and absorption are normal. Doses of 1 to 20 mg per day are necessary in patients with malabsorption. Treatment with folic acid rapidly corrects the anemia. Improvement of neurological abnormalities may occur over several months; complete recovery may not occur. Parenteral therapy with folinic acid may be needed in patients with methotrexate induced encephalopathy.[49]

Vitamin A

Biology

Vitamin A refers to retinol (vitamin A alcohol), whereas the term retinoids is used to describe the various derivatives of vitamin A. These include retinal (vitamin A aldehyde), retinoic acid (vitamin A acid), and the carotenoids. The latter are precursor molecules, such as beta-carotene, which are converted to retinol. Beta-carotene is available in many plant sources such as carrots, leafy green vegetables, papayas, and oranges. Preformed vitamin A (retinol) is derived in the diet from numerous animal sources. Liver and internal organs have high concentrations of vitamin A. The highest sources of retinol are liver oils of the shark, marine fish, and polar bear.[50]

The absorption, transportation, and storage of vitamin A have been thoroughly reviewed.[50] Both vitamin A (retinol) and beta-carotene are absorbed by the intestinal mucosa. Beta-carotene is cleaved within the intestinal mucosa, forming two retinol molecules. Retinol is esterified, forming retinyl palmitate, which is incorporated into chylomicrons and transported to the general circulation. The liver provides the major store of vitamin A in the form of retinyl palmitate. Retinol released from the liver by hydrolysis binds to apo-retinal binding protein (RBP), forming holo-RBP, which in turn forms a complex with transthyretin. Cell surface receptors which bind holo-RPB have been identified in several tissues, with the best studied being the retinal pigment epithelium. Within cells, retinol binds to tissue-specific cellular retinal binding proteins, which transport retinol or the oxidized form, retinoic acid, to intranuclear binding sites, where vitamin A may influence gene expression.

The recommended daily adult requirement for vitamin A is 1000 retinol equivalents. A retinol equivalent is equal to 6 µg of beta-carotene, 1 µg of retinol, or 10 international units (IU) of beta-carotene and 3.33 IU of retinol. However, when adult daily requirements are expressed in international units, the quoted amount is 5000 IU, which reflects an assumption that the U.S. diet contains roughly equal amounts of retinol and beta-carotene.

symptomatic hypocalcemia. The lack of vitamin D leads to decreased calcium absorption from the intestine. The loss of small bowel surface further reduces the ability of the intestine to absorb calcium. The lack of vitamin D and resultant hypocalcemia leads to secondary hyperparathyroidism, with excessive PTH secretion. The increased PTH drives the hydroxylation of 25 (OH) vitamin D to the active form. Hence, in many cases, the level of 1,25 (OH) vitamin D is normal, while the immediate precursor may be extremely low. Advanced renal or liver disease can lead to defective metabolism of vitamin D to its active form. Certain drugs can also interfere with the absorption or metabolism of the vitamin D. Chief among these are anticonvulsants, phenobarbital and phenytoin, which not only inhibit 25 (OH) hydroxylation in the liver, but additionally inhibit calcium absorption in the intestine. Institutionalized patients with little sun exposure who are taking anticonvulsants are especially prone to osteomalacia and myopathy.

Diagnosis of Vitamin D Deficiency

The possibility of vitamin D deficiency should be considered in any patient with known fat malabsorption, short intestine, extensive small intestinal Crohn's disease, cholestatic liver disease, severe renal disease, or in patients who present with proximal weakness, bone pain, or pathologic fractures. The diagnosis of vitamin D deficiency can usually be made by demonstrating low serum 25 (OH) vitamin D, and evidence of the metabolic consequences of the low vitamin D. These include a high alkaline phosphatase of bone origin, raised serum PTH, hypocalcemia, hypophosphatemia, a low urine calcium excretion (a 24 hour urine calcium <100 mg/24 hours), and raised urinary hydroxyproline. Radiological changes include osteopenia, pseudofractures (especially in the hip and shoulder girdles), compression fractures of the spine in adults, and rickets in children. Bone biopsy with prior tetracycline labeling may confirm osteomalacia, but this is not often required, as the clinical, laboratory, and radiographic findings usually provide sufficient information for diagnosis. Kidney disease may result in low 1,25 (OH) vitamin D, but normal 25 (OH) vitamin D. Electrophysiology in patients with myopathy due to vitamin D deficiency does not show abnormal spontaneous activity, but motor unit potentials show changes consistent with a myopathic process.[65] Muscle biopsy may show type-2 fiber atrophy.[66]

Treatment

Treatment of vitamin D deficiency is mandated by the demonstration of a low serum vitamin D level and some metabolic consequence. Of course, the underlying disease causing the vitamin D deficiency should be identified and treated concomitantly with vitamin D replacement. Vitamin D can be given by mouth as vitamin D2 or vitamin D3; 400 IU of vitamin D per day is usually adequate to prevent deficiency in individuals with minimal sun exposure. 2 to 3 hours of moderate sun exposure to 20% of body surface area, 2 to 3 days per week, is an alternative method. The sun exposure should not be great enough to cause skin erythema. This may be ineffective in the presence of smog, age >75 years, high content of melanin in the skin, latitude above 47°, and in winter time. In clinically deficient individuals, complete repletion can also be obtained by oral ingestion of 4000-8000 IU daily for several weeks if absorption is normal, or 50,000 IU weekly is sometimes used.

In malabsorptive disorders, larger doses of vitamin D and parenteral administration may be needed. Treatment with intramuscular vitamin D improves bone pain in 2 to 4 weeks, but improvement of muscle strength is much slower, sometimes taking 3 months to begin to improve. An important consideration is the presence of secondary hyperparathyroidism, which can cause very rapid hydroxylation of vitamin D, with resultant hypercalcemia, hypercalcuria and nephrolithiasis. This can usually be avoided by insuring that there is adequate calcium repletion and avoiding stimulation of PTH secretion. Secondary hyperparathyroidism can be suspected when there is an inappropriately high phosphate level. Close monitoring is important in patients given very high doses, such as 50,000 IU 3 times a week, as the threshold for toxicity is reached at 5000 IU per day. Toxicity includes hypercalcuria, hypercalcemia, and renal failure that may be only slowly reversible. These can be avoided by monitoring the serum and urine calcium and, when urinary calcium excretion exceeds 100 mg/24 hours, cutting back on the vitamin D dose. The 25 (OH) vitamin D level may also be monitored. An artificial analogue of vitamin D, called 1, alpha vitamin D, is metabolized in the liver to the active 1,25 (OH) vitamin D form, and is used frequently in Europe. In patients with severe liver dysfunction, 25 (OH)-vitamin D (calciferol) can be used, and is rapidly metabolized in the kidney.

Vitamin E Deficiency

Biology

Vitamin E is a naturally occurring substance found in many plants. The richest dietary sources include wheat germ, certain nuts, and vegetable oils. Vitamin E consists of at least eight different chemical structures, known as tocopherols and tocotrienols, which all have a 6-chromanol ring and a variable side chain.[67] The form called alpha-tocopherol has the greatest biologic activity. The synthetic form of vitamin E is *dl*-alpha-tocopherol acetate (also called all-*rac*-alpha-tocopherol), and the natural form is *d*-alpha-tocopherol acetate, also called RRR-alpha-tocopherol acetate.[68] Quantities of vitamin E are usually expressed in IU, with one IU equal to the activity of 1 mg of alpha-tocopherol acetate.

Vitamin E is absorbed predominantly in the small intestine, as a mixed micelle, together with other fat-soluble vitamins, free fatty acids, cholesterol, and monoglycerides. The ester forms of vitamin E, e.g., tocopherol acetate, are hydrolyzed before absorption. Absorption of vitamin E depends upon bile salts and the lipases in pancreatic juices for lipolysis. Vitamin E absorption is influenced by dietary lipid, such that medium chain triglycerides facilitate vitamin E absorption, while polyunsaturated fatty acids inhibit absorption.[67] There is a high correlation between total serum lipid or cholesterol levels and the serum vitamin E level.[67–69]

After absorption by the luminal epithelial cell, vitamin E is incorporated into chylomicrons which enter the mesenteric lymphatics.[67] From the mesenteric lymphatics, vitamin E in chylomicrons travels in the circulation to be distributed to the body tissues. Vitamin E is bound to various lipoproteins, with most associated with the low density lipoproteins. The main absolute stores of vitamin E are in adipose tissue, liver, and muscle. Other tissues with high concentrations of vitamin E include the adrenal gland, testis, pituitary gland, and platelets. Vitamin E is concentrated in cell fractions rich in membranes such as mitochondria and microsomes.

Cytosolic binding proteins facilitate transport of vitamin E into mitochondria and microsomal membranes.[70,71] The α-tocopherol-transfer protein is a cytosolic liver protein of critical importance for hepatic incorporation of α-tocopherol into very low density lipoproteins.[72,73] The phytyl side chain of α-tocopherol is believed to interact with the fatty acyl chain of polyunsaturated phospholipids in membranes.[67,74] There is little metabolism of vitamin E, with the major excretion being fecal.[67] A mechanism for regenerating vitamin E is described below.

Functions

The major function of vitamin E is as an antioxidant. Free radicals generated during cellular metabolic processes can interact with membrane polyunsaturated fatty acids to form peroxides. Peroxidation of lipids leads to decomposition of membranes and cellular damage. It is believed that the phytyl side chain of vitamin E is incorporated in the lipid bilayer of membranes and reacts with free radicals to protect polyunsaturated fatty acids from oxidative damage.[67,74–77] Other antioxidants, such as superoxide dismutase, catalase, glutathione peroxidase, glutathione reductase, and vitamin C, also help protect cells from oxidative degradation; however, vitamin E is felt to be critically important because of its specific location within cell membranes and its ability to remain in tissues.[67] A unique role of vitamin E in protecting against free radicals is its ability to be regenerated from the tocopheroxy radical by interacting with vitamin C.[67] The ascorbate radical formed can be reduced back to ascorbate by an NADH-dependent system. Thus, vitamin E is an essential antioxidant due to its location within membranes and the fact that it can be regenerated after reacting with free radicals. Vitamin E also appears to have the ability to inhibit platelet aggregation, secretion, and internal contraction.[78,79]

Clinical Features of Vitamin E Deficiency

Vitamin E deficiency in animals often causes a necrotizing myopathy of varying severity.[67] Other species-specific disorders caused by vitamin E deficiency are: liver necrosis in the pig, rat, and mouse; encephalomalacia in the chicken; testes degeneration; and organ-specific lipofuscin accumulation in many different species.[67]

In humans, vitamin E deficiency may be subclinical,[68] with manifestations of hemolytic anemia being clinically silent. Vitamin E is incorporated in the red blood cell membrane, and deficiency of vitamin E results in increased susceptibility of the red cell membrane to oxidative hemolysis in vitro, and a decreased life span in vivo.[67] A form of hemolytic anemia in the newborn has been attributed to use of commercial formulas high in polyunsaturated fatty acids, and low in vitamin E.[80,81] Modification of commercial formulas to increase the vitamin E content has eliminated the need for supplemental vitamin E to prevent this form of hemolytic anemia in the newborn.[67,81]

Vitamin E deficiency in humans is uncommon, but may occur under several circumstances outlined in Table 12.1. The most common cause of vitamin E deficiency is impaired fat absorption. This has been described in children with chronic cholestatic liver disease[82–86] and cystic fibrosis,[87,88] and also in adults with Crohn's disease, bowel resection,[89,90] chronic pancreatitis,[90] or bacterial overgrowth.[91] Rarely, selective impairment of vitamin E absorption may occur in the absence of fat malabsorption.[73,92–96] Such patients with isolated vitamin E deficiency have been found to have mutations in the gene encoding for the α-tocopherol-transfer protein.[73,97]

Absence of serum apolipoprotein B, known as abetalipoproteinemia, also causes vitamin E deficiency.[98–100]

Neurologic Manifestations.   Chronic vitamin E deficiency may lead to development of a serious neurologic disorder.[101] A syndrome of spinocerebellar degeneration due to vitamin E deficiency has been described in children with chronic cholestatic liver disease.[83–86] Major manifestations have included cerebellar ataxia, posterior column dysfunction, and peripheral neuropathy. Specific features reported in various combinations have included ataxic gait, dysmetria, ophthalmoplegia, areflexia, distal weakness, and sensory loss involving vibration, position, pain, and light touch sensations.[83–86] Skeletal muscle involvement has been observed, consisting of both neurogenic and myopathic components.[83,102]

A similar disorder may occur in adults with chronic fat malabsorption syndromes secondary to Crohn's disease, celiac disease, bowel resection, chronic pancreatitis, and blind loop syndrome with bacterial overgrowth.[89–91] As in the syndrome seen in children with cholestatic liver disease, gait ataxia, proprioceptive loss, and weakness are the most consistent features. In adults or children, some features of the syndrome are variable, e.g., preserved reflexes were seen in seven of nine patients in one series,[90] and extensor plantar responses are occasionally seen.[90] Although infrequently reported, retinal pigmentary degeneration and abnormal electroretinograms may occur with this disorder.[85,90,91] Somatosensory evoked potential studies may be abnormal, indicating abnormal conduction in central sensory pathways, even when peripheral nerve conduction studies are normal.[90]

A rare cause of the syndrome of spinocerebellar degeneration due to vitamin E deficiency is a selective impairment of vitamin E absorption.[73,92–96] One patient with undetectable serum vitamin E levels had evidence of familial hypercholesterolemia.[92] The patient's serum vitamin E level rose to normal with a large oral load of vitamin E. However, prolonged treatment offered little clinical improvement, presumably due to irreversible central nervous system injury. Other patients have shown mild improvement with prolonged vitamin E treatment.[73] In these patients, intestinal absorption of vitamin E and transport to the liver are normal, but hepatic incorporation of α-tocopherol into very low density lipoproteins is defective,[73,94] due to a mutation in the α-tocopherol-transfer protein.[73,97]

Another uncommon disorder with similar neurologic manifestations is abetalipoproteinemia, or Bassen-Kornzweig disease.[98–100] In this autosomal recessive condition, a complete absence of apolipoprotein-B results in inability to synthesize low-density and very-low-density lipoproteins, and resultant malabsorption of fat and fat-soluble vitamins. Acanthocytes are present, due to the lipid deficiency in the red cell membrane. Retinitis pigmentosa occurs in virtually all patients, and usually develops by the second decade. Night blindness may begin in the first or second decade. The major neurologic manifestations of abetalipoproteinemia are cerebellar ataxia, areflexia, and proprioceptive loss. Other features which may occur include ophthalmoplegia, proximal or distal weakness, and cutaneous sensory loss. The fact that the neurologic abnormalities of abetalipoproteinemia are essentially the same as those reported in vitamin E deficiency associated with other intestinal fat malabsorption syndromes, has led to speculation that the deficiency of vitamin E is the critical factor for development of the neurologic syndrome.[89,99] This association is further supported by the occurrence of a spinocerebellar syndrome in patients with mutations in the α-tocopherol-transfer protein.[73,97]

The duration of vitamin E deficiency before development of neurologic manifestations is variable. Some children with chronic cholestasis have developed neurologic manifestations as early as age two,[83] while some adults developed neurologic manifestations as late as 15 to 32 years after onset of malabsorption syndromes.[89,91,103] Patients with abetalipoproteinemia have undetectable levels of vitamin E from birth, but in some individuals, neurologic manifestations may not become apparent until the mid-teen years.[98,99]

Pathologic studies in children with the syndrome of spinocerebellar degeneration associated with biliary atresia revealed degeneration of the posterior columns and the spinocerebellar tracts. In addition, reduction of dorsal root ganglion cells, and loss of large myelinated sural nerve fibers occurred.[83] Sural nerve pathology in abetalipoproteinemia revealed reduction in fibers in the 8 to 12 micron range, with preservation of the total number of myelinated fibers. Internodal length was shorter and more variable than controls, suggesting a component of demyelinative nerve injury.[99]

Diagnosis of Vitamin E Deficiency

Serum vitamin E levels can be determined by a variety of methods including bioassays, spectrophotometric or fluorometric analysis, and chromatography (thin layer gas-liquid, and high-performance liquid).[67] High-performance liquid chromatography can also be used to determine vitamin E levels from tissue samples.[89,104]

There is evidence that the serum vitamin E level may not adequately represent the levels in tissues.[78] The serum content of vitamin E is highly correlated with the total serum lipid or cholesterol levels. Thus, disorders associated with high serum lipid levels, such as diabetes mellitus, hypothyroidism, and hypercholesterolemia, have high vitamin E levels regardless of the vitamin E stores or intake.[84] Conditions associated with low serum lipids, for example, cystic fibrosis and malabsorption syndromes, have low vitamin E levels.

In some children with vitamin E deficiency secondary to chronic cholestasis, the serum vitamin E level determination was normal as was the ratio of vitamin E to cholesterol.[84] In these children the diagnosis of vitamin E deficiency was supported by the presence of the typical neurologic syndrome known to be associated with vitamin E deficiency, and evidence of impaired intestinal absorption of vitamin E with an oral vitamin E tolerance test.[74,84] In these children, the ratio of serum vitamin E to total serum lipids was abnormally low. This information suggests that a normal serum vitamin E level does not exclude vitamin E deficiency, and that detection of vitamin E deficiency is best accomplished by evaluating the ratio of vitamin E to total serum lipids, rather than the vitamin E level in isolation or the ratio of vitamin E to cholesterol.[84]

Therapy

Treatment of vitamin E deficiency involves oral ingestion of vitamin E. The dose which is given and the success at achieving normal serum levels varies with the underlying condition causing vitamin E deficiency. Likewise, the success of improving or stabilizing the neurologic disorder varies with the underlying condition and the stage of the illness when vitamin E therapy is instituted. In general, correcting vitamin E deficiency soon after the neurologic syndrome develops is more likely to permit stabilization or improvement. Treatment of vitamin E deficiency before neurologic sequelae develop may serve to prevent the neurologic disorder from occurring.[98]

In disorders associated with insufficient bile salts to form micelles, the results of oral replacement of vitamin E are variable.[89] One patient, with mild cerebellar ataxia attributed to vitamin E deficiency and fat malabsorption secondary to multiple intestinal resections, was treated with 1.6 gm per day of DL-α-tocopheryl acetate, and showed normalization of serum vitamin E levels, and gradual improvement in walking and hand coordination.[89] Patients with blind loop formation may have fat malabsorption and vitamin E deficiency due to bacterial overgrowth that impairs normal bile-salt metabolism. Treatment of such patients includes antibiotics to reduce bacterial overgrowth, supplementation of bile salts and pancreatic enzymes, as well as high dose oral vitamin E. In some patients with blind loop syndrome, these treatments may result in correction of vitamin E levels and improvement of the neurologic syndrome.[91] In patients with isolated vitamin E deficiency, treatment with high dose oral vitamin E raises vitamin E levels from undetectable or low, to normal.[73,92] Treatment appears to stop further neurologic deterioration; however, improvement in the prominent cerebellar ataxia and sensory loss may be limited.[73,92] Excessive vitamin E intake produces few side effects, although it may exacerbate the coagulation defect associated with vitamin K deficiency.[67]

Use of Vitamin E as an Anti-Oxidant in Neurologic Syndromes.   Whilst vitamin E has been shown to be effective in animal models of neurological diseases,[105] the benefits in humans have been less definite.[106] These trials have included refractory epilepsy, Alzheimer's disease, and Parkinson's disease.

Vitamin B6 (Pyridoxine)

Biology

Vitamin B6, commonly called pyridoxine, refers to three major related chemical structures: pyridoxine, pyridoxal, and pyridoxamine, and their phosphate derivatives. Pyridoxine is a naturally occurring substance found in plants, with common dietary sources including wheat, corn, nuts, beans, fruits, and green leafy vegetables. Ingested pyridoxine is converted to the more biologically active forms, pyridoxal phosphate and pyridoamine phosphate, which are also available from animal sources such as liver, meats, eggs, and milk.

Pyridoxine is absorbed predominantly in the upper gastrointestinal tract. The mechanism of absorption is believed to be a nonsaturable passive diffusion process. Vitamin B6 is transported in the circulation in different forms with some binding to albumin and some transported in erythrocytes. Interconversion of the various forms of vitamin B6 occurs in the liver, and selected conversions occur in other tissues. Vitamin B6 is widely distributed in the body where pyridoxal phosphate is bound to tissue proteins. The major metabolite of pyridoxine is 4-pyridoxic acid, which is excreted in urine. The daily adult requirement for vitamin B6 is 2 mg for women and 2.2 mg for men. There is an increased demand for vitamin B6 during pregnancy and breastfeeding. High temperature, including pressure cooking and autoclaving, may significantly reduce the activity of vitamin B6.

Functions

Vitamin B6 functions as a major coenzyme in the intermediary metabolism of several amino acids. It acts as a coenzyme for decarboxylation, deamination, transamination, transulfuration, and desulfuration of specific amino acids. Vitamin B6 also acts as a coenzyme for kynureninase, which converts kynurenine to anthranilic acid.[107] Other actions of vitamin B6 include transfer of amino acids into cells, which may include absorption of amino acids from the intestine. Vitamin B6 is also involved in the biosynthesis of hemoglobin and sphingosine.

In the central nervous system, vitamin B6 is a codecarboxylase in the metabolism of glutamic acid to succinic acid, with the important intermediary, gamma-amino-butyric acid (GABA), produced by decarboxylation of glutamic acid. GABA is found in high concentrations in the brain and spinal cord, where it functions as an inhibitory neurotransmitter.[108]

Clinical Disorders Involving Pyridoxine

Deficiency. Because vitamin B6 is adequately supplied in most diets, nutritional deficiency is uncommon. Nutritional vitamin B6 deficiency may occur in chronic alcoholics with an inadequate diet, or in pregnant women or their newborn infants when the diet is not supplemented. Vitamin B6 deficiency is not a uniform complication of malabsorption syndromes, as only roughly 50% of patients with biopsy-proven celiac disease have reduced vitamin B6 levels.[109,110] Even following extensive distal small bowel resection, vitamin B6 absorption may remain normal.[109]

Several drugs are known to antagonize the effect of vitamin B6, leading to a deficiency state unless vitamin B6 supplementation is given. Examples include use of isoniazid or cycloserine for treatment of tuberculosis. Isoniazid forms a hydrazone complex with pyridoxal phosphate that interferes with the vitamin activity. Other drugs which may interfere with vitamin B6 function include oral contraceptives, penicillamine, and L-DOPA.[111]

Manifestations of pyridoxine deficiency may include those commonly seen with other B vitamin deficiencies such as glossitis, stomatitis, cheilosis, and dermatitis. Patients with chronic vitamin B6 deficiency may develop secondary hyperoxaluria, and thus are at a higher risk of nephrolithiasis.

In infants, pyridoxine deficiency may manifest as irritability, increased startle response, and seizures. Seizures may also occur in newborns of mothers treated with isoniazid. Seizures have occurred in adults treated with isoniazid[112] and in experimental pyridoxine deficiency produced by desoxypyridoxine, a pyridoxine antagonist.[113]

In adults, peripheral neuropathy may occur with vitamin B6 deficiency. This is usually related to treatment with isoniazid. The peripheral neuropathy complicating isoniazid use is a distal sensorimotor axonal polyneuropathy, which begins with paresthesias in the feet, followed by gradually progressive distal weakness and sensory loss. Nerve biopsy reveals axonal degeneration of myelinated and unmyelinated fibers.[114] The risk of developing neuropathy with isoniazid treatment is clearly related to vitamin B6 deficiency, as treatment with pyridoxine 100 mg/day usually prevents development of neuropathy. In addition, the risk of developing neuropathy is influenced by the individual's ability to metabolize isoniazid by acetylation. Slow acetylation is an autosomal recessively inherited trait, which predisposes to neuropathy as blood levels of isoniazid are maintained at higher levels for a longer time. Isoniazid inhibits pyridoxal phosphokinase, which is the enzyme responsible for phosphorylating pyridoxal.[115]

Dependency. Dependency syndromes refer to a number of conditions in which features of vitamin B6 deficiency are not present, but yet affected patients require pharmacologic doses of pyridoxine to maintain remission. Perhaps the best known of these syndromes is the syndrome of pyridoxine-dependent seizures which occurs in newborns or young children.[116] This is a rare autosomal recessive disorder in which seizures usually begin shortly after birth and progress to status epilepticus. The seizure type may be focal clonic, multifocal clonic, or generalized tonic-clonic. The seizures do not respond to anticonvulsant medications, but resolve promptly with intravenous injection of 50 to 100 mg of pyridoxine. Daily dietary B6 supplementation prevents recurrence.

Other vitamin B6 dependency syndromes include pyridoxine-dependent anemia, homocystinuria due to cystathionine synthetase deficiency, cystathioninuria, and xanthurenic aciduria.[117]

Pyridoxine Excess. A severe ataxic sensory polyneuropathy has been observed in individuals taking excessive amounts of vitamin B6.[118] Clinically, patients lose large fiber sensory function (vibration and position sensory modalities), and consequently become ataxic. Strength is preserved, as are pain and temperature sensory modalities. Nerve conduction studies show loss of sensory nerve action potentials with preserved motor responses and normal motor nerve conduction velocities. Experimental studies indicate this disorder is a neuronopathy due to injury of the dorsal root ganglia.[119,120]

The initial reports indicated this disorder occurred in individuals taking megadoses of pyridoxine, on the order of 2 to 6 grams per day.[118] However, subsequent reports have suggested that prolonged use of lower doses, e.g., 50 to 200 mg/day for a year, can cause a similar but less severe neuropathy.[121,122] This information, together with experimental evidence that the neuronal dysfunction from megadoses of pyridoxine is reversible within the first few days, suggests that pyridoxine is toxic to the dorsal root ganglion, and when present in excessive amounts causes neuronal dysfunction at low doses and neuronal death at high doses.

Diagnosis. Pyridoxine deficiency can be determined by a number of means. The most straightforward and commonly used method is direct assay of vitamin B6 levels in blood, with the normal value greater than 50 ng per milliliter. The lower limits of normal have been called into question.[123] Other methods of measuring vitamin B6 deficiency include: the tryptophan load test; functional enzyme assays, e.g., activity of aspartate aminotransferase in red cell hemolysates with and without pyridoxal phosphate; and urinary excretion of 4-pyridoxic acid, the major metabolite of pyridoxine. Excretion of less than 1 mg/day of 4-pyridoxic acid suggests pyridoxine deficiency. The tryptophan load test involves oral ingestion of tryptophan and measurement of urinary xanthurenic acid, which is increased in vitamin B6 deficient individuals.

MALABSORPTIVE DISEASES AND THEIR NEUROLOGIC ASSOCIATIONS

Celiac Disease

Celiac disease is an inflammatory condition of the small intestine due to an intolerance of the cereal proteins (glutens) derived from wheat, barley and rye. Celiac disease is primarily caused by an immunologically-mediated inflammation in the small intestine when exposed to gluten in the diet. Dermatitis herpetiformis (DH) is an intensely itchy, blistering skin rash affecting the extensor surfaces of the arms, legs, buttocks, and back, that is the skin manifestation of gluten sensitivity. Seventy to 80% of the DH patients have coexisting damage in the intestine. However, most patients with celiac disease do not develop the skin disease.

Pathogenesis of Celiac Disease

While it has long been recognized that celiac disease is precipitated by the exposure of the intestine to gluten, the development is the result of the concurrence of three factors: immunological, genetic, and environmental.

Immunological Processes.   There are both a cell-mediated and humoral responses evident in patients with celiac disease; however, the intestinal inflammation is predominantly a T-cell-mediated delayed hypersensitivity reaction that results in a characteristic, but not specific, pathologic abnormality in the small intestine. The pathology reveals a loss of absorptive villi, proliferation of the secretory epithelium (crypt hyperplasia), and an inflammatory infiltration of the lamina propria and surface layers (Figure 12.7).

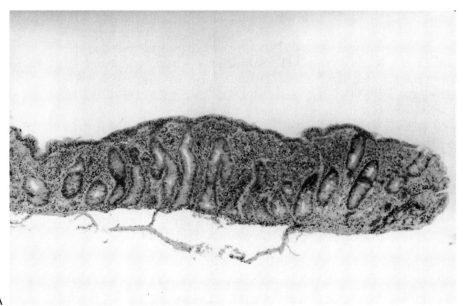

A

Figure 12.7. A. Photomicrograph of the small intestinal mucosa showing villous atrophy, crypt hyperplasia, and an inflammatory infiltrate of untreated celiac disease.

Figure continued on following page

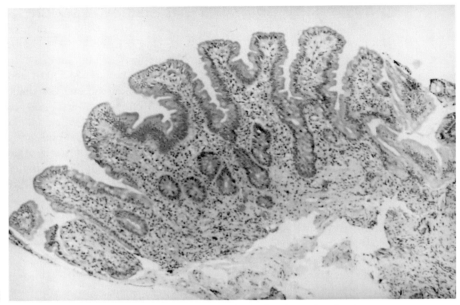

B

Figure 12.7 *Continued*. **B.** A biopsy taken from the same individual after 6 months of a gluten free diet showing significant healing.

These pathologic findings are not specific for celiac disease, but celiac disease is the common explanation in developed nations. There is a pathologic spectrum of celiac disease, and lesser degrees of damage may occur and can cause some diagnostic uncertainty, or even be discounted entirely by pathologists not familiar with the more subtle findings of celiac disease. Other immunologically-mediated disorders are also common, and include autoimmune thyroid disease, connective tissue disease, inflammatory arthropathies, Addison's disease, and juvenile onset diabetes. There is also a potent humoral response to gluten-derived peptides and to connective tissue autoantigens, recently identified as tissue transglutaminase.[124] The pathogenetic role of the antibodies is not clear, but exclusion of gluten from the diet results in loss of the measurable antibodies.

Genetics.   Although the disorder itself is not inherited, there appears to be a genetic predisposition to develop celiac disease. Celiac disease or dermatitis herpetiformis in one family member increases the risk that other family members have one condition. The familial prevalence of this disease is approximately 10 to 20% in first degree family members of a patient with celiac disease. Both dermatitis herpetiformis and celiac disease may be seen in the same family. The closer the relationship to the affected person, the higher is the risk. The highest risk, that for identical twins, is 70%, that for HLA identical sibs 30 to 40%, non-HLA identical sibs 10 to 20%, parents <10%, children <10%, others not known. About 50% of the family members so-affected are asymptomatic, in that they have a flat small intestine but no gastrointestinal symptoms.[125,126] Celiac disease susceptibility is closely associated with the major histocompatibility complex (MHC) class 2 antigen DQ2. These are encoded on chromosome 6 by the gene haplotype DRB1*0301 and DQB1*0201. Between 90 to 97% of all celiacs express this antigen. It is thought that these MHC antigens are required to present the gliadin derived peptides to reactive T-cells in the gut mucosa.[127] Twenty percent of the healthy population also expresses the same MHC antigen, suggesting that the MHC molecules are necessary, but not sufficient, for celiac disease to occur.[128] In some Southern European populations, 5 to 10% of celiacs possess DQ8 instead of DQ2. It appears that the possession of DQ2 contributes only 30% of the genetic risk for celiac disease and DQ8 even less.

Environmental Factors.   Celiac disease is unique among autoimmune diseases in that there is a known environmental precipitant, the dietary protein, gluten. What is not clear is when or why the disease presents at a specific point in time. Infant feeding practices such as early introduction of gluten and no or curtailed breast feeding, and the amount of gluten in the diet seem to be associated with a higher risk of childhood presentation.[129] Several events may precipitate symptomatic disease, including gastrointestinal surgery, parturition, viral infections, and possibly a high dose gluten challenge. It is not at all clear that these events are precipitating the sensitivity or merely interfering with the body's ability to compensate for damage that is already present.

Epidemiology

Celiac disease affects not only those peoples of Northern Europe, but also Southern Europe, the Near East, and North Africa. Case series have also been reported from Cuba, Kuwait, Sudan, and India. The reported prevalence of celiac disease varies widely from 352 per 100,000 in western Ireland to 27 per 100,000 in Portugal. Celiac disease is very rare in African-Americans and Asians. Epidemiological studies done in the USA suggest that there is a marked discrepancy between the rate of diagnosis and the actual prevalence when screening is done. One revealed the prevalence of diagnosed celiac disease in Olmsted County in Minnesota to be 1:5000.[130] The other suggested a prevalence of dermatitis herpetiformis to be 1:10,000 in Utah.[131] By contrast, a multicenter study in healthy subjects from the USA suggested a prevalence of 1:133 based on serology.[132] These likely represent only a portion of those patients with celiac disease, as in other countries the rate of diagnosis of celiac disease seems to be related to the level of suspicion for its presence. Indeed a more recent study from Olmsted County demonstrated a substantial increase in detection of celiac disease.[132a] Seemingly healthy individuals may harbor celiac disease at a significantly high rate, suggesting that the diagnosed cases are just the tip of the celiac iceberg.[133,134]

Clinical Features

Patients with celiac disease may be asymptomatic for many years prior to developing clinical features. This condition can present at any age, except for infants who have never had exposure to wheat, barley, rye, or their derivatives. However, now most cases are diagnosed in adulthood, with age at diagnosis ranging from 6 months to over 85 years.

   Celiac disease has been conceived of as a malabsorptive disease whose classic symptoms are steatorrhea, diarrhea, failure to thrive in children, and malnutrition in adults. However, the clinical features are quite variable. Symptoms include either gastrointestinal dysfunction, such as diarrhea, steatorrhea, or abdominal pain, or symptoms secondary to the malabsorption or maldigestion. Symptoms from the latter problems may be diverse, relating to anemia, malnutrition, or fat-soluble vitamin deficiencies. Many affected patients deny gastrointestinal symptoms. Some patients with complete villous atrophy may be entirely asymptomatic, with the diagnosis of celiac disease determined when screening family members of affected celiac patients.[125] Recently, atypical presentations of celiac disease have been increasingly recognized[135] (Table 12.8). Such atypical presentations may be monosymptomatic, rather than presenting with definite features of malabsorption. Celiac disease in children can result in stunting of growth and intellectual development, as well as the more classic malabsorptive symptoms. Celiac disease is also seen in greater frequency than the general population in insulin-dependent diabetes mellitus, Sjögren's syndrome, systemic lupus erythematosis, Down's syndrome, and Addison's disease.[136,137]

Neurologic Associations of Celiac Disease.   The estimated prevalence of neurologic abnormalities in celiac disease varies widely. One series of 603 cases revealed no patient with neurologic abnormalities,[138] whereas Senser reported that 52% of patients had neurologic abnormalities.[139] The reported prevalence of neurologic syndromes in these patients is undoubtedly affected by extent of evaluation, the manner of definition of neurologic abnormalities, as well as the methods used to confirm the diagnosis of celiac disease. Approximately 5% of adult patients with celiac disease may have significant neurologic disturbances. These neurologic manifestations are quite diverse (Table 12.9). The neurologic syndromes associated with celiac disease may be divided etiologically into syndromes resulting from: 1) malabsorption of specific nutrients that are recognized as causing neurologic damage; 2) autoimmune processes that can be seen in increased frequency in patients with celiac disease, such as systemic lupus, and; 3) other processes of uncertain etiology. Although most patients who develop a neurologic disorder in association with celiac disease have obvious symptoms, signs and/or laboratory evidence of malabsorption, this is not always the case. Indeed, neurologic symptoms may be the sole or major presentation of celiac disease.[140–142] Hadjivassiliou reported that covert celiac disease may be responsible for a significant proportion of neurologic syndromes for which prior investigation had not revealed a cause. Because the relationship between celiac disease and neurologic symptoms is not obvious or well-appreciated, the patient may neglect to mention the prior diagnosis of celiac disease or its associated skin condition dermatitis herpetiformis. The neurologic

Table 12.8. Atypical Presentations of Celiac Disease

Iron deficiency anemia
Lactose intolerance
Constipation
Nutritionally compensated
Osteopenia
Fatigue
Arthralgias
Brittle diabetes
Short stature
Neurological disorders
Dental enamel defects

Table 12.9. Neurologic Associations of Celiac Disease

Deficiency states	
Vitamin E	Spinocerebellar syndrome, brown bowel syndrome
Vitamin D	Proximal myopathy
Vitamin B12	Multiple problems (see text)
Vitamin A	Night blindness
Vitamin B6	Peripheral neuropathy, depression/fatigue
Calcium	Tetany
Folic acid	Combined system degeneration, dementia
Psychiatric associations	Dementia
	Depression
	Anxiety/neurosis
	Schizophrenia
	Autism
Unknown etiology	Axonal neuropathy
	Mononeuritis multiplex
	Spinocerebellar syndromes
	Headache
	Ocular myopathy
	Vasculitis
	Polymyositis
	Myoclonus
	Central demyelination
Seizure disorder	Intracerebral calcifications
Bacterial meningitis	Possibly secondary to hyposplenism

abnormalities of celiac disease may be divided into two broad categories: those due to an identifiable deficiency state relating to malabsorption, or to some other uncertain etiology.

Celiac disease leads to malabsorption of fat soluble vitamins D, E, A, and K. Pyridoxine (B6), B12, and folate deficiencies are also common. Occasionally the presentation of celiac disease consists of the neurological sequelae of deficiency of one or more of these nutrients. Parenteral thiamine and other B-complex vitamins have been given to celiac patients with poorly defined central nervous system disease with occasional improvement.[143]

In most patients with celiac disease who develop neurologic abnormality, it cannot be ascribed to an identifiable nutritional defect. These abnormalities can also be divided into central or peripheral sites of nervous system involvement. Central nervous system abnormalities include epilepsy, dementia, neuropsychiatric syndromes, spinocerebellar syndromes, chronic headaches, and subacute combined system degeneration of the cord. The peripheral nervous system is affected most commonly by a distal sensory neuropathy, but other features have also included tetany, restless leg syndrome, and myopathy. Neuropathological examination of peripheral nerves reveals demyelination, inflammation, and axonal degeneration (Figure 12.8). Autopsies have revealed variable cortical degeneration, demyelination in the spinal tracts and nerve roots, and changes suggestive of Wernicke's encephalopathy.

An increase in the prevalence of epilepsy has been reported in adult patients with celiac disease.[144] Chapman and colleagues described 9 of 185 patients with celiac disease as having epileptic symptoms, and they described the majority of these as having temporal lobe epilepsy on clinical grounds. Subsequently, Ambrosetto et al.

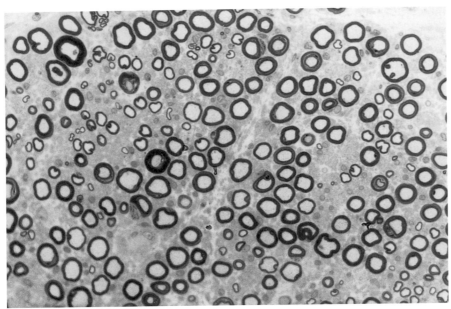

Figure 12.8. Biopsy from nerve to ancoveus showing degeneration in a patient with celiac disease (courtesy of S. Moore).

described four patients with celiac disease who also had epilepsy.[145] More recently, Fois discovered celiac disease in 9 of 783 children who presented with various forms of seizures.[146] Patients with the syndrome of celiac disease, seizures, and intracranial calcification had visual manifestations as well as ictal EEG abnormalities arising from the occipital region.[147] The calcifications were apparent on computed tomography, but not magnetic resonance imaging. A similar pattern of predominantly occipital lobe epilepsy and intracranial calcification has been described in patients with congenital folate deficiency.[148] It is more than coincidental that phenytoin interferes with folate metabolism and can exacerbate a folate deficiency.[145,149–151] Methotrexate inhibition of folic acid metabolism may result in intracranial calcification.[151] Gluten ingestion in celiac children may induce electroencephalographic changes. While the association between celiac disease and epilepsy seems unlikely to be a coincidence, the lack of a consistent benefit of a gluten free diet on the epilepsy leaves a direct causal effect in some doubt. A recent report suggested that the association, among children with childhood partial epilepsy, was confined to those with occipital paroxysms.[152] It has been suggested that by the time the celiac disease has been recognized, irreversible damage has occurred. Heightened suspicion for celiac disease in epilepsy, especially with an occipital focus, may reveal a number of hitherto undiagnosed cases, and possibly earlier dietary intervention may alter the natural history of the syndrome.[146] Patients with celiac disease diagnosed in childhood, who do not adhere to a gluten free diet, may be more likely to develop the syndrome of epilepsy with intracranial calcifications.[153,154]

Dr. William Dicke, who first recognized the pathologic nature of gluten in celiac disease, noted that children challenged with gluten often became morose, withdrawn, and depressed, often hours after the ingestion of gluten.[155] Psychiatric illness has been associated with celiac disease in several ways. It has been reported as the most frequent cause of disability in a group of celiacs in Sweden. Patients with celiac disease have a high rate of divorce (prior to diagnosis). In one Swedish study, 8 of 42 patients with celiac disease had attended a psychiatrist—5 for depression and 2 for anxiety neurosis—whereas, only 1 of 42 controls had attended a psychiatrist. The mechanism for the depression is uncertain. It seems unlikely that an adjustment reaction to the imposition of a gluten free diet is responsible, as most patients had attended a psychiatrist for an average of 15 years prior to the diagnosis of celiac disease. Metabolic abnormalities have been shown in tryptophan metabolism and monoamine metabolism. Kynurenic compounds are increased, and these may interfere with 5-HT elaboration in the brain.[156] One study has suggested that there is a therapeutic benefit to be gained in patients with depression and celiac disease with pyridoxine.

Recent reports from England have described neurologic syndromes associated with circulating gliadin antibodies and possession of the same MHC class II molecule DQ2 found in celiac disease, without any gut evidence of actual celiac disease.[157,158] These have included ataxic syndromes, and more recently migraine. The pathogenetic role of dietary gluten, the actual gliadin antibodies detected, and the benefit of a gluten free diet remain unproven in many of these syndromes.

Several connections have been suggested between schizophrenia, autism, and gluten ingestion.[159,160] Epidemiologic evidence had suggested that the population rates of admission to hospital for schizophrenia were lower in countries in which gluten was not a staple, but increased following the introduction of a western diet.[161,162] Other studies suggested that patients who were treated with a gluten free diet following admission with schizophrenia were discharged faster from the hospital.[163] Other studies did not confirm these findings.[164,165] Interestingly enough, most of these patients do not have demonstrable celiac disease on biopsy. The mechanism for the effect has been suggested to be disordered metabolism of peptide fragment derived from the wheat gliadin, which accumulate in the CSF and act as partial opioid receptor agonists.[166] A similar but unproved association has been made for autism and gluten.[167] Studies addressing the occurrence of biopsy-proven celiac disease in schizophrenia are mixed, with some suggesting a prevalence of at least 38/1000, and others very much less than that.

Investigation

Celiac disease may be suspected by the presence of a prior diagnosis of celiac disease in childhood that the individual "grew out of," or dermatitis herpetiformis. If the patient has symptoms such as steatorrhea, diarrhea, post-prandial abdominal bloating, lactose intolerance, or chronic anemia, specific investigation for malabsorption should be undertaken. Multiple biopsies taken from the proximal small intestine should suffice to confirm the diagnosis of celiac disease. In patients in whom there are no specific history or laboratory findings to suggest the presence of malabsorption, then serologic screening tests may be done to detect celiac disease. A combination of antigliadin and antiendomysial or tissue transglutaminase antibodies seem to maximize the sensitivity of the testing strategy.[168] Antiendomysial antibodies have been claimed to be highly sensitive and specific for celiac disease; however, false negatives occur in those celiacs with IgA deficiency, and perhaps in others with lesser degrees of damage. The autoantigen recognized in the endomysial test is tissue transglutaminase. This has been used as a substrate for ELISA tests that are both sensitive and almost as specific for celiac disease.[124] The gliadin antibodies are not specific for celiac disease. A single positive gliadin antibody in the absence of endomysial or tissue transglutaminase is unlikely to be due to true celiac disease.

Treatment

The primary treatment of celiac disease is a gluten free diet. While this is not an easy diet to learn and follow, it is possible, with informed dietary counseling, to both motivate and educate patients to achieve complete gluten removal from the diet. If a specific nutritional deficit is identified, it should be treated. In otherwise healthy patients with celiac disease, supplements may not be necessary, as with healing of the intestine there should be adequate absorption from dietary sources. Some patients may so restrict their diet in adapting to a gluten free diet that a regular multivitamin may help ensure an adequate intake of vitamins and minerals. It is still prudent to correct any symptomatic deficiency state. This may occasionally require parenteral therapy.

Whipple's Disease

Biology

Whipple's disease is a chronic multisystem disease caused by *Tropheryma whippelii* that affects predominantly the gastrointestinal, rheumatological, neurological, and lymphatic systems.[169] It affects males more than females, with a tendency to occur in the 5th and 6th decades of life. It is a rare disease, with no more than a few hundred cases reported in the literature. However, this is probably an underestimation, as many cases no longer are reported. Whipple's disease differs from other malabsorptive diseases in that the neurologic disease is usually the result of direct infection of the central nervous system, rather than as a consequence of deficiency of some nutrient. In addition, non-gastrointestinal symptoms predominate. These include arthralgias, fever, generalized malaise, and lymphadenopathy. The organism that has long been suspected as the cause of the disease, *Tropheryma whippelii*, a gram positive, PAS positive rod-shaped bacteria, has been characterized using molecular techniques and has been successfully cultured in a human fibroblast culture line with a shell vial assay.[170] Several recent reports have applied modern molecular techniques to identify the ribosomal RNA sequences extracted from involved tissues.[171–173] The organisms have been classified as part of the *Actinomycetes* family though they have similarities to other organisms.

Pathology

The small intestinal disease is characterized by: 1) the presence of large foamy macrophages in the lamina propria along with dilated lymph channels packed with lipid material; 2) small intracellular rod-shaped bacteria (*Tropheryma whippelii*); and 3) engorgement of the mesenteric lymphatics. Remarkably similar features are seen in the intestine in association with infection with *Mycobaterium avium intercellulare* in patients with the acquired immunodeficiency syndrome. The intestinal

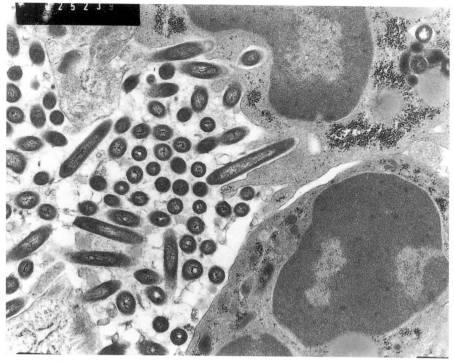

Figure 12-9. Electron microscopic picture of Whipple organism (courtesy of S. Bonsib).

changes may be patchy. Other features of the disease include involvement of serosal membranes, including the peritoneum, pleura, pericardia, synovium, myocardium, endocardium, and lymphedema.

Central nervous system involvement is, typically, a diffuse patchy involvement of the brain. There may occasionally be multiple mass lesions.[174] Involved areas of the brain usually show the bacterium. Whipple organisms have not been identified in peripheral nerves, even though peripheral neuropathy has been reported. In contrast, Whipple's organisms have been identified in skeletal muscle in patients with myopathy in association with Whipple's disease.[175]

Clinical Features

Whipple's disease affects predominantly males in the 5th and 6th decades; however, cases involving women and children have been described. Most cases of Whipple's disease present with gastrointestinal and systemic manifestations, most typically weight loss, arthralgias, fevers, and steatorrhea. Physical examination may reveal evidence for malabsorption, with malnutrition often accompanied by hyperpigmentation and diffuse lymphadenopathy. Abdominal distension and steatorrheic stool may also be identified. Anemia, dyspnea, bipedal edema, and erythema nodosum have occasionally been described. There are rare cases of central nervous system Whipple's disease presenting in the absence of gastrointestinal involvement. However, frequently the gastrointestinal symptoms may not be obvious. Symptoms relating to nervous system involvement of Whipple's are protean. Most commonly, these include disorders of mentation, characterized by psychosis, amnesia, depression, or dementia. The neurologic syndrome associated with Whipple's disease typically consists of impaired cognition and a peculiar slow (1 Hz) convergent divergent high amplitude pendular nystagmus. This is often associated with arrhythmic movements of the masticatory muscles and occasionally of the limbs. Indeed, the finding of so-called oculofacial myorhythmia is a pathognomonic feature of central involvement of Whipple's disease.[176] Cerebellar ataxia, myoclonus, progressive nerve deafness, ocular involvement,[177] and papilledema have also been described. Pyramidal tract signs and Parkinsonian features have also been identified. Disorders of eye movement, as well as direct involvement of the structures of the eye, have all been identified. Non-specific symptoms of headache, disturbed sleep patterns, and increased appetite have also been identified. Spasticity, loss of vibration, and proprioception may also be seen. Peripheral neuropathy and proximal myopathy have also been described. Eye examination may reveal vertical nystagmus. Papilledema may also be present, and vitreous opacities have been described.[178] Whipple's bacilli have been identified in the eye using molecular techniques.

Neurologic involvement has also been described in patients without evident intestinal symptoms, and indeed rarely in patients who have no evidence for Whipple's disease affecting the intestine. The central nervous system may also be the site of symptomatic relapse following seemingly successful treatment for intestinal involvement, often with antibiotics which have poor penetration to the central nervous system, such as tetracycline.

Diagnosis

The diagnosis of Whipple's disease is often suspected on the basis of a history of chronic illness, features of malnutrition or malabsorption, and atypical manifestations like pigmentation, arthropathy, and lymphadenopathy. Laboratory abnormalities include markedly raised white cell count, often with lymphocytosis, and anemia which may be microcytic, macrocytic, or combined. Laboratory features of malabsorption can also be seen with hypoproteinemia, excessive fat in the stool, and diminished serum folate.

Brain imaging, while not specific, may be suggestive of Whipple's disease. CT scans have been, on the whole, relatively unhelpful, being normal in most patients with Whipple's disease. Magnetic imaging will often demonstrate high signal intensity in the hypothalamus, uncus, and medial temporal lobes on T2 weighted images. A CSF examination will often reveal a moderately raised protein and IgG. A PAS stain may reveal positively staining macrophages in the CSF.

Definitive diagnosis is usually readily obtained by examining biopsies from the duodenum which reveal the characteristic pathological findings. The PAS positive inclusions in foamy macrophages are easily identified if multiple biopsies are taken from the small intestine. The bacteria can be easily differentiated from the intracellular inclusions of mycobacterium avium intracellulare (MAI) by acid fast staining. The Whipple bacterium is acid fast negative, while the MAI is positive. Electron microscopy of the small bowel biopsies also may reveal the organisms with a characteristic rod-like shape (Figure 12.9). Recent developments using molecular analysis have allowed PCR amplification of the 16s ribosomal RNA sequences that seem to be specific for Whipple's organism.[179] This provides a powerful molecular tool that will allow precise identification of the infection, either from tissue or even in peripheral blood.[172,180]

There are rare cases in which small intestinal involvement is absent, in which case tissue from the affected organ may reveal the presence of PAS staining macrophages. Brain biopsy has a relatively low yield, probably due to the patchy nature of the lesions in the brain. Hence, most would advocate the use of empiric antibiotic therapy in patients in whom there is a high suspicion for Whipple's disease.

The differential diagnosis includes celiac disease, small bowel ischemia, or *mycobacterium avium intracellulare,* occurring in the setting of HIV infection, sarcoidosis, or endocarditis.[181] Most are readily differentiated from Whipple's disease. Occasionally lipophages (lipid laden macrophages) may be mistaken for the macrophages of Whipple's disease; however, the PAS stain should readily differentiate between these.

Treatment

The treatment essentially is antibiotic treatment, preferably an agent with penetration into the central nervous system, such as ceftriaxone or trimethoprim/sulfamethoxazole. Alternatives such as ceftriaxone intravenously, or chloramphenicol and trimethoprim/sulfamethoxazole have also been moderately efficacious. The tetracycline of choice is probably minocycline. Neurologic relapse is common in patients who initially have responded to prior antibiotic therapy; hence, long-term suppressive therapy is probably indicated.[182] Dementia, while often arrested by antibiotic therapy, is usually not improved, whereas more acute confusional states may respond, emphasizing the importance of prompt therapy. The ocular and facial myorhythmias usually respond to antibiotic therapy. The response to therapy is primarily monitored by clinical improvement. Typically, fever, arthralgias, and gastrointestinal involvement respond first, with an often slower response of neurological deficits. If there are mass-like abnormalities seen on MRI, these will usually respond and often clear completely. Long-term follow up should be planned, as there is a definite chance of relapse, often in the central nervous system. It may be possible to use molecular techniques to monitor response to therapy and possibly identify relapse before serious complications occur.

Post-Gastrectomy Syndromes

The surgical removal of part or all of the stomach[183] and a now abandoned bariatric operation, the jejuno-ileal bypass,[184] frequently result in malabsorption. The Billroth II distal partial gastrectomy with gastrojejunostomy is especially prone to result in steatorrhea, iron, B12, and folic acid deficiency. This is the result of a combination of rapid gastric emptying, less than adequate bile acid and pancreatic secretions for fat emulsification and digestion, rapid intestinal transit due to vagotomy, and bacterial overgrowth in the afferent loop syndrome. Reduced food intake is common due to early satiety caused by reduction in the size of the stomach.

Clinical Features

The gastrointestinal manifestations can include early satiety, weight loss, steatorrhea, post prandial diarrhea, and dumping syndrome. Dumping syndrome is hypoglycemia and hypotension due to the rapid emptying of gastric contents into the unprepared intestine.[185] These syndromes have been associated with a wide range of neurologic perturbations. These may be the result of B12 deficiency, folate deficiency, or steatorrhea, with consequent depletion of fat soluble vitamins, including vitamins D and E.[186] The diagnosis is easily made by identifying the surgery, usually apparent from the patients history and by identifying the abdominal scar, usually an upper midline incision. In uncertain cases where the original surgical record is unavailable, upper endoscopy or contrast radiology should readily disclose the post surgical anatomy. Treatment consists of surgical correction in the case of the jejunal ileal bypass, and nutritional replacement in the post-gastrectomy situation.

REFERENCES

1. Craig RM, Atkinson AJ Jr. D-xylose testing: a review. Gastroenterology 1988;95: 223–231.
2. Cano N. Disorders of cobalamin metabolism. Crit Rev Oncol Hematol 1995;3:1–34.
3. Poston JM. Leucine 2,3-aminomutase, an enzyme of leucine catabolism. J Biol Chem 1976; 251:1859–1863.
4. Stabler SP, Lindenbaum J, Allen RH. Failure to detect beta-leucine in human blood or leucine 2,3-aminomutase in rat liver using capillary gas chromatography-mass spectrometry. J Biol Chem 1988;263:5581–5588.
5. Kinsella LJ, Green R. `Anesthetic Paresthetica' nitrous oxide-induced cobalamin deficiency. Neurology 1995;45:1608–1610.
6. Layzer RB. Myeloneuropathy after prolonged exposure to nitrous oxide. Lancet 1979; 2:1227–1230.
7. Saltzman JR, Kemp JA, Golner BB, et al. Effect of hypochlorhydria due to omeprazole treatment or atrophic gastritis on protein-bound vitamin B12 absorption. J Am Coll Nutr 1994; 13:584–591.
8. Marcuard SP, Albernaz L, Khazanie PG. Omeprazole therapy causes malabsorption of cyanocobalamin (vitamin B12). Ann Int Med 1994;120:211–215.
9. Kittang E, Aadland E, Schjonsby H, Rohss K. The effect of omeprazole on gastric acidity and the absorption of liver cobalamins. Scand J Gastroenterol 1987;22:156–160.
10. Koop H, Bachem MG. Serum iron, ferritin, and vitamin B12 during prolonged omeprazole therapy. J Clin Gastroenterol 1992;14:288–292.
11. Healton EB, Savage DG, Brust JC, et al. Neurologic aspects of cobalamin deficiency. Medicine 1991;70:229–245.
12. Karnaze DS, Carmel R. Neurologic and evoked potential abnormalities in subtle cobalamin deficiency states, including deficiency without anemia and with normal absorption of free cobalamin. Arch Neurol 1990;47:1008–1012.
13. Lindenbaum J, Healton EB, Savage DG, et al. Neuropsychiatric disorders caused by cobalamin deficiency in the absence of anemia or macrocytosis. N Engl J Med 1988; 318:1720–1728.
14. Louwman MW, van Dusseldorp M, van de Vijver FJ, et al. Signs of impaired cognitive function in adolescents with marginal cobalamin status. Am J Clin Nutr 2000;72:762–769.
15. Shovron SD, Carney MWP, Chanarin I, Reynolds EH. The neuropsychiatry of megaloblastic anaemia. Brit Med J 1980;281:1036–1038.
16. Regland B, Gottfries CG, Lindstedt G. Dementia patients with low serum cobalamin concentration: relationships to atrophic gastritis. Aging Clin Exp Res 1992;4:35–41.
17. Shemesh Z, Attias J, Ornan M, et al. Vitamin B12 deficiency in patients with chronic-tinnitus and noise-induced hearing loss. Am J Otolaryngol 1993;14:94–99.
18. Blunt SB, Silva M, Kennard C, Wise R. Vitamin B12 deficiency presenting with severe pseudoathetosis of upper limbs. Lancet 1994;343:550.
19. Areekul S, Roongpisuthipong C, Churdchu K, Thanomsak W. Optic neuropathy in a patient with vitamin B12 deficiency: a case report. J Med Assoc Thailand 1992;75:715–718.
20. Wilhelm H, Grodd W, Schiefer U, Zrenner E. Uncommon chiasmal lesions: demyelinating disease, vasculitis, and cobalamin deficiency. German J Ophthalmol 1993;2:234–240.

21. Schilling RF. Intrinsic factor studies II: the effect of gastric juice on the urinary excretion of radioactivity after the oral administration of radioactive vitamin B12. J Lab Clin Med 1953; 42:860–866.
22. Katz JH, Dimase J, Donaldson RM Jr. Simultaneous administration of gastric juice bound and free radioactive cyanocobalamin: rapid procedure for differentiating between factor deficiency and other causes of vitamin B12 malabsorption. J Lab Clin Med 1963;61:266–269.
23. Briedis D, McIntyre PA, Judisch J. An evaluation of a dual isotope method for the measurement of B12 absorption. J Nucl Med 1973;14:135.
24. Lucas MH, Elgazzar AH. Detection of protein bound vitamin B12 malabsorption. A case report and review of the literature. Clin Nucl Med 1994;19:1001–1003.
25. Doscherholmen A, Silvis S, McMahon J. Dual isotope Schilling test for measuring absorption of food bound and free vitamin B12 simultaneously. Am J Clin Pathol 1984;80:490–499.
26. Magnus E, Muller C. A new peroral non-radioactive vitamin B12 absorption test compared with the Schilling test. Eur J Haemat 1995;54:117–119.
27. Carmel R, Perez-Perez GI, Blaser MJ. Helicobacter pylori infection and food-cobalamin malabsorption. Dig Dis Sci 1994;39:309–314.
28. Jones BP, Broomhead AF, Kwan YL, Grace CS. Incidence and clinical significance of protein-bound vitamin B12 malabsorption. Eur J Haematol 1987;38:131–136.
29. Carmel R, Aurangzeb I, Qian D. Associations of food-cobalamin malabsorption with ethnic origin, age, Helicobacter pylori infection, and serum markers of gastritis. Am J Gastroenterol 2001;96:63–70.
30. Bastrup-Madsen P, Helleberg-Rasmussen I, Norregaard S, et al. Long term therapy of pernicious anemia with depot cobalamin preparation betolvex. Scand J Haematol 1983; 31:57.
31. Berlin H, Berlin R, Brante G. Oral treatment of pernicious anemia with high doses of vitamin B12 without intrinsic factor. Acta Med Scand 1968;184:247–258.
32. Slot WB, Merkus FW, Van Deventer SJ, Tytgat GN. Normalization of plasma vitamin B12 concentration by intranasal hydroxocobalamin in vitamin B12-deficient patients. Gastroenterology 1997;113:430–433.
33. Delpre G, Stark P, Niv Y. Sublingual therapy for cobalamin deficiency as an alternative to oral and parenteral cobalamin supplementation. Lancet 1999;354:740–741.
34. Elia M. Oral or parenteral therapy for B12 deficiency. Lancet 1998;352:1721–1722.
35. Hall CA, Begley JA, Green-Colligan PD. The availability of therapeutic hydroxycobalamin to cells. Blood 1984;63:335–341.
36. Schulman R. Psychiatric aspects of pernicious anemia: a prospective controlled investigation. Brit Med J 1967;3:266–270.
37. Czeilel AE, Dudas I. Prevention of the first occurrence of neural tube defects by periconceptual vitamin supplements. N Engl J Med 1992;327:1832–1835.
38. Gerson CD, Hepner GW, Brown N, et al. Inhibition by diphenylhydantoin of folic acid absorption in man. Gastroenterology 1972;63:246–251.
39. Rivey MP, Schottelius DD, Berg MJ. Phenytoin-folic acid: a review. Drug Intell Clin Pharm 1984;18:292–301.
40. Ogawa Y, Kaneko S, Otani K, Fukushima Y. Serum folic acid levels in epileptic mothers and their relationship to congenital malformations. Epilepsy Res 1991;8:75–78.
41. Dansky LV, Rosenblatt DS, Andermann E. Mechanisms of teratogenesis: folic acid and antiepileptic therapy. Neurology 1992;42 (4 Suppl 5):32–42.
42. Bramanti P, Ricci RM, Bagala S, et al. Does folic acid exert a provocative action on the EEG of epileptic patients? A preliminary report. Acta Neurologica 1987;9:250–255.
43. Pincus JH. Folic acid in neurology, psychiatry and internal medicine. In MI Botez, EH Reynolds (eds), Folic Acid Deficiency: a Cause of Subacute Combined System Degeneration. New York: Raven Press, 1979;427–434.
44. Pincus JH, Reynolds EH, Glaser GH. Subacute combined system degeneration with folate deficiency. JAMA 1972;221:496–497.
45. Manzoor M, Runcie J. Folate responsive neuropathy: report of 10 cases. Br Med J 1976; 1:1176–1178.
46. Grant HC, Hoffbrand AV, Wells DG. Folate deficiency and neurological disease. Lancet 1965;2:763–767.

47. Ventura A, Bouquet F, Sartorelli C, et al. Coeliac disease, folic acid deficiency and epilepsy with cerebral calcifications. Acta Paediatr Scand 1991;80:559–562.

48. Garwicz S, Mortensson W. Intracranial calcification mimicking the Sturge-Weber syndrome: a consequence of cerebral folic acid deficiency. Pediatr Radiol 1976;5:5–9.

49. Kay HE, Knapton PJ, O'Sullivan JP, et al. Encephalopathy in acute leukemia associated with methotrexate therapy. Arch Dis Child 1972;47:344–354.

50. Olson JA. Vitamin A. In LJ Machlin (ed), Handbook of Vitamins, 2nd Edition. New York: Marcel Dekker, 1991;1–57.

51. Ong DE, Chytil F. Vitamin A and cancer. Vitam Horm 1983;40:105–144.

52. Sporn MB, Roberts AB. The role of retinoids in differentiation and carcinogenesis. Cancer Res 1983;43:3034–3040.

53. Scrimshaw NS, Behar M. Protein malnutrition in young children. Science 1961; 133:2039–2047.

54. Henry HL, Norman AW. Vitamin D: metabolism and metabolic actions. Annu Rev Nutr 1984;4:493–520.

55. Stio M, Lunghi B, Iantomasi T, et al. Effect of vitamin D deficiency and 1,25-dihydroxy-vitamin D3 on metabolism and D-glucose transport in rat cerebral cortex. J Neurosci Res 1993;35:559–566.

56. Saporito MS, Wilcox HM, Hartpence KC, et al. Pharmacological induction of nerve growth factor mRNA in adult rat brain. Exp Neurol 1993;123:295–302.

57. Naveilhan P, Neveu I, Baudet C, et al. Expression of 25(OH) vitamin D3 24-hydroxylase gene in glial cells. Neuroreport 1993;5:255–257.

58. Bidmon HJ, Stumpf WE. Distribution of target cells for 1,25-dihydroxyvitamin D3 in the brain of the yellow bellied turtle Trachemys scripta. Brain Res 1994;640:277–285.

59. Cai Q, Tapper DN, Gilmour RF Jr, et al. Modulation of the excitability of avian peripheral nerves by vitamin D: relation to calbindin-D28k, calcium status and lipid composition. Cell Calcium 1994;15:401–410.

60. Rimaniol JM, Authier FJ, Chariot P. Muscle weakness in intensive care patients: initial manifestation of vitamin D deficiency. Intensive Care Med 1994;20:591–592.

61. Gilchrist JM. Osteomalacic myopathy. Muscle Nerve 1995;8:360–361.

62. Martinelli P, Giuliani S, Ippoliti M, et al. Familial idiopathic strio-pallido-dentate calcifications with late onset extrapyramidal syndrome. Mov Disord 1993;8:220–222.

63. Gloth FM 3rd, Lindsay JM, Zelesnick LB, Greenough WB 3rd. Can vitamin D deficiency produce an unusual pain syndrome? Arch Intern Med 1991;151:1662–1664.

64. Leichtmann GA, Bengoa JM, Bolt MJ, Sitrin MD. Intestinal absorption of cholecalciferol and 25-hydroxycholecalciferol in patients with both Crohn's disease and intestinal resection. Am J Clin Nutr 1991;54:548–552.

65. Skaria J, Katiger BC, Srivastava TP, Dube B. Myopathy and neuropathy associated with osteomalacia. Acta Neurol Scand 1975;51:37–58.

66. Isenberg DA, Newham D, Edwards RH, et al. Muscle strength and pre-osteomalacia in vegetarian Asian women. Lancet 1982;1:55.

67. Machlin LJ. Vitamin E. In LJ Machlin (ed), Handbook of Vitamins. 2nd ed. New York: Marcel Dekker, 1991;99–144.

68. Bieri JG, Corash L, Hubbard VS. Medical uses of vitamin E. N Engl J Med 1983; 308:1063–1071.

69. Horwitt MK, Harvey CC, Dahm CH, Searcy MT. Relationship between tocopherol and serum lipid levels for determination of nutritional adequacy. Ann NY Acad Sci 1972;203: 223–236.

70. Mowri H, Nakagawa Y, Inoue K, Nojima S. Enhancement of the transfer of alpha-tocopherol between liposomes and mitochondria by rat-liver protein(s). Eur J Biochem 1981;117: 537–542.

71. Murphy DJ, Mavis RD. Membrane transfer of alpha-tocopherol. Influence of alpha-tocopherol-binding factors from the liver, lung, heart and brain of the rat. J Biol Chem 1981; 256:10464–10468.

72. Traber MG, Sokol RJ, Burton GW, et al. Impaired ability of patients with familial isolated vitamin E deficiency to incorporate alpha-tocopherol into lipoproteins secreted by the liver. J Clin Invest 1990;85:397–407.

73. Gotoda T, Arita M, Arai H, et al. Adult-onset spinocerebellar dysfunction caused by a mutation in the gene for the alpha-tocopherol-transfer protein. N Engl J Med 1995; 333:1313–1318.

74. Sokol RJ, Heubi JE, Iannaccone ST, et al. Mechanism causing vitamin E deficiency during chronic childhood cholestasis. Gastroenterology 1983;85:1172–1182.

75. Lucy JA. Structural interaction between vitamin E and polyunsaturated phospholipids. In E deDuve, O Hayaishi (eds), Tocopherol, Oxygen, and Biomembranes. New York: Elsevier/North Holland Biomedical Press, 1978;109–120.

76. Zappel AL. Vitamin E and selenium protection from in vitro lipid peroxidation. Ann NY Acad Sci 1980;55:18–31.

77. Burton GS, Ingold KU. Auto-oxidation of biological molecules: the antioxidant activity of vitamin E and related chain-breaking phenolic antioxidants in vitro. J Am Chem Soc 1981; 103:6472–6477.

78. Fong JS. Alpha-tocopherol: its inhibition on human platelet aggregation. Experientia 1976;32:639–641.

79. Steiner M, Anastasi J. Vitamin E: an inhibitor of the platelet release reaction. J Clin Invest 1976;57:732–737.

80. Williams ML, Shot RJ, O'Neal PL, Osaka FA. Role of dietary iron and fat on vitamin E deficiency anemia of infancy. N Engl J Med 1975;292:887–890.

81. Ehrenkranz RA. Vitamin E and the neonate. Am J Dis Child 1980;134:1157–1186.

82. Alagille D, Odievre M, Gautier M. Hepatic ductular hypoplasia associated with characteristic facies, vertebral malformations, retarded physical, mental, and sexual development, and cardiac murmur. J Pediatrics 1975;86:63–71.

83. Rosenblum JL, Keating JP, Prensky AL, Nelson JS. A progressive neurologic syndrome in children with chronic liver disease. N Engl J Med 1981;304:503–508.

84. Sokol RJ, Heubi JE, Iannaccone ST, et al. Vitamin E deficiency with normal serum vitamin E concentrations in children with chronic cholestasis. N Engl J Med 1984;310: 1209–1212.

85. Tomasi LG. Reversibility of human myopathy caused by vitamin E deficiency. Neurology 1979;29:1183–1185.

86. Guggenheim MA, Ringel SP, Silverman A, Grabert BE. Progressive neuromuscular disease in children with chronic cholestasis and vitamin E deficiency: diagnosis and treatment with alpha tocopherol. J Pediatr 1982;100:51–58.

87. Farrell PM, Bieri JG, Fratantoni JF, et al. The occurrence and effects of human vitamin E deficiency: a study in patients with cystic fibrosis. J Clin Invest 1977;60:233–241.

88. Geller A, Gilles F, Schwachman H. Degeneration of fasciculus gracilis in cystic fibrosis. Neurology 1977;27:185–187.

89. Harding AE, Muller DPR, Thomas PK, Willison HJ. Spinocerebellar degeneration secondary to chronic intestinal malabsorption: a vitamin E deficiency syndrome. Ann Neurol 1982; 12:419–425.

90. Satya-Murti S, Howard L, Krohel G, Wolf B. The spectrum of neurologic disorder from vitamin E deficiency. Neurology 1986;36:917–921.

91. Brin MF, Fetell MR, Green PH, et al. Blind loop syndrome, vitamin E malabsorption, and spinocerebellar degeneration. Neurology 1985;35:338–342.

92. Harding AE, Matthews S, Jones S, et al. Spinocerebellar degeneration associated with a selective defect of vitamin E absorption. N Engl J Med 1985;313:32–35.

93. Krendel DA, Gilchrist JM, Johnson AO, Bossen EH. Isolated deficiency of vitamin E with progressive neurologic deterioration. Neurology 1987;37:538–540.

94. Laplante P, Vanesse M, Michaud J, et al. A progressive neurological syndrome associated with an isolated vitamin E deficiency. Can J Neurol Sci 1984;11(Suppl):561–564.

95. Sokol RJ, Kayden HJ, Bettis DB, et al. Isolated vitamin E deficiency in the absence of fat malabsorption-familial and sporadic cases: characterization and investigation of causes. J Lab Clin Med 1988;111:548–559.

96. Stumpf DA, Sokol R, Bettis D, et al. Friedreich's disease: V. Variant form with vitamin E deficiency and normal fat absorption. Neurology 1987;37:68–74.

97. Ouahchi K, Arita M, Kayden H, et al. Ataxia with isolated vitamin E deficiency is caused by mutations in the α-tocopherol transfer protein. Nat Genet 1995;9:141–145.

 98. Herbert PN, Gotto AM, Fredrickson DS. Familial lipoprotein deficiency. In JH Stanbury, DS Wyngaarden, DS Fredrickson (eds), The Metabolic Basis of Inherited Disease. New York: McGraw-Hill, 1978;544–588.

 99. Miller RG, Davis CJ, Illingworth DR, Bradley W. The neuropathy of abetalipoproteinemia. Neurology 1980;30:1286–1291.

100. Sobrevilla LA, Goodman ML, Kane CA. Demyelinating central nervous system disease, macular atrophy and acanthocytosis (Bassen-Kornzweig syndrome). Am J Med 1964; 237:823–828.

101. Muller DP, Lloyd JK, Wolff OH. Vitamin E and neurological function. Lancet 1983; 1:225–227.

102. Neville HE, Ringel SP, Guggenheim A, et al. Ultrastructural and histochemical abnormalities of skeletal muscle in patients with chronic vitamin E deficiency. Neurology 1983;33:483–488.

103. Weder B, Meienberg O, Wildi E, Meier C. Neurologic disorder of vitamin E deficiency in acquired intestinal malabsorption. Neurology 1984;34:1561–1565.

104. Kayden HJ, Hatam LJ, Traber MG. The measurement of nanograms of tocopherol by HPLC from needle aspiration biopsies of adipose tissue: normal and abetalipoproteinemic subjects. J Lipid Res 1983;24:652–656.

105. Gurney ME, Cutting FB, Zhai P, et al. Benefit of vitamin E, riluzole, and gabapentin in a transgenic model of familial amyotrophic lateral sclerosis. Ann Neurol 1996;39:147–157.

106. Delanty N, Dichter MA. Antioxidant therapy in neurologic disease. Arch Neurol 2000; 57:1265–1270.

107. Harper HA. The water-soluble vitamins. In HA Harper, VW Rodwell, PA Mays (eds), Review of Physiological Chemistry, 16th ed. Los Altos, CA: Harper Lange, 1977;156–181.

108. Cooper JR, Bloom FE, Roth RH. Amino Acids. The Biochemical Basis of Neuropharmacology, 4th ed. New York: Oxford University Press, 1982;249–256.

109. Brain MC, Booth CC. The absorption of tritium-labeled pyridoxine HCl in control subjects and in patients with intestinal malabsorption. Gut 1964;5:241–247.

110. Morris JS, Ajdukiewicz AB, Read AE. Neurological disorders in adult coeliac disease. Gut 1970;11:549–554.

111. Leklem JE. Vitamin B6. In LJ Machlin (ed), Handbook of Vitamins, 2nd Edition. New York: Marcel Dekker, 1991;376–377.

112. Reilly RH, Killam KF, Jenney EH, et al. Convulsant effects of isoniazid. JAMA 1953;152: 1317–1321.

113. Vilter RW, Mueller JF, Glazer HS, et al. The effect of vitamin B6 deficiency induced by desoxypyridoxine in human beings. J Lab Clin Med 1953;42:335–357.

114. Ochoa J. Isoniazid neuropathy in man: quantitative electron microscope study. Brain 1970;93:831.

115. Blakemore WF. Isoniazid. In PS Spencer, HH Schaumburg (eds), Experimental and Clinical Neurotoxicology. Baltimore: Williams & Wilkins, 1980;476–489.

116. Haenggeli CA, Girardin E, Paunier L. Pyridoxine-dependent seizures, clinical and therapeutic aspects. Eur J Pediatr 1991;150:452–455.

117. Mudd SH. Pyridoxine-responsive genetic disease. Fed Proc 1971;30:970–976.

118. Schaumburg HH, Kaplan J, Windebank A, et al. Sensory neuropathy from pyridoxine abuse: a new megavitamin syndrome. N Engl J Med 1983;309:445–448.

119. Krinke G, Naylor DC, Skorpil V. Pyridoxine megavitaminosis: an analysis of the early changes induced with massive doses of vitamin B6 in rat primary sensory neurons. J Neuropathol Exp Neurol 1985;44:117–129.

120. Krinke G, Schaumburg HH, Spencer PS, et al. Pyridoxine megavitaminosis produces degeneration of peripheral sensory neurons (sensory neuronopathy) in the dog. Neurotoxicology 1981;2:13–24.

121. Parry GJ, Bredesen DE. Sensory neuropathy with low-dose pyridoxine. Neurology 1985; 35:1466–1468.

122. Dalton K, Dalton MJ. Characteristics of pyridoxine overdose neuropathy syndrome. Acta Neurol Scand 1987;76:8–11.

123. Bailey AL, Wright AJ, Southon S. High performance liquid chromatography method for the determination of pyridoxal-5-phosphate in human plasma: how appropriate are cut-off values for vitamin B6 deficiency? Eur J Clin Nutr 1999;53:448–455.

124. Dieterich W, Ehnis T, Bauer M, et al. Identification of tissue transglutaminase as the autoantigen of celiac disease. Nat Med 1997;3:797–801.
125. Stokes PL, Ferguson R, Holmes GK, Cooke WT. Familial aspects of coeliac disease. Q J Med 1976;180:567–582.
126. Mylotte M, Egan-Mitchell B, Fottrell PF, et al. Family studies in coeliac disease. Q J Med 1974;171:359–369.
127. Sollid LM. Molecular basis of celiac disease. Ann Rev Immunol 2000;18:53–81.
128. Marsh MN. Gluten, major histocompatibility complex, and the small intestine. Gastroenterology 1992;102:330–354.
129. Ivarsson A, Persson LA, Nystrom L, et al. Epidemic of coeliac disease in Swedish children. Acta Paediatrica 2000;89:165–171.
130. Talley NJ, Valdovinos M, Petterson TM, Carpenter HA. Epidemiology of celiac sprue: a community-based study. Am J Gastroenterol 1994;89:843–846.
131. Smith JB, Tulloch JE, Meyer LJ, Zone JJ. The incidence and prevalence of dermatitis herpetiformis in Utah. Arch Dermatol 1992;128:1608–1610.
132. Fasano A, Berti I, Gerarduzzi T, et al. Prevalence of celiac disease in at-risk and not-at-risk groups in the United States: a large mutlicenter study. Arch Intern Med 2003;163:286–292.
132a. Murray JA, van Dyke C, Plevak MF, et al. Trends in the identification and clinical features of celiac features of celiac disease in a North American community 1950-2001. Clin Gastroenterol Hepatol 2003;1:19–27.
133. Grodzinsky E, Franzen L, Hed J, Strom M. High prevalence of coeliac disease in healthy adults revealed by antigliadin antibodies. Ann Allergy 1992;69:66–69.
134. Catassi C, Ratsch IM, Fabiani E, et al. Coeliac disease in the year 2000: exploring the iceberg. Lancet 1994;343:200-203.
135. Ferguson A, Arranz E, O'Mahony S. Clinical and pathological spectrum of celiac disease, active, silent, latent and potential. Gut 1993;34:150–151.
136. Collin P, Reunala T, Pukkala E, et al. Coeliac disease – associated diseases and survival. Gut 1994;35:1215–1218.
137. Hilhorst MI, Brink M, Wauters EA, Houwen RH. Down syndrome and coeliac disease: five new cases with a review of the literature. Eur J Pediatr 1993;152:884–887.
138. Haas SV, Haas MP. Diagnosis and treatment of celiac disease: report of 603 Cases. Post Grad Med 1950;7:239–250.
139. Senser W. Neurologic manifestations and the malabsorption syndrome. J Mt Sinai Hosp 1957;24:331–345.
140. Viader F, Chapon F, Dao T, et al. Adult celiac disease revealed by a sensory-motor neuropathy. Presse Medicale 1995;24:222–224.
141. Hadjivassiliou M, Gibson A, Davies-Jones GA, et al. Does cryptic gluten sensitivity play a part in neurological illness? Lancet 1996;347:369–371.
142. Hadjivassiliou M, Chattopadhyay AK, Davies-Jones GA, et al. Neuromuscular disorder as a presenting feature of coeliac disease. J Neurol Neurosurg Psychiatr 1997;63:770–775.
143. Cooke WT. Neurologic manifestations of malabsorption. In PJ Vinken, GW Bruyn (eds), Metabolic and Deficiency Diseases of the Nervous System, Part II. Handbook of Clinical Neurology. Amsterdam: North-Holland Publishing, 1976;28:225–241.
144. Chapman RW, Laidlow JM, Colin-Jones D, et al. Increased prevalence of epilepsy in coeliac diseases. Brit Med J 1978;2:250–251.
145. Ambrosetto G, Antonini L, Tassinari CA. Occipital lobe seizures related to clinically asymptomatic celiac disease in adulthood. Epilepsia 1992;33:476–481.
146. Fois A, Vascotto M, Di Bartolo RM, Di Marco V. Celiac disease and epilepsy in pediatric patients. Childs Nerv Syst 1994;10:450–454.
147. Magaudda A, Dalla Bernardina B, De Marco P, et al. Bilateral occipital calcification, epilepsy and coeliac disease: clinical and neuroimaging features of a new syndrome. J Neurol Neurosurg Psych 1993;56:885–889.
148. Gobbi G, Sorrenti G, Santucci M, et al. Epilepsy with bilateral occipital calcifications: a benign onset with progressive severity. Neurology 1988;38:913–920.
149. Gobbi G, Bouquet F, Greco L, et al. Coeliac disease, epilepsy, and cerebral calcifications. The Italian Working Group on Coeliac Disease and Epilepsy. Lancet 1992;340:439–443.

150. Goggin T, Gough H, Bissessar A, et al. A comparative study of the relative effects of anti-convulsant drugs and dietary folate on the red cell folate status of patients with epilepsy. Q J Med 1987;65:911–919.
151. Garwicz S, Mortensson W. Cerebral calcification associated with intrathecal methotrexate therapy in acute lymphocytic leukemia. J Pediatr 1977;90:496–497.
152. Labate A, Gambardella A, Messina D, et al. Silent celiac disease inpatients with childhood localization-related epilepsies. Epilepsia 2001;42:1153–1155.
153. Piattella L, Zamponi N, Cardinali C, et al. Endocranial calcifications, infantile celiac disease, and epilepsy. Childs Nerv Syst 1993;9:172–175.
154. Bardella MT, Molteni N, Prampolini L, et al. Need for follow up in coeliac disease. Arch Dis Child 1994;70:211–213.
155. Dicke WK, Weijers HA, van de Kamer JH. Coeliac disease. II-The presence in wheat of a factor having a deleterious effect in cases of coeliac disease. Acta Paediatr 1952;42:34–42.
156. Green R, Kinsella LJ. Current concepts in the diagnosis of cobalamin deficiency. Neurology 1995;45:1435–1440.
157. Hadjivassiliou M, Grunewald RA, Chattopadhyay AK, et al. Clinical, radiological, neuro-physiological, and neuropathological characteristics of gluten ataxia. Lancet 1998;352:1582–1585.
158. Hadjivassiliou M, Grunewald RA, Lawden M, et al. Headache and CNS white matter abnormalities associated with gluten sensitivity. Neurology 2001;56:385–388.
159. Rice JR, Ham CH, Gore WE. Another look at gluten in schizophrenia. Amer J Psychiat 1978;135:1417–1418.
160. Singh MM, Kay SR. Wheat gluten as a pathogenic factor in schizophrenia. Science 1976;191:401–402.
161. Dohan FC. More on celiac disease as a model for schizophrenia. Biol Psychiatr 1983;18:561–564.
162. Dohan FC, Harper EH, Clark MH, et al. Is schizophrenia rare if grain is rare? Biol Psychiatr 1984;19:385–399.
163. Dohan FC, Grasberger JC. Relapsed schizophrenics: earlier discharge from the hospital after cereal-free, milk-free diet. Am J Psychiatr 1973;130:685–688.
164. Storms LH, Clopton JM, Wright C. Effects of gluten on schizophrenics. Arch Gen Psychiat 1982;39:323–327.
165. Vlissides DN, Venulet A, Jenner FA. A double-blind gluten-free/gluten load controlled trial in a secure ward population. Brit J Psychiat 1986;148:441–452.
166. Reichelt KL, Landmark J. Specific IgA antibody increases in schizophrenia. Biol Psychiatr 1995;37:410–413.
167. Wakefield AJ, Puleston JM, Montgomery SM, et al. Review article: the concept of entero-colonic encephalopathy, autism and opioid receptor ligands. Aliment Pharmacol Ther 2002;16:663–674.
168. Chorzelski TP, Beutner EH, Sulej J, et al. IgA antiendomysium antibody: a new immuno-logical marker of dermatitis herpetiformis and celiac disease. Brit J Dermatol 1984;111:395–402.
169. Whipple GH. A hitherto undescribed disease characterized anatomically by deposits of fat and fatty acids in the intestinal and mesenteric lymphatic tissues. Bull Johns Hopkins Hosp 1907;18:382–391.
170. Raoult D, Birg ML, La Scola B, et al. Cultivation of the bacillus of Whipple's disease. N Engl J Med 2000;342:620–625.
171. Wilson KH, Blitchington R, Frothingham R, Wilson JA. Phylogeny of the Whipple's-disease-associated bacterium. Lancet 1991;338:474–475.
172. Relman DA, Schmidt TM, MacDermott RP, Falkow S. Identification of the uncultured bacillus of Whipple's disease. N Engl J Med 1992;327:293–301.
173. Muller C, Stain C, Burghuber O. Tropheryma whippelii in peripheral blood mononuclear cells and cells of pleural effusion. Lancet 1993;341:701.
174. Wroe SJ, Pires M, Harding B, et al. Whipple's disease confined to the CNS presenting with multiple intracerebral mass lesions. J Neurol Neurosurg Psychiatr 1991;54:989–992.
175. Swash M, Schwartz MS, Vandenburg MJ, Pollock CJ. Myopathy in Whipple's disease. Gut 1977;18:800–804.

176. Adler CH, Galetta SL. Oculo-facial-skeletal myorhythmia in Whipple disease: treatment with ceftriaxone. Ann Intern Med 1990;112:467–469.

177. Rickman LS, Freeman WR, Green WR, et al. Uveitis caused by Tropheryma whippelii (Whipple's bacillus). N Engl J Med 1995;332:363–366.

178. Selsky EJ, Knox DL, Maumenee AE, Green WR. Ocular involvement in Whipple's disease. Retina 1984;4:103–106.

179. Lowsky R, Archer GL, Fyle SG, et al. Brief report: diagnosis of Whipple's disease by molecular analysis of peripheral blood. N Engl J Med 1994;331:1343–1346.

180. Ramzan NN, Loftus E Jr, Burgart LJ, et al. Diagnosis and monitoring of Whipple disease by polymerase chain reaction. Ann Intern Med 1997;126:520–527.

181. Southern JF, Moscicki RA, Magro C, et al. Lymphedema, lymphocytic myocarditis, and sarcoid-like granulomatosis: manifestations of Whipple's disease. JAMA 1989;261:1467–1470.

182. Cooper GS, Blades EW, Remler BF, et al. Central nervous system Whipple's disease: relapse during therapy with trimethoprim-sulfamethoxazole and remission with cefixime. Gastroenterology 1994;106:782–786.

183. Rege RV, Jones DB. Current Role of Surgery in Peptic Ulcer Disease. In M Feldman, LS Friedman, MH Sleisenger (eds), Sleisenger and Fordtran's Gastroenterology and Liver Disease. Pathophysiology/Diagnosis/Management, 7th Ed. Philadelphia: WB Saunders, 2002;797–809.

184. Quigley EMM, Thompson JS. Surgery for Obesity. In JM Nightingale (ed), Intestinal Failure. London: Greenwich Medical Media, 2001;165–176.

185. Brooke-Cowden GL, Braash JW, Gibb SP, et al. Post-gastrectomy syndromes. Am J Surg 1976;131:464–470.

186. Blake J, Rechnitor PA. The hematological and nutritional effects of gastric operations. Q J Med 1953;22:419–442.

187. Ehrenpreis ED, Carlson SJ, Boorstein HL, Craig RM. Malabsorption and deficiency of vitamin B12 in HIV-infected patients with chronic diarrhea. Dig Dis Sci 1994;39:2159–2162.

Chapter 13
Anorectal and Pelvic Floor Dysfunction

Arnold Wald

The main functions of colonic and anorectal motor activity are to mix and promote dehydration of fecal material, to store fecal wastes, and to eliminate them in a socially acceptable manner. The first is achieved by colonic segmentation and motor activity, which propels colonic material forward and backward over relatively short distances, the second is facilitated by colonic and rectal compliance and accommodation, whereas the third is regulated by the coordination of anorectal and pelvic floor mechanisms with behavioral and cognitive responses. These functions can be evaluated by a variety of diagnostic techniques: anorectal and colonic manometry; radiographic, scintigraphic, and sonographic studies; movement of radiopaque markers through the large intestine; and neurophysiologic methods to study striated pelvic floor muscles and pudendal nerve function. These techniques have allowed investigations of anorectal physiology, which have characterized neuromuscular and afferent dysfunction in a number of neurological disorders associated with fecal incontinence and constipation. The enhanced understanding of anorectal dysfunction in neurological diseases allows a more rational approach to the treatment of those patients with bowel dysfunction.

This chapter reviews anorectal anatomy and function during normal defecation and bowel control, the diagnostic studies of anorectal and colonic function, and summarizes current knowledge concerning the pathophysiology of disorders of continence and defecation associated with neuromuscular diseases.

ANORECTAL ANATOMY DURING CONTINENCE AND DEFECATION

The major structures of the anorectum are the rectum, the puborectalis muscle which forms the anorectal angle, and the internal (IAS) and external (EAS) anal sphincters surrounding the anal canal (Figure 13.1). The internal anal sphincter consists of thickened circular smooth muscle which is innervated by autonomic and enteric nerves; the puborectalis and external anal sphincter muscles are striated muscles whose innervation is provided from the sacral nerves. The efferent innervation of the external anal sphincter is from S-2 and travels via the pudendal nerves, whereas that of the puborectalis muscle is from the direct branches of the S3 and 4.[1,2] Sensory mechanoreceptors in the perirectal tissues allow awareness

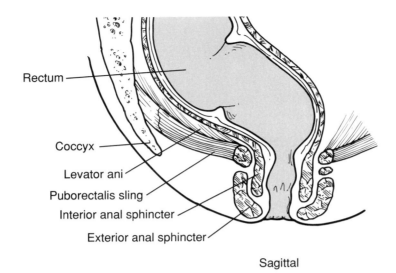

Sagittal

Figure 13.1. Sagittal view of the anorectum, illustrating the important anatomical structures. (Reproduced with permission from Sun WM, Rao SS. Manometric assessment of anorectal function. Gastroenterol Clin North Am 2001;30:15–32.)

of rectal filling or distension, although the precise location of these receptors is not established,[2] whereas anal nerve endings permit discrimination of gas, liquid, or solid rectal contents. The neural pathways for rectal sensation are at present unresolved.

At rest, the anorectal angle approximates 85 to 105°, and normally is at the level of a line drawn from the symphysis pubis to the tip of the coccyx. About 75 to 80% of the resting pressure in the anal canal is derived from the internal anal sphincter,[3] and this exceeds intrarectal pressure. The movement of fecal wastes to the rectum triggers a reflex which temporarily relaxes the internal anal sphincter; defecation is deferred by simultaneous contraction of the puborectalis muscle and external sphincter (Figure 13.2), narrowing the anorectal angle and increasing resistance pressures in the anal canal until the rectum accommodates to the increased contents and propulsive forces are diminished. During defecation, increased intraabdominal pressures help to propel bowel contents toward the anal canal, the internal anal sphincter is tonically inhibited and relaxation of striated muscles results in perineal descent, widening of the anorectal angle, and decreased pressures in the anal canal (Figure 13.2). After defecation is completed, anorectal structures return to their normal positions at rest.

STUDIES OF COLONIC AND ANORECTAL FUNCTION

Motility studies may provide useful information in many patients with fecal incontinence and in some patients with constipation.[4,5] They may also be used therapeutically in biofeedback retraining in selected patients with incontinence and defecation disorders.[6]

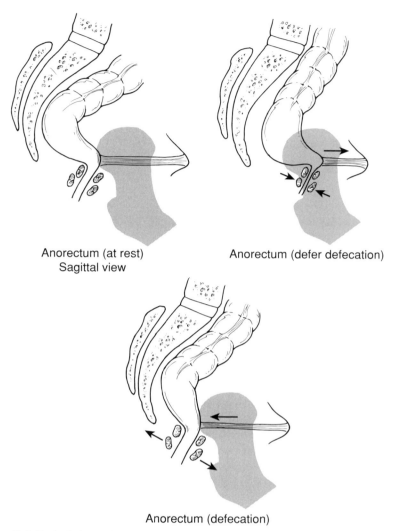

Anorectum (at rest)
Sagittal view

Anorectum (defer defecation)

Anorectum (defecation)

Figure 13.2. Sagittal views of the anorectum at rest, when defecation is being deferred and during defecation. Arrows indicate muscle vector forces when the striated muscles are contracted *(center)* or relaxed *(right)*. (Reproduced with permission from Sun WM, Rao SS. Manometric assessment of anorectal function. Gastroenterol Clin North Am 2001;30:15–32.)

Anorectal Manometry

Satisfactory measurements of anal sphincter responses can be obtained with open-tipped perfused catheters, direct on-line pressure transducers, or air-filled balloons of various sizes and configurations.[7] If rectal sensation is impaired, as it is in many patients with severe constipation and fecal incontinence, it is helpful to know whether it is associated with increased rectal compliance or megarectum. Compliance can be measured by inflating a balloon placed in the rectum with increasing volumes of air, and measuring pressures at each level of distention. Pressures should be corrected by subtracting those obtained by inflation outside the patient.

Colonic Manometry

Techniques have been developed to permit prolonged recordings of contractile activity through the colon, using perfused catheters or solid-state transducers.[8] Most activity appears to be of the segmental type, with propagation over a few centimeters at most in either direction. Less frequently, contractions of high amplitude migrate distally over long segments of bowel (HAPCs), and have been shown to be associated with the mass movements.[9–11] Colonic motor activity occurs most often upon awakening, after meals, and is more frequent during the day.[12]

Colonic motility studies are time intensive and present formidable technical difficulties. As colonic motor activity appears to be intermittent and highly variable, studies must be carried out over prolonged time periods, and considerable overlap with normal values has been reported. Intraluminal catheters may underestimate contractile activity, which itself may be altered by the bowel preparations necessary to place the catheter. Ambulatory systems have been developed to overcome some of these limitations.[13–15] These studies remain largely investigational and are confined to a few centers.

Pelvic Floor Neurophysiology

In pelvic floor electromyography, a ground electrode is strapped to the thigh of the patient and a standard concentric needle electromyographic (EMG) electrode is inserted, without anesthesia, into the superficial portion of the external sphincter or the puborectalis muscle. Alternatively, surface electrodes are placed on the skin over the superficial part of the external anal sphincter. The myoelectric activity recorded by the concentric needle electrode is displayed on an oscilloscope, either at rest with voluntary squeeze, or after a supramaximal stimulus is applied to the terminal portion of the pudendal nerves, which supply the external anal sphincter. In addition to evaluating neurogenic or myopathic damage in patients with fecal incontinence,[16] EMG recordings may be used to complement manometry in the diagnosis of rectoanal dyssynergia by detecting increased EMG activity of the external anal sphincter during attempted defecation.[17]

To determine pudendal nerve terminal motor latency, a stimulus is applied to the right and left pudendal nerves at the level of the ischial tuberosities, and motor unit potentials are recorded from the external anal sphincter. Pudendal nerve conduction is measured by calculating the time between application of the stimulus and the sphincter muscle response, and is called the latency period. A prolonged latency is highly suggestive of pudendal nerve damage, which is characteristic of many patients with "idiopathic" fecal incontinence.[18]

Anal Endosonography

This is a technique which has been shown to accurately delineate the layers of the rectal wall, the internal and external anal sphincters, and the levator muscles.[19,20] Early studies indicate that endosonography is useful in evaluating pelvic floor structures in patients with fecal incontinence,[21] and is capable of detecting occult sphincter injuries related to childbirth or other conditions where there is potential for injury to continence mechanisms.[22]

Defecography/Proctography

Defecation can be evaluated using either radiographic and scintigraphic techniques, which have been advocated as clinically useful in patients who complain of excessive straining during defecation (dyschezia), or who employ digital manipulation to facilitate evacuation.[23,24] These tests vary in their complexity and the information provided, and have potential limitations.[25,26] Defecography is theoretically helpful to evaluate rectal emptying, but a number of deficiencies render its clinical usefulness uncertain.[27] Optimally, these studies are best performed by those with an interest and training in these techniques. Recently, magnetic resonance imaging (MRI) techniques have been applied to this area.[28,29]

DISORDERS ASSOCIATED WITH FECAL INCONTINENCE

During the last 15 years, our knowledge of the pathophysiology of incontinence associated with "idiopathic fecal incontinence," diabetes mellitus, and multiple sclerosis has been advanced by investigations of anorectal continence mechanisms in patients with these disorders.

Idiopathic Fecal Incontinence

This condition occurs predominantly in middle aged and elderly women who have no history of overt anorectal injury or disease. There is evidence that such patients may have occult anal sphincter injuries and/or a peripheral neuropathic injury to the striated muscles important to the maintenance of continence.

Manometric and radiographic studies demonstrate that many patients have decreased resting and/or squeeze anal canal pressures, and many exhibit a widened anorectal angle, suggestive of impairment of puborectalis muscle function.[30] Whether incontinence occurs appears to depend more upon a competent anal canal mechanism, although continence for solid stool is usually maintained if the puborectalis is intact, even when the anal sphincter mechanism is weakened.[31]

The mechanism(s) by which neuropathic muscle injury occurs is somewhat speculative. EMG studies (both single fiber and concentric needle studies) of the puborectalis muscle and external anal sphincter frequently exhibit findings consistent with a denervation-reinnervation injury of the striated muscles.[18,32] Pudendal nerve studies have found delayed terminal motor latencies of one or both nerves in patients with idiopathic fecal incontinence, compared to age and sex matched control subjects.[18,33] Occasionally, a patient will manifest such changes due to a cauda equina lesion, but most studies indicate a peripheral nerve conduction delay.

Occult damage to the peripheral nerves subserving pelvic floor striated muscles may occur during vaginal delivery, especially with forceps assistance or with prolonged and difficult labor.[32] Chronic repetitive damage to the pudendal nerves may be associated with stretch injury during repeated straining at defecation after multiple vaginal deliveries[18,34]; this may weaken the pelvic floor, resulting in the syndrome of perineal descent.[35] Other studies done with anal endosonography demonstrate the presence of occult internal and/or external anal sphincter injuries, which may contribute to incontinence in such patients.[22] However, such injuries are associated with fecal incontinence only if anal sphincter pressures are abnormal.

Finally, manometric studies have shown that resting pressure is reduced in some patients with idiopathic fecal incontinence.[36–38] Studies on a comparatively small number of patients indicate that in idiopathic fecal incontinence, the internal anal sphincter is less sensitive to noradrenaline than in control subjects.[39,40] The major abnormality appears to reside in α-adrenoreceptors, which mediate contractile activity, whereas β-adrenoreceptors are not significantly affected. It has been hypothesized that the abnormality is of extrinsic sympathetic innervation, perhaps caused by injury to the sympathetic nerve supply which travels via the hypogastric and lumbar colonic nerves. Thus, although the resting tone of the internal anal sphincter appears to be derived from the myogenic properties of the smooth muscle, adrenergic receptors may play an important role in the modulation of resting tone of the sphincter muscles.

Diabetes Mellitus

Fecal incontinence occurs in about 4 to 5% of diabetic patients, most of whom have diarrhea associated with peripheral and autonomic neuropathy. The prevalence of fecal incontinence in diabetes has been underestimated, since patients often do not volunteer this symptom because of embarrassment at their loss of bowel control.[41] Although much remains unknown about the pathogenesis of diabetic incontinence, considerable progress has been made in delineating anorectal abnormalities which occur in this disorder.

Contrary to earlier teaching, it is unusual for voluminous diarrhea to overwhelm normal continence mechanisms in diabetic patients. Indeed, most diabetics with fecal incontinence have frequent passage of loose stools, with daily stool volumes either within the normal range or only moderately increased.[42] Rather, there appear to be multiple abnormalities of anorectal function in the vast majority of incontinent diabetic patients (Figure 13.3); these include increased threshold of the perception of rectal sensation,[43,44] decreased resting anal canal pressures,[42,44] decreased

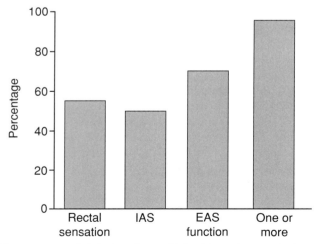

Figure 13.3. The percentage of diabetic patients with fecal incontinence who have exhibited abnormalities of anorectal function when evaluated by anorectal manometry at the University of Pittsburgh Medical Center.

squeeze anal canal pressures,[44] impaired phasic contraction of the external anal sphincter in response to rectal distension,[43] and impaired anal sensation.[45] In contrast, continent diabetic patients have subtle changes in anomucosal sensitivity, but otherwise exhibit normal anorectal neuromuscular function.[42–44,46,47]

The relative importance of anorectal abnormalities, and the volume and consistency of diarrheal stools to fecal incontinence, is unclear, but as liquid stools are more difficult to perceive and retain, there is undoubtedly an additive effect. However, it does not appear that most diabetics have latent abnormalities of anorectal function which become manifest only when continence mechanisms are stressed by loose stools. Rather, the available evidence suggests that diarrhea and fecal incontinence may be due to a common defect; that is, whatever produces diarrhea in diabetics may simultaneously affect anorectal sensory and motor function. There is some evidence that rectal sensory thresholds and responsiveness of the external anal sphincter can be improved with biofeedback techniques.[43] Biofeedback conditioning in 11 diabetic patients with fecal incontinence resulted in normal thresholds of rectal sensation in 6 of 7 patients with pretreatment thresholds above 20 ml; of these, 5 became continent. Biofeedback also improved responsiveness of external anal sphincter phasic contraction to rectal distension in 9 diabetics, 8 of whom became continent. Three patients were retested at 7, 18, and 30 months after biofeedback; all maintained improvement of both sensory and motor parameters, and all were continent. There are no controlled studies of biofeedback, nor is the mechanism by which biofeedback alters bowel continence certain. Nevertheless, biofeedback therapy remains a risk-free treatment for diabetics with fecal incontinence who exhibit evidence of abnormal anorectal sensorimotor function.

Multiple Sclerosis

Multiple sclerosis is a common neurological disease that affects approximately one-quarter million Americans. The characteristic pathologic feature in multiple sclerosis is focal demyelination of axons, with plaque formation in the white matter of the central nervous system. Both constipation and fecal incontinence occur frequently in multiple sclerosis; in one large survey, approximately two-thirds of randomly selected patients had constipation and/or fecal incontinence, complaints that were common even in mildly disabled subjects.[48]

Alterations of anorectal sensory and motor function occur frequently in multiple sclerosis patients with fecal incontinence.[44,49] These include an increased threshold of conscious rectal sensation, an increased threshold of phasic contraction of the external anal sphincter in response to rectal distension, and reduced contractile strength of the external anal sphincter. In contrast to diabetes with fecal incontinence, internal anal sphincter function appears to be normal.[44] Others have shown that multiple sclerosis alone has an effect on external anal sphincter function, characterized by increased fiber density in the external anal sphincter and normal pudendal nerve latencies.[50] One explanation for these findings could be demyelination of that segment of the lower motor neuron between the anterior horn cell and its exit from the spinal cord. However, pudendal nerve injury or occult anal sphincter defects associated with childbirth may have an additive effect in some women with multiple sclerosis and fecal incontinence.[16] In addition, the chronic use of baclofen, an analogue of the inhibitory neurotransmitter gamma-aminobutyric acid (GABA), theoretically could alter responses to rectal distension and therefore the threshold of conscious rectal sensation.

In contrast to diabetic patients, continent multiple sclerosis patients often exhibit decreased contractile strength of the external anal sphincter and increased fiber densities of the sphincter muscle.[44] However, these are not as frequent nor as severe as in multiple sclerosis patients with incontinence. Certainly, the low incidence of diarrhea in multiple sclerosis provides a degree of protection from fecal incontinence, and constipation should not be vigorously treated in these patients for this reason.

Spinal Cord Injury

Although profound changes in anorectal functions occur with spinal cord injuries, fecal incontinence is an uncommon cause of chronic disability.[51] This is due, in large part, to the development of constipation and fecal impaction, related, in turn, to decreased motility,[52] which may act as a counter effect to loss of continence mechanisms.[53] Thus, with good bowel management programs, incontinence can be minimized.

In patients with sacral cord lesions, there is absence of a sensation of rectal filling, modest or no changes in resting anal sphincter tone, and loss of voluntary contraction of the external anal sphincter.[54] Reflex defecation and warning of impending defecation are also absent. Fecal incontinence can be prevented by manual evacuation of the rectum on a regular basis and stimulant laxative suppositories to promote evacuation. Continuous weak electrical stimulation of the sacral roots, especially S4, theoretically could enhance fecal continence.[55]

In contrast to sacral injuries, suprasacral lesions are associated with preservation of reflex defecation, normal resting anal pressures, and not uncommonly, autonomic signs of impending defecation.[56] Thus, despite absence of rectal sensation and voluntary muscle control, prevention of incontinence is often achieved by planned defecation by puborectalis or rectal stimulation.[57]

Idiopathic Fecal Impaction

Fecal impaction can occur at any age, but is found with increased frequency in children with functional soiling (encopresis) and in the elderly who are hospitalized or otherwise institutionalized.[58] Indeed, the most common cause of fecal incontinence in these two age groups is fecal impaction, which often occurs with megarectum.

While the effects of aging on colonic and anorectal physiology remain poorly documented, the balance of evidence suggests that the aging process, per se, cannot explain the predilection of the elderly to impaction and incontinence.[59,60] It is more likely that their occurrence is related to associated disease processes. Physiologic abnormalities may, however, be important in perpetuating this condition and predisposing to its recurrence. Indeed, physiologic studies have documented several abnormalities of anorectal function in recently disimpacted patients; these include impairment of anal, perianal, and rectal sensation, a hypotonic rectum, and diminished anal canal pressures, findings typical of patients with sacral cord damage.[61] These findings may persist for up to one year after successful treatment of encopretic children, providing one explanation as to why there is such a high frequency of relapse in these children.[62] Any or all of these findings could promote fecal retention in the rectum.

DISORDERS ASSOCIATED WITH CONSTIPATION

Chronic functional constipation may be associated with abnormally slow transit through the colon or by disorders of defecation. As the distal colon, rectum, and anal sphincters receive autonomic and somatic innervation via the same sacral spinal roots, it is not unexpected that neurologic disorders may be associated with an increased frequency of constipation and defecatory disorders. The mechanisms which may produce functional disorders of defecation include those associated with impaired propulsion and those associated with increased resistance to the evacuation of rectal contents through the anal canal (Table 13.1).

Weak Rectal Propulsion

During defecation, increased intraabdominal pressures help to move bowel contents toward and through the anal canal. In patients who are weakened due to neuromuscular disorders or inanition, who are unable to ambulate, or in those in whom intraabdominal or spinal cord pain inhibits straining efforts, defecation may be inhibited or completely prevented. Alternatively, propulsive vector forces in the rectum may be blunted or diffused in patients with megarectum.[63] This may be characterized by measuring the height and duration of intrarectal pressures during straining (pseudodefecation) (Figure 13.4).

Misdirected Propulsion

Rectal examination or defecography may lead to the discovery of a rectocele, intussusception, or rectal prolapse. As rectoceles are common in older nonconstipated women, care must be taken before attributing defecatory difficulties to this entity. Preferably, one should demonstrate improved evacuation when pressure is exerted transvaginally in order to implicate a rectocele as a cause of dyschezia. This is important since rectocele repairs frequently do not alleviate dyschezia.

Table 13.1. Mechanisms Which Produce Disordered Defecation

Mechanisms	Disorders
Weak propulsion	Neuromuscular diseases
	Pain syndromes
	Megarectum
Misdirected propulsion	Rectocele (occasional)
Failure of IAS relaxation	Hirschsprung's disease
Failure of muscle relaxation	Pelvic floor dyssynergia

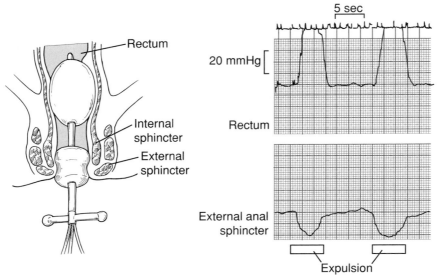

Figure 13.4. Anorectal balloon manometry in which the rectal balloon and the external anal sphincter balloon record pressures during attempted expulsion of the manometer (pseudodefecation). At right is a normal expulsion pattern, in which increased pressures are recorded from the rectal balloon whereas decreased pressures are observed on the external balloon. In patients with weak expulsion efforts, rectal pressures are greatly diminished and/or are of short duration. (Reproduced with permission from Wald A: Manometry. In MM Schuster, MD Crowell, KL Koch [eds], Schuster Atlas of Gastrointestinal Motility in Health and Disease. Philadelphia: BC Decker, 2002;289-303.)

Similarly, as intussusceptions not uncommonly occur in nonconstipated patients, their presence in constipated patients does not imply causation. Symptoms that suggest an intussusception include a sensation of continual rectal fullness or incomplete rectal emptying, despite intense and prolonged straining.

Hirschsprung's Disease

Children and young adults with severe constipation from birth should always be assessed for Hirschsprung's disease. There is a strong male predominance and a significant minority of patients (~ 7%) have a familial pattern. Recent studies have identified specific mutations in association with this disorder.[64] Most cases are recognized during the first year of life, but a small number remain undiagnosed until childhood or young adulthood.[65]

Functional obstruction of the distal bowel is suggested radiographically by a spastic nonpropulsive segment of distal bowel with colonic dilatation proximally (Figure 13.5). The primary pathogenetic defect is absence of intramural ganglion cells of the submucosal and myenteric plexuses as a result of arrest of neural crest cell migration during embryonic development. In addition, there is hyperplasia of the extramural parasympathetic and postganglionic adrenergic fibers in the narrowed segment of colon, including the internal anal sphincter. Anorectal manometry shows the characteristic absence of internal anal sphincter relaxation after rectal distension (Figure 13.6); a rectal biopsy to document the characteristic histopathology or increased acetylcholinesterase levels using histochemical techniques[66] should be done to confirm the diagnosis. In short segment disease, the form seen in

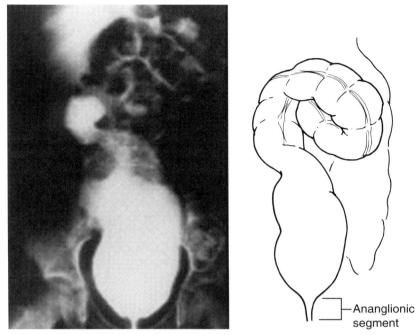

Figure 13.5. Hirschsprung's disease. An 11-year-old boy with involvement of only the distal 1 to 2 cm of rectum, i.e., short segment disease. It is imperative to remove the insertion catheter used to instill barium in order to avoid missing short segment disease. It is also preferable not to cleanse the colon prior to barium studies so as to accentuate the transition from aganglionic to normally innervated bowel (Reproduced with permission from Wald A: Manometry. In MM Schuster, MD Crowell, KL Koch [eds], Schuster Atlas of Gastrointestinal Motility in Health and Disease. Philadelphia: BC Decker, 2002;289-303.)

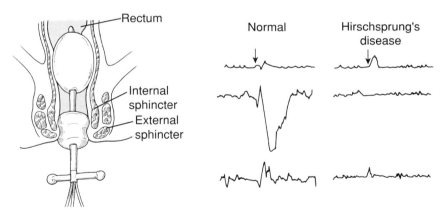

Figure 13.6. Hirschsprung's disease. Internal anal sphincter responses to rectal distension in a patient with Hirschsprung's disease are compared with those in a normal subject using the Schuster-type balloon manometer. The congenital aganglionosis of Hirschsprung's disease invariably affects the internal anal sphincter. In contrast to normal reflexive relaxation of the internal anal sphincter following rectal distension (arrows), no such relaxation occurs in patients with Hirschsprung's disease (Reproduced with permission from Wald A: Manometry. In MM Schuster, MD Crowell, KL Koch [eds], Schuster Atlas of Gastrointestinal Motility in Health and Disease. Philadelphia: BC Decker, 2002;289-303.)

adults, the only abnormality may be absence of internal anal sphincter relaxation and failure of expulsion of contrast during defecography. The presence of internal anal sphincter relaxation, as demonstrated by anorectal manometry, excludes a diagnosis of Hirschsprung's disease.[67]

Surgery is the treatment of choice for Hirschsprung's disease. In patients with short segment disease, posterior rectal myectomy, with incision of the internal anal sphincter and a varying portion of rectal smooth muscle, is the preferred procedure.[68] In the classic form of the disease, more extensive procedures to remove or bypass the aganglionic segment are required.[69]

Pelvic Floor Dyssynergia

The concept that obstructed defecation could be associated with failure to relax, or the inappropriate contraction of the striated muscles of the pelvic floor during attempted defecation, was first reported in 1985.[70] The clinical findings in these patients include inability to initiate defecation, incomplete evacuation, manual disimpactions and assumption of contorted postures during defecation, laxative and enema abuse, and rectal discomfort.[30,71] The manometric and radiographic findings include inappropriate contraction or failure to relax the external anal sphincter, lack of pelvic floor descent and straightening of the anorectal angle, and inability to expel rectal contents during attempted defecation. EMG studies confirm that the external sphincter and puborectalis muscle exhibit an inappropriate increase in myoelectrical activity during attempted defecation (Figure 13.7).

Pelvic floor dyssynergia ("Anismus") has been observed in 36 to 52% of children with fecal impactions and overflow soiling,[17,72] as well as a minority of adults with defecatory difficulty. Electrophysiological and radiological evidence of dyssynergia were found in five of six patients with Parkinson's disease and chronic constipation[73]; these findings were subsequently confirmed by others.[74] Functional improvement following administration of apomorphine, a dopamine receptor agonist, was noted in the earlier study, but this was not tested against a placebo.

At present, many issues concerning this disorder remain unclear.[75] These include the correlation between manometric, EMG, and radiographic findings, and the possible influence of psychological factors in producing this pattern when testing occurs in a laboratory setting.[76] It has been hypothesized that dyssynergia may arise as a learned behavior in response to avoiding the discomfort associated with defecating large hard stools. Clearly, this pattern also has been observed in healthy controls and in patients who are not constipated.[25,77]

Multiple Sclerosis

Studies of colonic dysfunction in multiple sclerosis were performed in seven men with severe spastic quadriparesis who also were severely constipated and had bladder dysfunction.[78] Somatosensory-evoked potentials, cystometrograms, colonmetrograms, and studies of colonic motor and myoelectric activity were carried out. All seven patients exhibited "hyperreflexic," or high pressure/volume, colonmetrograms, which were felt to be analogous to the hyperreflexic cystometrograms present in most of these patients. Colonic motor and myoelectrical activity were also abnormal in all seven patients. The baseline mean amplitude of colonic motor activity in the multiple sclerosis patients was significantly lower than in normal controls. In addition, patients

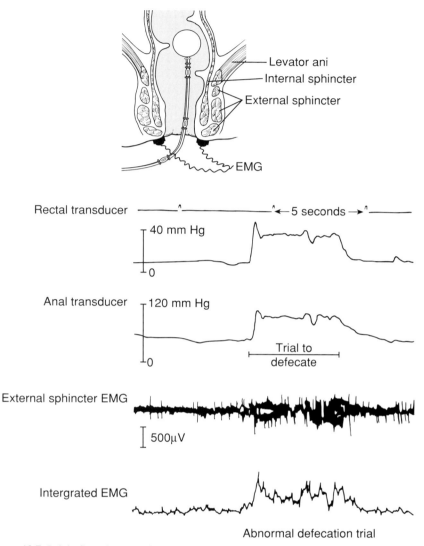

Figure 13.7. Pelvic floor dyssynergia. Pressure changes in rectum and anal canal and EMG recordings from the external anal sphincter during pseudodefecation. Normal defecation is characterized by increased rectal (intraabdominal) pressure, decreased anal pressure, and decreased direct and integrated EMG activity, as measured by surface electrodes. In this patient with pelvic floor dyssynergia, there is increased anal pressure and EMG activity of the external sphincter during attempted defecation (courtesy of Dr. Vera Loening-Baucke, University of Iowa Hospitals, Iowa City, IA).

had no demonstrable postprandial increase in colonic motility, as was observed in the controls (Figure 13.8). All patients had abnormal cortical somatosensory-evoked responses, demonstrating lesions in the central neural pathways.

In another study, 16 patients with multiple sclerosis and urinary bladder dysfunction were evaluated using anorectal manometry and colonic transit studies.[79] Fifteen described themselves as constipated, and six also complained of fecal incontinence. Prolonged colonic transit was demonstrated in 14 patients, 7 had left-sided

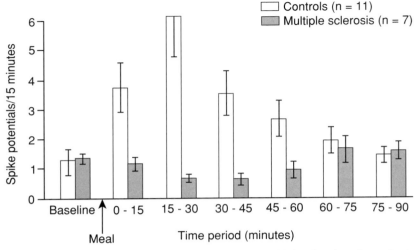

Figure 13.8. Colonic myoelectric activity in 7 patients with multiple sclerosis and constipation compared to control subjects (Reproduced from Glick ME, Meshkinpour H, Haldeman S, et al. Colonic dysfunction in multiple sclerosis. Gastroenterology 1982;83:1002–1007.)

delay only, whereas the others had a more generalized colonic slowing. Ten exhibited manometric criteria suggestive of so-called "outlet obstruction," defined as hypertonia in the upper anal canal, with or without ultraslow waves; the presence of an "overshoot" contraction after the rectoanal inhibitory reflex (RISR); and an RISR which was absent or of insufficient amplitude. On the basis of these results, the authors suggested that the prolonged colonic transit and anorectal dysfunction were secondary to the neurological disorder, and hypothesized the existence of "rectoanal dyssynergia" causing problems of rectal evacuation in the same way that detrusor urethral dyssynergia causes abnormal bladder emptying.

SUMMARY

Colonic and anorectal dysfunction are not uncommon in patients with neurological disorders and are characterized by constipation, defecatory difficulties, and/or fecal incontinence. The development of more sophisticated techniques to study large bowel function has advanced our knowledge of the pathogenesis of these disorders, and in some instances has resulted in new therapeutic strategies to deal with these often socially disabling problems.[80,81]

ACKNOWLEDGMENT

The author wishes to thank Helen Gibson for her expert preparation of the manuscript.

REFERENCES

1. Snooks SJ, Henry MM, Swash M. The innervation of the muscles of continence. Ann R Coll Surg Engl 1986;68:45–49.

2. Whitehead WE, Schuster MM. Anorectal physiology and pathophysiology. Am J Gastroenterol 1987;82:487–497.

3. Bennett RC, Duthie HL. The functional importance of the internal anal sphincter. Brit J Surg 1964;51:355–357.

4. Azpiroz F, Enck P, Whitehead WE. Anorectal function testing: review of collective experience. Am J Gastroenterol 2002;97:232–240.

5. Sun WM, Rao SS. Manometric assessment of anorectal function. Gastroenterol Clin North Am 2001;30:15–32.

6. Enck P. Biofeedback training in disordered defecation: a critical review. Dig Dis Sci 1993;38:1953–1960.

7. Wald A. Anorectum. In MM Schuster (ed), Atlas of Gastrointestinal Motility in Health and Disease. Baltimore: Williams and Wilkins, 1993;229–249.

8. Bassotti G, Crowell MD, Whitehead WE. Contractile activity of the human colon: lessons from 24 hour studies. Gut 1993;34:129–133.

9. Hertz AF, Newton A. The normal movements of colon in man. J Physiol 1913;47:57–65.

10. Cook IJ, Furukawa Y, Panagopoulos V, et al. Relationships between spatial patterns of colonic pressure and individual movements of content. Am J Physiol 2000;278:G329–G341.

11. Bampton PA, Dinning PG, Kennedy ML, et al. Spatial and temporal organization of pressure patterns throughout the unprepared colon during spontaneous defecation. Am J Gastroenterol 2000;95:1027–1035.

12. Narducci F, Bassotti G, Gaburri M, Morelli A. Twenty-four hour manometric recordings of colonic motor activity in healthy man. Gut 1987;28:17–25.

13. Soffer EE, Scalabrini P, Wingate DL. Prolonged ambulant monitoring of human colonic motility. Am J Physiol 1989; 257:G601–G606.

14. Crowell MD, Bassotti G, Cheskin LJ, et al. Method for prolonged ambulatory monitoring of high-amplitude propagated contractions from colon. Am J Physiol 1991;261:G263–G268.

15. Bampton PA, Dinning PG, Kennedy ML, et al. Prolonged multi-point recording of colonic manometry in the unprepared human colon: providing insight into potentially relevant pressure wave parameters. Am J Gastroenterol 2001;96:1838–1848.

16. Swash M, Snooks SJ, Chalmers DH. Parity as a factor in incontinence in multiple sclerosis. Arch Neurol 1987;44:504–508.

17. Loening-Baucke VA, Cruikshank BM. Abnormal defecation dynamics in chronically constipated children with encopresis. J Pediatrics 1986;108:562–566.

18. Kiff ES, Swash M. Normal proximal and delayed distal conduction in the pudendal nerves of patients with idiopathic (neurogenic) faecal incontinence. J Neurol Neurosurg Psychiatry 1984;47:1269–1273.

19. Law PL, Bartram CI. Anal endosonography: technique and normal anatomy. Gastrointest Radiology 1989;14:349–353.

20. Tjandra JJ, Milsom JW, Stolfi VM, et al. Endoluminal ultrasound defines anatomy of the anal canal and pelvic floor. Dis Colon Rectum 1992;35:465–470.

21. Cuesta MA, Meijer S, Derksen EJ, et al. Anal sphincter imaging in fecal incontinence using endosonography. Dis Colon Rectum 1992;35:59–63.

22. Sultan AH, Kamm MA, Hudson CN, et al. Anal sphincter disruption during vaginal delivery. N Engl J Med 1993;329:1905–1911.

23. Mahieu P, Pringot J, Bodart P. Defecography: I. Description of a new procedure and results in normal patients. Gastrointest Radiol 1984;9:247–252.

24. Mahieu P, Pringot J, Bodart P. Defecography: II. Contribution to the diagnosis of defecation disorders. Gastrointest Radiol 1984;9:253–261.

25. Wald A, Caruana BJ, Freimanis MG, et al. Contributions of evacuation proctography and anorectal manometry to the evaluation of adults with constipation and defecatory difficulty. Dig Dis Sci 1990;35:481–487.

26. Wald A, Jafri F, Rehder J, Holeva K. Scintigraphic studies of rectal emptying in patients with constipation and defecatory difficulty. Dig Dis Sci 1993: 38:353–358.

27. Diamant NE, Kamm MA, Wald A, Whitehead WE. AGA technical review on anorectal testing techniques. Gastroenterol 1999;116:735–760.

28. Dohke M, Mitchell DG, Vasavada SP. Fast magnetic resonance imaging of pelvic organ prolapse. Tech Urol 2001;7:133–138.

29. Stoker J, Halligan S, Bartram CI. Pelvic floor imaging. Radiology 2001;218:621–641.
30. Pemberton JH. Anorectal and pelvic floor disorders: putting physiology into practice. J Gastroenterol Hepatol 1990;Suppl 1:127–143.
31. Varma RJ, Stephens D. Neuromuscular reflexes of rectal continence. Aust N Z J Surg 1972;41:263–272.
32. Snooks SJ, Setchell M, Swash M, Henry MM. Injury to the pelvic floor sphincter musculature in childbirth. Lancet 1984;2:546–550.
33. Womack NR, Morrison JFB, Williams NS. The role of pelvic floor denervation in the aetiology of idiopathic fecal incontinence. Brit J Surg 1986;73:404–407.
34. Snooks SJ, Barnes PR, Swash M, Henry MM. Damage to the innervation of the pelvic floor musculature in chronic constipation. Gastroenterology 1985;89:977–981.
35. Parks AG, Porter NH, Hardcastle J. The syndrome of the descending perineum. Proc Roy Soc Med 1966;59:477–482.
36. Neill ME, Parks AG, Swash M. Physiological studies of the pelvic floor in idiopathic faecal incontinence and rectal prolapse. Brit J Surg 1981;68:531–536.
37. Lubowski DZ, Nicholls RJ, Burleigh DE, Swash M. Internal anal sphincter in neurogenic fecal incontinence. Gastroenterology 1988;95:997–1002.
38. Sun WM, Read NW, Donnelly TC. Impaired internal anal sphincter in a subgroup of patients with idiopathic fecal incontinence. Gastroenterology 1989;97:130–135.
39. Speakman CT, Hoyle CH, Kamm MA, et al. Adrenergic control of the internal anal sphincter is abnormal in patients with idiopathic fecal incontinence. Brit J Surg 1990;77:1342–1344.
40. Speakman CT, Hoyle CH, Kamm MA, et al. Abnormalities of innervation of internal anal sphincter in fecal incontinence. Dig Dig Sci 1993;38:1961–1969.
41. Feldman M, Schiller LR. Disorders of gastrointestinal motility associated with diabetes mellitus. Ann Intern Med 1983;98:378–384.
42. Schiller LR, Santa Ana CA, Schmulen AC, et al. Pathogenesis of fecal incontinence in diabetes mellitus: evidence for internal-anal-sphincter dysfunction. N Engl J Med 1982;307:1666–1671.
43. Wald A, Tunuguntla AK. Anorectal sensorimotor dysfunction in fecal incontinence and diabetes mellitus. N Engl J Med 1984;310:1282–1287.
44. Caruana BJ, Wald A, Hinds JP, Eidelman BH. Anorectal sensory and motor function in neurogenic fecal incontinence: comparison between multiple sclerosis and diabetes mellitus. Gastroenterology 1991;100:456–470.
45. Aitchison M, Fisher BM, Carter K, et al. Impaired anal sensation and early diabetic faecal incontinence. Diabet Med 1991;8:960–963.
46. Cazzolini D, Salvatore T, Giugliano D, et al. Sensorimotor evaluation of ano-rectal complex in diabetes mellitus. Diabete Metabolisme (Paris) 1991;17:520–524.
47. Rogers J, Levy DM, Henry MM, Misiewicz JJ. Pelvic floor neuropathy: a comparative study of diabetes mellitus and idiopathic faecal incontinence. Gut 1988;29:756–761.
48. Hinds JP, Eidelman BH, Wald A. Prevalence of bowel dysfunction in multiple sclerosis: a population survey. Gastroenterol 1990;98:1538–1542.
49. Wiesel PH, Norton C, Glickman S, Kamm MA. Pathophysiology and management of bowel dysfunction in multiple sclerosis. Eur J Gastroenterol Hepatol 2001;13:441–448.
50. Jameson JS, Rogers J, Chia YW, et al. Pelvic floor function in multiple sclerosis. Gut 1994;35:388–390.
51. Stone JM, Nino-Murcia M. Wolfe VA, Perkash I. Chronic gastrointestinal problems in spinal cord injury patients: a prospective analysis. Am J Gastroenterol 1990;85:1114–1119.
52. Fajardo NR, Pasiliao RV, Modeste-Duncan R, et al. Decreased colonic motility in persons with chronic spinal cord injury. Am J Gastroenterol 2003;98:128–134.
53. Menardo G, Bausano G, Corazziari E, et al. Large bowel transit in paraplegic patients. Dis Colon Rectum 1987;30:924–928.
54. Wheatly IC, Hardy KJ, Dent J. Anal pressure studies in spinal patients. Gut 1977;18:488–490.
55. Binnie NR, Smith AV, Creasey GH, Edmond P. Motility effects of electrical anterior sacral nerve root stimulation of the parasympathetic supply of the left colon and anorectum in paraplegic subjects. J Gastrointest Motil 1990;2:12–17.

56. Sun WM, Read NW, Donnelly TC. Anorectal function in incontinent patients with cerebrospinal disease. Gastroenterol 1990;99:1372–1379.

57. Miner PB. Fecal Incontinence. In TM Bayless (ed), Current Therapy in Gastroenterology and Liver Disease III. Philadelphia: BC Decker, 1990;363–369.

58. Wrenn K. Fecal impaction. N Engl J Med 1989;321:658–662.

59. Orr WC, Chen CL. Aging and neural control of the GI tract: IV. Clinical and physiological aspects of gastrointestinal motility and aging. Am J Physiol 2002;283:G1226–G1231.

60. O'Mahony D, O'Leary P, Quigley EMM. Aging and intestinal motility. Drugs Aging 2002; 19:515–527.

61. Read NW, Abouzekry L. Why do patients with faecal impaction have faecal incontinence? Gut 1986;27:283–287.

62. Loening-Baucke VA. Sensitivity of the sigmoid colon and rectum in children treated for chronic constipation. J Ped Gastro and Nutr 1984;3:454–459.

63. Gattuso JM, Kamm MA. Clinical features of idiopathic megarectum and megacolon. Gut 1997;41:93–99.

64. McCabe EB. Hirschsprung's disease: dissecting complexity in a pathogenic network. Lancet 2002;359:1169–1170.

65. Metzger PP, Alvear DT, Arnold GC, Stoner RR. Hirschsprung's disease in adults: report of a case and review of the literature. Dis Colon Rectum 1978;21:113–117.

66. Boston VE, Dale G, Riley KW. Diagnosis of Hirschsprung's disease by quantitative biochemical assay of acetylcholinesterase in rectal tissue. Lancet 1975;2:951–953.

67. Tobon F, Reid NC, Talbert JL, Schuster MM. Nonsurgical test for the diagnosis of Hirschsprung's disease. N Engl J Med 1968;278:188–193.

68. Lynn HB, van Heerden JA. Rectal myectomy in Hirschsprung's disease. Arch Surg 1975; 110:991–993.

69. Martin LW, Torres AM. Hirschsprung's disease. Surg Clin North America 1985; 65:1171–1180.

70. Preston DM, Lennard-Jones JE. Anismus in chronic constipation. Dig Dis Sci 1985; 30:413–418.

71. Rao SS. Dyssynergic defecation. Gastroenterol Clin North Am 2001;30:97–114.

72. Wald A, Chandra R, Chiponis D, Gabel S. Anorectal function and continence mechanisms in childhood encopresis. J Ped Gastro Nutr 1986;5:346–351.

73. Mathers SE, Kempster PA, Swash M, Lees AJ. Constipation and paradoxical puborectalis contraction in anismus and Parkinson's disease: a dystonic phenomenon? J Neurol Neurosurg Psychiatry 1988;51:1503–1507.

74. Edwards LL, Quigley EMM, Harned RK, et al. Characterization of swallowing and defecation in Parkinson's disease. Am J Gastroenterol 1994;89:15–25.

75. Jones PN, Lubowski DZ, Swash M, Henry MM. Is paradoxical contraction of the puborectalis muscle of functional importance? Dis Colon Rectum 1987;30:667–670.

76. Duthie GS, Bartolo DC. Anismus: the cause of constipation? Results of investigations and treatment. World J Surg 1992;16:831–835.

77. Voderholzer WA, Neuhaus DA, Klauser AG, et al. Paradoxical sphincter contraction is rarely indicative of anismus. Gut 1997;41:258–262.

78. Glick ME, Meshkinpour H, Haldeman S, et al. Colonic dysfunction in multiple sclerosis. Gastroenterol 1982;83:1002–1007.

79. Weber J, Grise P, Roquebert M, et al. Radiopaque markers transit and anorectal manometry in 16 patients with multiple sclerosis and urinary bladder dysfunction. Dis Colon Rectum 1987;30:95–100.

80. Wiesel PH, Norton C, Brazzelli M. Management of fecal incontinence and constipation in adults with central neurological diseases. Cochrane Database Syst Rev 2001;(4):CD002115.

81. Clinical practice guidelines: Neurogenic bowel management in adults with spinal cord injury. Spinal Cord Medicine Consortium. J Spinal Cord Med 1998;21:248–293.

PART IV
Management Issues

Chapter 14
Management of Swallowing Disorders

Kia Saeian and Reza Shaker

Swallowing, a highly coordinated physiologic event, requires sequential and overlapping contractions of the facial, cervical, oral, pharyngeal, laryngeal, and esophageal muscular apparatus, all culminating in transit of the ingested material and oral secretions from the mouth into the stomach. Neurologic disorders adversely affecting any portion of this coordinated sequence may lead to oropharyngeal dysphagia (OPD).

Swallowing may be divided into four consecutive phases: 1) preparatory, 2) oral, 3) pharyngeal, and 4) esophageal.[1,2] These phases roughly correlate with the anatomic regions traversed by an ingested bolus. During the preparatory phase, the bolus essentially remains in the oral cavity, is altered physically by being subjected to mastication, and altered chemically by mixing with saliva, all resulting in a bolus with suitable characteristics allowing for safe transit through the aerodigestive tract. It is during this phase that the bolus is sized, shaped, and positioned on the dorsum of the tongue for initiation of the upcoming oral phase of swallowing.

During the oral phase, a sequential contraction of the tongue against the hard and soft palates, a peristaltic pressure wave,[3,4] is generated that propels the bolus from the oral cavity into the pharynx. It is in the pharyngeal phase that the pharynx, upper esophageal sphincter (UES), and larynx[1,5] are all elevated, and three of the four routes for exit from the pharynx (namely the nasal cavity, oral cavity, and larynx), become sealed off, while the fourth route, the upper esophageal sphincter, opens. Contraction of the superior pharyngeal constrictor and elevation of soft palate and its contact with the posterior pharyngeal wall (velopharyngeal closure) close off the nasopharynx. The oral cavity is closed by elevation of the tongue base and its contact with the hard and soft palate.[3] The bolus is then transported into the esophagus by rapid forceful posterior tongue movements which persist from the oral phase, as well as the peristaltic contraction of the pharyngeal constrictors against the soft palate, base of the tongue, and the larynx.

It is during the oropharyngeal swallow that important biomechanical events involving intrinsic glottic, as well as supra- and infra-hyoid muscles, take place that result in the closure of the airway,[5–7] as well as in the opening of the upper esophageal sphincter[8–10] (Figure 14.1). These events include: 1) adduction of the true vocal cords and arytenoids (first tier of airway closure), followed by vertical

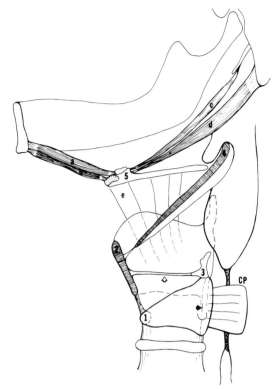

Figure 14.1. Schematic representation of suspension of hyoid and larynx. Hyoid (**5**) is suspended from mandible and skull by four suprahyoid muscles: anterior pair - geniohyoid (**b**) and
anterior digastric (**a**); posterior pair - stylohyoid (**c**) and posterior digastric (**d**). These muscles
generate a superior and anterior movement of hyoid during swallowing. Larynx is attached to
hyoid by paired thyroglossus muscles (**e**) and thyrohyoid membrane (not shown). Larynx consists of following cartilages: epiglottic (**4**), thyroid (**2**), cricoid (**1**), and arytenoid (**3**). Epiglottis
is attached anteriorly to thyroid cartilage, just superior to ventral attachment of vocal cords (*open
arrow*) on thyroid cartilage. Posteriorly, vocal cords attach to vocal process of arytenoids.
Arytenoids sit on superior margin of cricoid plate. Posterior border of trachea is indicated by
solid arrow. Just below this arrow is a hinge joint between inferior cornu of thyroid cartilage and
cricoid cartilage. Shortening of cricothyroid muscle (not shown) approximates anterior thyroid
cartilage to anterior rim of cricothyroid muscle. This movement passively tenses vocal cords and
tucks introitus of laryngeal vestibule ventrally under free margin of epiglottis. During swallowing, larynx makes a superoanterior excursion because of its attachment to hyoid. Thyrohyoid
muscles (**e**) contract so that larynx approximates and becomes locked to hyoid. Thus, superior
movement of the larynx exceeds that of the hyoid. Shortening of the thyrohyoid muscles also
rotates epiglottis into a horizontal position. Because of its attachment to cricoid, cricopharyngeus
(CP) moves superiorly about 1.5 cm during swallow-induced orad excursion of larynx.
(Reproduced by permission from Dodds WJ, Stewart ET, Logemann JA. Physiology and radiology of the normal oral and pharyngeal phases of swallowing. Am J Roentgenol
1990;154:953–963.)

approximation of the adducted arytenoids to the base of epiglottis (second tier of
closure) (Figure 14.2); 2) descent of the epiglottis covering the closed glottis,
thereby closing the laryngeal vestibule (third tier of closure); and 3) the entire larynx is pulled upwards and forward by the contraction of the suprahyoid muscle
group at the time of vocal cord closure or shortly thereafter. This displacement
results in the positioning of the closed larynx under the tongue base, away from the

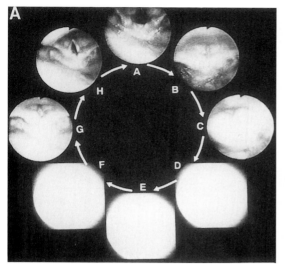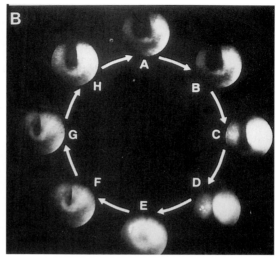

Figure 14.2. Examples of still frames of deglutitive vocal cord closure seen by transnasal videoendoscopy in (**A**) a normal volunteer and (**B**) by transtracheal videoendoscopy in a patient with tracheostomy. (**A**) (*A*) Glottis immediately before initiation of swallow. Vocal cords are open at their resting position. (*B*) Complete deglutitive vocal cord and arytenoid adduction. (*C*) Adducted arytenoids have approximated the base of the epiglottis. (*D–F*) Obscured view because of pharyngeal contraction and laryngeal elevation. (*G*) Vocal cords can be seen still adducted following the descent of the larynx and opening of the pharynx after passage of the bolus. (*H*) Vocal cords are beginning to open at the completion of swallow. (**B**) (*A*) Inferior view of glottis at rest. The introitus to the trachea is wide open immediately before the initiation of swallow. (*B* and *C*) Vocal cords are in the process of adduction narrowing the introitus. (*D*) Cords are in contact with each other in the anterior part. However, the posterior gap (*arrow*) is still open. (*E*) Posterior gap is now closed, resulting in complete closure of the introitus to the trachea. (*F*) Posterior gap is partially reopened while anterior part of the cords are still in contact. (*G* and *H*) Cords are further opened returning to resting position. Please note that contrary to the transnasal view, in the transtracheal view, the introitus to the trachea remained visible during the entire period of swallowing. (Reproduced by permission from Shaker R, Milbrath M, Ren J, et al. Deglutitive aspiration in patients with tracheostomy: effect of tracheostomy on the duration of vocal cord closure. Gastroenterology 1995;108:1357–1360.)

path of the bolus, thereby providing additional protection against aspiration[11,12] (Figure 14.3).

During oropharyngeal swallowing, the UES transiently relaxes and is subsequently pulled upward/forward by the contraction of the same suprahyoid muscles that displace the larynx. This traction results in active opening of the UES, which is also modified by the bolus size.[2,10,13,14] The temporal relationship of the events that take place during the oropharyngeal phase of swallowing is shown in Figure 14.4. Under normal conditions, oropharyngeal swallowing begins with the closure of the vocal cords, marking the initiation of airway protection,[7] and ends when the cords return to their resting positions. During this time, respiration is reflexively inhibited[15–18] and the protective mechanisms of swallowing are fully activated. Finally, the esophageal phase of swallowing transports the bolus further into the esophagus and stomach.

The elaborate mechanism of oropharyngeal swallowing ensures two important functions: 1) transit of the bolus, and 2) protection of the airway. Normal oropharyngeal swallowing is therefore defined as complete transit of the ingested material from the mouth into the esophagus, without compromising the airway. Oropharyngeal dysphagia may result when the efficacy and/or coordination of either transport or protective aspect of oropharyngeal swallowing are compromised.

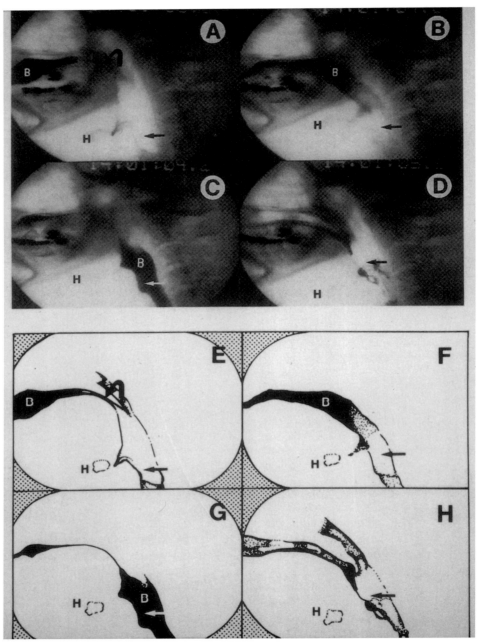

Figure 14.3. Example of the sequence of events during primary swallows. The primary swallow (**A–D**) resulted in bolus transport from the mouth into the pharynx and esophagus. Straight arrows indicate pharyngeal lumen. (**A** and **E**) Bolus of 5 ml of barium is held in the oral cavity immediately before the onset of swallowing. Tongue base and soft palate are in contact (*curved arrow*), segregating the oral bolus from the pharyngeal cavity. (**B** and **F**) Tongue base is depressed and soft palate has elevated and is in contact with the posterior pharyngeal wall. This resulted in closing off the nasopharynx and allowing the bolus to enter the pharynx (**C** and **G**). Bolus traversing the pharynx while the nasopharynx and oral cavity are sealed off by approximation of the soft palate and posterior pharyngeal wall, and apposition of the tongue base and soft palate, respectively. The hyoid bone has moved upward and forward (**D** and **H**). The barium bolus has cleared the pharynx, the oral cavity and nasopharynx are open, and the larynx and hyoid bone have returned to the resting position. (B = barium bolus; H = hyoid bone.) (Reproduced by permission from Shaker R, Ren J, Zamir Z, et al. Effect of aging, position, and temperature on the threshold volume triggering pharyngeal swallows. Gastroenterology 1994;107:396–401.)

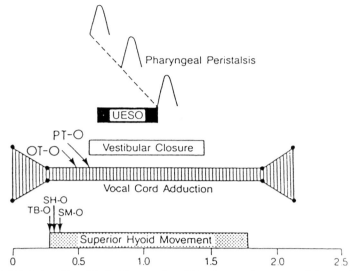

Figure 14.4. Relationship of deglutitive vocal cord kinetics to other events of the oropharyngeal phase of swallowing during 5-ml barium swallows. Bolus transit through the pharynx and across the UES begins and ends while the vocal cords are at maximal adduction. (TB-O = onset of tongue base movement; SH-O = onset of superior hyoid movement; SM-O = onset of submental myoelectrical activity; UESO = UES opening; OT-O = onset of bolus movement from the mouth; PT-O = arrival of bolus into pharynx.) (Reproduced by permission from Shaker R. Oropharyngeal dysphagia: practical approach to diagnosis and management. Semin Gastrointest Dis 1992;3:115–128.)

Although, the true prevalence of oropharyngeal dysphagia is unknown, studies have shown a 10 to 30% prevalence in general medical wards[19,20] and up to a 50 to 60% prevalence in nursing homes.

CONTROL OF SWALLOWING

Neural control of swallowing consists of three major components: 1) sensory afferent fibers contained in the cranial nerves, 2) central organizing centers, and 3) efferent motor fibers contained in the cranial nerves and ansa cervicalis.

Sensory Afferent Signals

Sensory afferent signals originating from the oral-pharyngeal cavity are carried by the branches of glossopharyngeal (IX) and vagus nerves (X) to the nucleus tractus solitarius (NTS) in the medulla. These afferent sensory fibers also carry sensory information from the pulmonary stretch receptors, as well as chemoreceptors located in carotid and aortic bodies. They also play a role in the control of the respiratory system.

Central Organizing Center

The medulla oblongata houses paired swallowing centers responsible for processing afferent sensory signals and programming the motor swallowing sequences.[21–23]

These centers are poorly defined areas and are comprised of the nucleus tractus solitarius (NTS), ventromedian reticular formation (VMRF), and nucleus ambiguous (NA). There is increasing evidence that cortical structures have a significant influence on the brain stem swallowing centers.[24] Cortical areas in the preorbital gyrus and lateral precentral gyrus have been implicated in modulation of deglutition. Cortical projections have been found connecting the cortical and medullary swallowing centers. Although poorly understood, some experimental evidence suggests the presence of a close functional, structural, and physiologic interaction between deglutitive and respiratory centers and their afferent and efferent inputs.

Motor Efferent Signals

Motor output to the muscular apparatus of the oropharynx for swallowing is transmitted by axons, whose cell bodies are located in the brain stem swallowing centers. These include motor nuclei of the trigeminal (V), facial (VII), and hypoglossal (XII) nerves. It also includes the NA, which not only consists of premotor commanding neurons, but also houses large motor neurons that are distributed to striated muscles innervated by the glossopharyngeal (IX) and vagus (X) nerves.

SWALLOWING MUSCULATURE

The muscular apparatus of oropharyngeal swallowing consists of a total of 30 paired striated muscles, which are shown along with their innervation in Table 14.1. Briefly, cranial nerve XII and the ansa cervicalis (C1-C2) control the tongue, while the vagus nerve exerts predominant control over the muscles of the palate, pharynx, and larynx, as well as the cricopharyngeus muscle. Deglutitive orad movement of the hyoid bone, larynx, and upper esophageal sphincter, and active opening of the UES following its relaxation, are induced by the supra- and infra-hyoid muscles that are innervated by the ansa cervicalis (C1-C2), cranial nerve V3, and cranial nerve VII.

PRESENTATION OF OROPHARYNGEAL DYSPHAGIA (OPD)

Most patients with oropharyngeal dysphagia (OPD) seek help because of symptoms, although a subset are silent aspirators who may present with recurrent

Table 14.1. Muscular Apparatus of Oral/Pharyngeal Swallowing

Muscle Group	Innervation
Mandibular muscles	Mandibular branch of trigeminal nerve (V3)
Facial muscles	Facial nerve (VII)
Intrinsic tongue muscles	Hypoglossal nerve (XII)
Extrinsic tongue muscles (except palatoglossus, X)	Ansa cervicalis (C1, C2)
Soft palate (except tensor veli palatini, V3)	Vagus (X)
Pharyngeal muscles and cricopharyngeus (except stylopharyngeus, IXn)	Vagus (X)
Intrinsic laryngeal muscles (except cricothyroid, SLN)	Vagus (X) recurrent laryngeal
Suprahyoid and infrahyoid muscles	V3, ansa cervicalis (C1, C2) and (VII)

pneumonias. Dysphagia symptoms reflect a breakdown in the transport or protective functions of oropharyngeal swallowing (Table 14.2). These symptoms are highly specific and should not be simply dismissed as functional or psychogenic. For instance, Ravitch et al. were able to document a reason for dysphagia in 15/23 (65%) of patients previously labeled as psychogenic dysphagia.[25] Every effort should be exerted to arrive at a specific diagnosis, but subtle abnormalities often escape detection.

A sensation of "food sticking in my throat" is often reported and reflects inadequate clearance of the bolus from the pharynx. Although this sensation may be caused by the presence of a large amount of residue in the pyriform sinus or valleculae, an obstructive lesion of the proximal or distal esophagus may lead to the very same complaint. Thus, patients with complaints of cervical dysphagia should undergo a thorough evaluation of the esophagus. Of course, careful direct visualization of the hypopharyngeal area must also rule out inflammation, abrasion, or tumors in this area.

Misdirection of the bolus into the airway leading to swallow-related coughing or choking is another common complaint. Invasion of the upper airway by the bolus may occur before initiation of, during, or after completion of oropharyngeal swallowing,[26] and result in a coughing or choking sensation. Aspiration into the airway may also occur prior to deglutition, because of the premature loss of the bolus into the hypopharynx from the mouth while the path to the airway is still open—a condition commonly encountered in post-stroke dysphagic patients. An inability to segregate the oral bolus from the pharynx by apposition of the tongue base and soft palate results in this premature spillage, called predeglutitive aspiration. If pharyngeal sensation is deranged, and swallowing is not initiated by entry of the prematurely passed bolus into the pharynx, predeglutitive aspiration and its concomitant complications follow. Deglutitive aspiration occurs either because of an incompetent glottis or one that does not close properly during the swallowing sequence, which leads to invasion of the airway by the bolus while it is being transported through the hypopharynx. Finally, post-deglutitive aspiration develops when the bolus transport is incomplete and a large residue remains in the pyriform sinus or valleculae—a condition encountered in parkinsonism, post stroke, myasthenia

Table 14.2. Symptoms of Oral/Pharyngeal Dysphagia

Inability to keep the bolus in the oral cavity
Difficulty gathering the bolus in the back of the tongue
Hesitation or inability to initiate the swallow
Food sticking in the throat
Nasal regurgitation
Inability to propel the food bolus caudad into the pharynx
Difficulty swallowing solids
Frequent repetitive swallowing
Frequent throat clearing
Gargly voice after meal
Hoarse voice
Nasal speech and dysarthria
Swallow related cough: before, during, or after swallowing
Avoidance from social dining
Weight loss
Recurrent pneumonia

gravis, and multiple sclerosis. When the glottis opens and respiration is resumed, the large residue is either inhaled or overflows into the trachea.

CAUSES OF OROPHARYNGEAL DYSPHAGIA (OPD)

A variety of disease entities may affect the muscular apparatus of the oropharynx and its related neuromuscular plate, as its well as its connections to the peripheral and central nervous system.[27–29] Oropharyngeal transport, deglutitive airway closure, or both may be affected and thus result in OPD. The causes of OPD are listed in Table 14.3. Neuromuscular diseases, which will be reviewed later in detail, account for approximately 80% of these cases, while local structural lesions make up the remainder.[14]

Structural Lesions

Structural lesions often present with solid food dysphagia and may have cervical symptoms and choking when bolus impaction occurs. Malignancies of the head and neck, which account for approximately 10% of all the cancers in North America, as well as their surgical resection or radiation therapy, result in considerable oropharyngeal dysphagia and present significant management problems.[30] Proximal

Table 14.3. Causes of Oral/Pharyngeal Dysphagia

Peripheral and Central Nervous System	Local Structural Lesions
Cerebrovascular accident	Surgical resection of oropharynx/larynx
Head injury	Oropharyngeal carcinoma
Parkinson's disease	Laryngeal carcinoma
Huntington's chorea	Zenker's diverticulum
Multiple sclerosis	Extrinsic compression
Amyotrophic lateral sclerosis	Enlarged thyroid gland
CNS tumor	Senile ankylosing hyperostosis of the cervical spine
Tabes dorsalis	Rheumatoid cricoarytenoid arthritis
Alzheimer's disease	Radiation injury, neuromuscular damage, salivary gland damage
Bulbar poliomyelitis	Cricopharyngeal abnormalities
Peripheral neuropathies	? Achalasia
Post traumatic	? Fibrosis
Friedreich's ataxia	Proximal esophageal webs and rings
Familial dysautonomia	
Muscular/neuromuscular	Pharmacologic agents
Inflammatory muscle diseases	Antihistamines
Polymyositis	Anticholinergics
Dermatomyositis	Phenothiazines
Inclusion body myositis	
Muscular dystrophies (myotonic oculopharyngeal)	
Kearns-Sayre syndrome	
Metabolic myopathy (thyroid associated myopathy)	
Alcoholic myopathy	
Myasthenia gravis	

esophageal webs, as seen in Plummer-Vinson or Paterson, Brown, Kelly syndrome, occur in the upper 2 to 4 cm of the esophagus and are associated with iron deficiency anemia, as well as some reports of post-cricoid carcinoma. Proximal esophageal webs may also be associated with graft versus host disease and Zenker's diverticulum, which itself may cause dysphagia and present with regurgitation, halitosis, a tracheoesophageal fistula, or bleeding. Proximal or distal esophageal strictures may occur as the result of lye ingestion, nasogastric tube placement, reflux disease, or malignancy.

Neuromuscular Etiologies

Oropharyngeal dysphagia following cerebrovascular accidents (CVA), a common clinical problem, has been attributed to a number of abnormalities in the swallowing sequence, including: diminished control of the tongue, abnormal closure of the larynx, and a delay in initiating a swallow.[28,31] Although a less commonly encountered type of CVA, brain-stem CVAs more commonly result in OPD.[29] Early studies of brain-stem CVA-associated dysphagia using cinefluorography characterized the abnormalities as pharyngeal dysmotility, pharyngeal asymmetry, or incomplete relaxation of the upper esophageal sphincter.[32] Subsequent work, however, has only found pharyngeal motility to be a significant factor in the occurrence of aspiration.[29] The same group found that while 15/23 (62%) patients with brain stem strokes developed dysphagia, 10 of those 15 patients were eventually able to resume full oral nutrition (mean 97.4 days) with aggressive therapy.

Dysphagia has also been noted in hemispheric lesions, especially in the acute stages, with studies reporting a prevalence of 23% to 43%,[33] depending on the makeup of the study population (increasing up to ~ 50% in series of bilateral hemispheric CVAs).[34] Of those patients who survive a hemispheric CVA, nearly 90% rapidly (within 14 days) regain their ability to swallow.[33] Following head injury, approximately 25% of adults develop oropharyngeal dysphagia, 94% of whom have been reported to recover within three months.[27]

Degenerative neuronal diseases commonly lead to dysphagia, with the prevalence of oropharyngeal dysphagia in this group ranging widely between 18% and 89%, depending on the specific disease entity.[29,35–45] Even though the presenting symptoms are often similar to those caused by other pathologies, the oropharyngeal dysphagia in this population is typically more pronounced for liquids than for solids. In addition, material that is granular/crumbly or of high viscosity may be more problematic for these patients. Objective findings on videofluoroscopic examination are indicative of discoordination of lingual function and oral/pharyngeal bolus transit, inadequate pharyngeal constrictor function, discoordination between bolus transit and protection of the airway during the oral/pharyngeal phase of swallowing, and abnormal upper esophageal sphincter opening (Table 14.4).

Now a well-recognized entity, post poliomyelitis syndrome (PPS) occurs three or four decades after the initial infection by the polio virus,[46] and typically presents with new neuromuscular findings in previously stable patients. These findings may include fatigue, cold intolerance, joint pain, new weakness, muscle pain and atrophy, respiratory insufficiency, dysphagia, and sleep apnea. It is estimated that half of all polio survivors (1.6 million in the USA) will develop this syndrome. The incidence of dysphagia among patients with this syndrome has been reported to be 18%.[47]

Table 14.4. Oral/Pharyngeal Dysphagia in Neuronal Diseases—Videofluoroscopic Findings

Parkinson's disease	Post-polio syndrome
Abnormal lip control	Unilateral/bilateral tongue weakness
Abnormal tongue control	Pharyngeal paralysis (paresis)
Abnormal soft palate movement	Absent/incomplete epiglottic tilt
Poor bolus manipulation/control	Poor laryngeal elevation
Abnormal triggering of pharyngeal phase	Poor laryngeal closure
Incomplete pharyngeal clearance time	Laryngeal penetration/aspiration
Tracheal aspiration	Incomplete UES opening
Dementia	Huntington's disease
Lingual dysfunction	Abnormal preparatory phase
Abnormal bolus control	Impaired mastication, bolus control
Dyscoordination of oral and pharyngeal phase	Premature spill
Epiglottal dysmotility	Incomplete oral bolus clearance
Pharyngeal constrictor paresis	Repetitive swallows
Incomplete pharyngeal clearance	Lingual chorea
Incomplete UES opening	Tracheal aspiration
Aspiration	Dyscoordination of swallowing and breathing
Closed head trauma	Brain stem stroke
Defective tongue control	Delayed initiation of swallow
Abnormal pharyngeal peristalsis	Pharyngeal residue
Abnormal laryngeal elevation/closure	Incomplete UES opening
Aspiration	Aspiration
Cerebrovascular accident	Alzheimer's disease
Incomplete oral bolus clearance	Abnormal preparatory phase
Abnormal lingual function	Abnormal initiation of pharyngeal phase
Delayed pharyngeal phase	Defective pharyngeal clearance
Pharyngeal residue	Incomplete UES opening
Aspiration	Aspiration
Multiple sclerosis	
Difficulty in mastication	
Difficulty manipulating/control of bolus	
Delay in pharyngeal phase	
Impaired pharyngeal contraction/clearance	
Aspiration	

The Kearns-Sayre syndrome (KSS) is a rare multisystem disorder caused by a mitochondrial disease with a deficiency of cytochrome c-oxidase. It is characterized by progressive external ophthalmoplegia, pigmentary retinopathy, and cardiac conduction defects. Swallowing difficulties occur late in the course of the disease and result in incomplete pharyngeal clearance and aspiration. This is due to ineffective pharyngeal peristalsis secondary to involvement of the striated muscles in bolus transit.[48]

It was Valsalva, who in 1707 proposed the designation "cricopharyngeal muscle" as the most distal muscle fibers of the pars cricopharyngea of the inferior pharyngeal constrictor, after he recognized its anatomical and functional identity. Dysfunction of the cricopharyngeal muscle, the main component of the upper esophageal sphincter (UES), is now becoming an increasingly recognized cause of dysphagia. Normal deglutitive UES opening is determined by 1) transient UES relaxation (i.e., loss of active cricopharyngeus tone); 2) persistence of minimal passive tension, namely, normal distensibility of the CP muscle; 3) active traction on the UES generated by anterior hyoid and laryngeal movement which, in turn, is induced by contraction of the suprahyoid muscles; and 4) pulsion forces imparted to the relaxed UES by the oncoming pharyngeal bolus. Disordered UES opening as a consequence of abnormalities in any of these opening factors results in a compromised transsphincteric flow, leading to the underlying basis for the majority of the disorders of the UES.

The term cricopharyngeal achalasia was originally used by radiologists upon observation of a prominent pharyngo-esophageal segment during swallowing, causing inadequate opening of the pharyngo-esophageal junction in patients with cervical dysphagia (Figure 14.5). However, comparing the mechanism of closure and opening of the CP (striated) muscle with that of the lower esophageal sphincter (smooth) muscle to which the term achalasia was first applied, as well as comparing the innervation and maintenance of basal tone by the two organs, the term cricopharyngeal achalasia needs to be viewed more critically.

Cricopharyngeal achalasia may develop due to primary neurogenic cricopharyngeous muscle dysfunction, causing disordered UES relaxation and/or dyscoordination with pharyngeal peristalsis. This may occur due to a variety of neurogenic causes (e.g., cerebrovascular hemorrhage, Parkinson's disease). Delayed or failure of cricopharyngeal muscle opening has been reported in 30 to 50%[49,50] of brain stem lesions, central degenerative disorders, posterior cerebellar artery thrombosis, as well as in bulbar paralysis. Primary myogenic cricopharyngeus dysfunction causing CP achalasia includes loss of elasticity, as well as fibrotic changes of the UES that prevent its adequate opening during swallowing. A variety of causes, including gastroesophageal reflux and aging, have been suggested to be responsible for these changes.

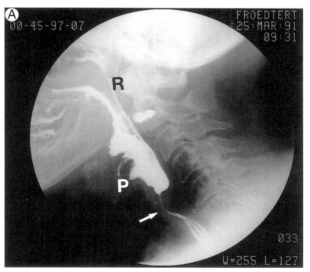

Figure 14.5. An example of a modified video barium swallow in a patient with cricopharyngeal achalasia resulting in a feeling of incomplete swallow, deglutitive cough and pharyngeal residue. **A.** Barium bolus is seen in the pharynx during the pharyngeal phase of swallowing immediately before the UES opens. A trace of barium from previous swallow is seen within the UES and proximal esophagus (*arrow*). Vestibular penetration (P) and nasal regurgitation (R) are also seen.

Figure continued on following page

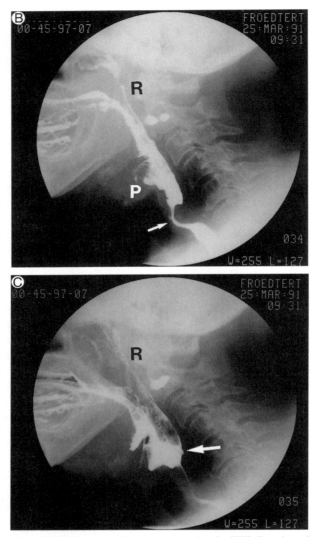

Figure 14.5 *Continued.* **B.** Barium bolus is seen transversing the UES. Prominent indentation induced by incomplete opening of the CP muscle is seen (*arrow*). The result is severe narrowing of the UES lumen. However, barium bolus has filled the proximal esophagus. Also present is nasal regurgitation (R) and vestibular penetration (P). **C.** Pharyngeal phase swallowing is now ended. UES has closed, however, a large amount of barium is left behind in the hypopharynx (*arrow*).

In secondary cricopharyngeus dysfunction causing CP achalasia, the pathology lies within the suprahyoid muscles, believed to be due to inflammatory changes such as those seen in inclusion body myositis. These patients are incapable of exerting an adequate traction force to pull the UES open during swallowing, and typically lack normal laryngeal elevation. In this condition, excitatory impulses to the cricopharyngeal muscle are indeed inhibited during swallowing, and result in manometric relaxation of the UES, but the UES itself does not open adequately due to insufficient traction. Depending on the severity of the condition, patients suffering from UES dysfunction may present with aspiration pneumonia, swallow-related cough, choking, repeated swallowing, food sticking in the throat, and weight loss.

Oropharyngeal dysphagia, associated with the disruption of the normal laryngeal innervation, ranges from minimal cough to severe frequent deglutitive aspiration with swallowing. These patients present with various degrees of hoarseness, aspiration pneumonia, and weight loss. The etiology of the laryngeal paralysis includes insults to the recurrent and/or superior laryngeal nerve due to a variety of surgical procedures, inflammatory disorders, and central nervous system diseases. On the average, 10% of the laryngeal paralysis, however, is reported to be idiopathic.[51]

EVALUATION OF OROPHARYNGEAL DYSPHAGIA

Oropharyngeal dysphagia (OPD) may result from a variety of abnormal conditions that extend across various disciplines. Although diagnostic modalities will often lead to the identification of a specific derangement in the oral or pharyngeal phase of swallowing, they rarely help in determination of the causative factors. Therefore, a multidisciplinary systematic approach is required, not only in identifying the cause(s) leading to OPD, but also for its management. Obtaining a detailed history of the problem should be followed by a focused physical and neurological examination. Special attention should be given to concomitant disorders that may be responsible for oropharyngeal dysphagia, such as thyroid disease, previous radiation therapy of the head and neck, neurologic disease or trauma, diabetes mellitus, Parkinson's disease, polymyositis, dermatomyositis, myotonia, myasthenia gravis, anemia, and connective tissue diseases, such as rheumatoid arthritis, scleroderma, Sicca syndrome, and Raynaud's phenomenon. History of recurrent pneumonia, weight loss, water and sour brash, regurgitation, and heartburn must be sought, and a careful account of the use of medications, including tranquilizers, ulcer, and cancer medications, needs to be taken. Since some symptoms of oropharyngeal dysphagia, such as hoarseness, could be either due to unilateral paralysis of the cords or inflammation of the glottis due to frequent aspiration of food, correct diagnosis requires a thorough laryngologic examination.

This, again, emphasizes the need for a multidisciplinary approach to the OPD patients. This team may consist of representatives from the following disciplines: 1) Gastroenterology, 2) Otolaryngology, 3) Radiology, 4) Dentistry, 5) Speech/ Language Pathology, and 6) Neurology. The role of individual members depends on the expertise available in respective institutions. However, the care of the oropharyngeal dysphagia patient, like any other patient, needs to be coordinated by a single managing physician. Multidisciplinary working conferences focused on diagnosis and management of unusual cases are most helpful.

DIAGNOSTIC MODALITIES

The approach to the oropharyngeal dysphagia patient is evolving. Until recently, barium studies were the only modality available and used for evaluation of OPD patients. During the past decade, several other modalities such as manometry, endoscopy, ultrasonography, and scintigraphy have been introduced into this field. Ongoing, intensive research by various disciplines is making the approach to the oropharyngeal dysphagia patient a dynamic and improving phenomenon. Quantitative normalcy data are becoming available, and study recordings and test substances are more standardized, allowing for interstudy comparison. With the advent of videorecorders and digitalization technology, endoscopic and fluoro-scopic images are videotaped and analyzed later, using the slow motion and frame-by-frame movements capability of the tape recorder. This technology permits the accurate timing of the events. Availability of specially designed timers allows syn-chronization of several investigative modalities. This synchronization allows deter-mination of temporal relationship of various events, such as bolus movement and airway closure during oropharyngeal swallowing. Since not all of the structures of the oropharynx during swallowing are adequately seen by one single modality, this multisystem recording is essential for studying the coordination of oropharyngeal swallowing events.

Modified Barium Swallow

Currently, videofluoroscopic recording of a modified barium swallow is the diag-nostic modality of choice for initial investigation of the patient with oropharyngeal dysphagia. During this study, recordings of a variety of boluses with different con-sistencies and volumes are made for subsequent analysis. These recordings may be used subsequently for future comparisons to evaluate progress. This technique not only provides adequate information about the movement of the barium bolus through the aerodigestive tract and documents misdirection of the bolus into the air-way, it also provides vital information about the anatomy and function of the indi-vidual anatomical components of the aerodigestive tract involved in swallowing.[50,52] Additionally, this modality is used to evaluate the effect of various postural and breathing techniques on the efficiency, as well as safety, of swallowing.[9,53] Normal and abnormal videofluoroscopic findings of swallowing (Table 14.5) have been published extensively.[2,9,54] On videofluoroscopy, abnormalities of the oral phase of swallowing may manifest themselves as inadequate clearance of the barium bolus from the mouth (leaving a barium residue behind), piece-meal swallowing due to inadequate tongue function, or difficulty initiating the swallowing sequence due to impaired cognitive or neural function.[9] Patients with difficulty controlling the labial or facial muscles will not be able to hold the barium bolus in their anterior

Table 14.5. Abnormalities of the Oropharyngeal Phase of Swallowing (Seen by Videofluoroscopy)

Oral Phase	Pharyngeal Phase
Anterior spill of the bolus from the mouth	Decreased or absent coupled antrocephalad movement of the hyoid bone and larynx
Inability to gather the bolus on the dorsum of the tongue	Lack of, or abnormal, epiglottal descent
Posterior spill into the pharynx	Lack of, or incomplete, palatal movement
Abnormal lingual palatal contact	Abnormal pharyngeal wall movement
Impaired tongue movement	Laryngeal aspiration
Repetitive	Abnormal unilateral/bilateral residue
Disorganized	Valeculae
Difficulty in initiating swallow	Pyrifrom sinus
Residue in the oral cavity	Incomplete opening of the upper esophageal sphincter
Sublingual	
Sulci	

mouth, and will end up drooling during swallow. Premature spilling of the oral contents into the pharynx before the pharyngeal phase is activated will catch the airway off guard, and may result in predeglutitive aspiration. This abnormality commonly occurs with impaired palatal and/or lingual control.

Abnormalities of the pharyngeal phase of swallowing documented by videofluoroscopy include concomitant absent or diminished upward/forward movement of the larynx and hyoid bone, indicating inadequate suprahyoid muscle contraction. This abnormality may be accompanied by entry of the barium into the airway beyond the level of the true vocal cords (aspiration). An incompetent velopharyngeal closure mechanism, due to inadequate elevation and/or weak posterior movement of the palate and uvula, may result in regurgitation of barium into the nasopharynx. This abnormality could develop after CVA in the setting of other neurogenic processes, inflammatory disorders of striated muscles, or following surgical excisions. Abnormalities of the oral phase of swallowing may or may not be accompanied by abnormalities of the pharyngeal phase of swallowing.

Abnormalities in transport function during oropharyngeal swallowing result in hypopharyngeal residue. Abnormal lingual, pharyngeal, or UES function, singularly or in combination, may be responsible. Unilateral involvement of the pharynx results in ipsilateral post-deglutitive bulging of the pharyngeal wall and residue on the same side.[2,6]

Misdirection of the barium into the airway may be due to intrinsic abnormalities of the glottal adductor muscles, resulting in an ineffective glottal sphincteric mechanism or lack of coordination between glottal closure and transport function of the oropharynx, commonly seen in neurologically impaired patients.

Abnormal opening of the upper esophageal sphincter during swallowing, seen by videofluoroscopy, may be due to lack of or impairment of its relaxation, decreased UES compliance, or inadequate traction by the suprahyoid muscles. Correct diagnosis requires manometric evaluation of the UES for its resting pressure and its swallow-induced relaxation. Diagnosis of cricopharyngeal achalasia cannot be made solely by its radiographic appearance.

Videoendoscopy

The chronic nature of oropharyngeal dysphagia requires assessment of therapeutic results and progress with repeat videofluoroscopic study. Because of the radiation exposure and also difficulty in moving some patients to the radiology suite, a videoendoscopic approach to the evaluation of oropharyngeal dysphagia has been developed.[26,55–57] In this technique, a small diameter endoscope, such as a laryngoscope or bronchoscope, is inserted through the nose and positioned at the level of posterior nares. In this position, the patient is asked to swallow. During this swallow, normal features of pharyngeal seal, namely the adduction of the superior constrictor and postero/orad elevation of palate seen as a bulging in the nasopharynx, is examined, then the scope is advanced to the level of free margin of the epiglottis. At this position the glottis is clearly seen (Figures 14.6–14.8) and its adduction function is examined by having the patient produce different vowels. Following this, a 5 to 10 ml water bolus colored with blue food dye is given through the mouth, and the patient is instructed to hold the bolus in the mouth for 20 seconds. During this time, the back of the tongue is observed videoendoscopically for presence or absence of unilateral or bilateral spill or entry of colored water into the airway

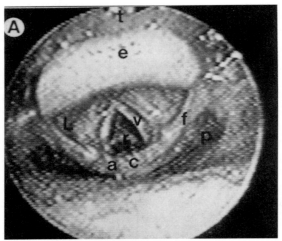
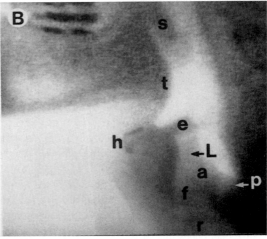

Figure 14.6. Hypopharynx and glottis viewed by videoendoscopy (**A**) and videofluroscopy (**B**). Although most of the anatomical structures involved in swallowing are visualized by both modalities, the hyoid bone is observed only by the x-ray technique, whereas vocal cords are visualized better by endoscopy. (a = arytenoid; c = posterior commissure; e = epiglottis; f = aryepiglottic fold; h = hyoid bone; L = laryngeal vestibule; p = pyriform sinus; r = trachea; v = vocal cord.) (Reproduced by permission from Shaker R. Oropharyngeal dysphagia: practical approach to diagnosis and management. Semin Gastrointest Dis 1992;3:115–128.)

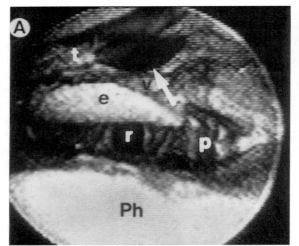
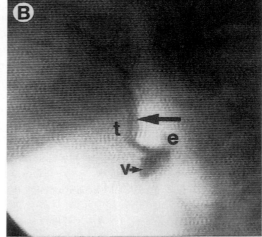

Figure 14.7. Still frames of videoendoscopic (**A**) and videofluoroscopic (**B**) views of premature spill (*arrow*) of oral bolus into the pharynx in the oropharyngeal dysphagic patient. On videofluoroscopy it is observed that the barium contrast spilled prematurely over the posterior aspect of the tongue and has filled the space between the posterior aspect of the tongue and anterior aspect of the free margin of the epiglottis (the valleculae). Similarly, on videoendoscopy it is observed that the blue-colored water has entered the pharynx prematurely and is over the posterior aspect of the tongue entering the valleculae. (e = epiglottis; p = pyriform sinus; ph = posterior pharyngeal wall; r = trachea; t = posterior aspect of the tongue; v = valleculae.) (Reproduced by permission from Shaker R. Oropharyngeal dysphagia: practical approach to diagnosis and management. Semin Gastrointest Dis 1992;3:115–128.)

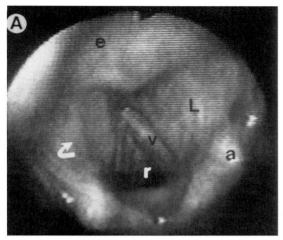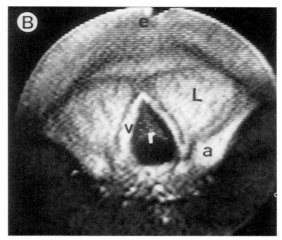

Figure 14.8. Endoscopic views of the glottis in a dysphagic patient (**A**) and a normal volunteer (**B**) after swallowing 5 ml of blue-colored water. As noted, the patient's vestibule is stained (*arrow*) after swallowing 5 ml of colored water, whereas, the healthy volunteer's vestibule is not, except for the staining edges. (a = arytenoids; e = epiglottis; L = laryngeal vestibule; r = trachea; v = vocal cord.) (Reproduced by permission from Shaker R. Oropharyngeal dysphagia: practical approach to diagnosis and management. Semin Gastrointest Dis 1992;3:115–128.)

(predeglutitive aspiration). The presence of spill is seen in patients with abnormalities of the tongue and/or palate control. Following this stage, the scope is withdrawn to the level of the posterior nares and the patient is asked to swallow once. The scope is immediately advanced to the level of the epiglottis. On the way toward the epiglottis, attention is given to the presence or absence of blue staining of the retro palatal pharynx, indicative of nasal regurgitation due to abnormalities of the velopharyngeal closure mechanism. This abnormality may be caused by inadequate elevation and posterior movement of the soft palate and uvula. Then the inner aspect of the epiglottis, aryepiglottic fold, posterior commissure, and true vocal cords are examined for the presence or absence of staining. In a study of normal volunteers in our laboratory, only the outer edges of the epiglottis and aryepiglottic-fold were stained with blue dye. Endotracheal coloring with blue dye is easily seen, proving aspiration. The patients are then asked to cough once and since, during cough the laryngeal vestibule remains open, expulsion of blue material from the trachea can be seen and is indicative of aspiration. Following this phase, the presence or absence of residue in the pyriform sinus and valleculae is determined, and overflow of residue into the trachea through the posterior commissure is sought.

Manometry

Although the use of intraluminal strain-gauges for pharyngeal manometry has resulted in a significant increase in our knowledge about the pharyngeal pressure phenomena, this modality still remains mainly a research tool, and its clinical application is limited to the evaluation of dysphagic patients with primary muscle diseases. An example of these disorders is the aforementioned Kearns-Sayre syndrome, where significant diminution of the pharyngeal peristaltic pressure wave amplitude is the prominent finding (Figure 14.9).

Because the pharynx is radially, as well as axially, an asymmetric cavity, orientation of the pressure transducers needs to be ascertained and preferably similar in all studies in order to obtain meaningful data. In our laboratory, the posterior orientation has been used, since it yields the most consistent results. Concurrent pharyngeal and UES manometry helps detect discoordination between the UES relaxation and arrival of pharyngeal peristalsis in the hyopharynx. Use of manometry to evaluate the oral phase in dysphagic patients has generally been unsuccessful, and this modality continues to be used for research purposes only.

As discussed previously, normal UES opening basically requires the existence of normal cricopharyngeal relaxation and distensibility, as well as normal contractile force of the suprahyoid muscles. Traditionally, UES resting tone and deglutitive relaxation have been studied by intraluminal manometry. Because of the orad displacement of the UES during swallowing and its to-and-fro movement during breathing, the use of a sleeve sensor has been advocated for this purpose. This 6 cm long sensor, which acts similar to a Sterling resistor, provides continuous measurement of the UES pressure,[58] and records maximal squeeze pressure regardless of the

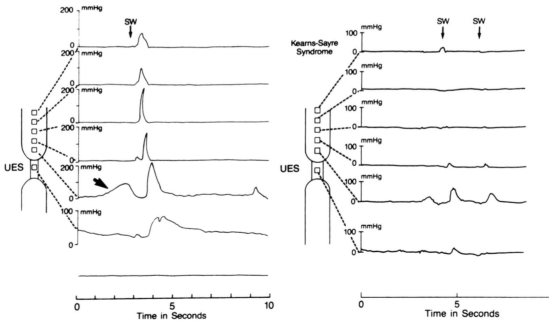

Figure 14.9. Pharyngeal peristalsis recorded using intraluminal strain-gauges in a patient with Kearns-Sayre syndrome and its comparison with age-matched control. The recording sites are 1.5 cm apart. During swallowing the bottom two sites record from the UES. The third from the bottom records the hypopharynx and the top three record from the proximal pharynx. As seen, the proximal pharyngeal pressure amplitude is significantly lower compared to the controls. However, the amplitude 1.5 cm above the UES (third from bottom) where the posterior tongue thrust is recorded, is similar to the control. (Reproduced by permission from Shaker R, Kupla JI, Kidder TM, et al. Manometric characteristics of cervical dysphagia in a patient with Kearns-Sayre syndrome. Gastroenterology 1992;103:1328–1331.)

axial sphincter movement along the length of the device. Shorter pressure sensors, either strain gauges or pneumohydraulic side holes, may remain within the sphincter at rest. However, during swallowing, they will drop into the cervical esophagus, due to the upward movement of the sphincter, and yield intraesophageal pressure which may be misinterpreted as UES relaxation (Figure 14.10).

Differentiating between deglutitive relaxation and opening of the CP muscle by intraluminal manometry is impossible. The sudden intraluminal UES pressure decline during swallowing, commonly referred to as UES relaxation, reflects the effect of (a) CP relaxation and (b) UES opening of various degrees. Concurrent manometry and fluoroscopy also provides information which is the summation of the two effects of relaxation and opening. For this reason, concurrent manometry, electromyography (Figure 14.11), and videofluoroscopy is essential to differentiate the effects of these phenomena.

A relatively common change in UES morphology, observed during pharyngoesophageal barium studies, is a prominent posterior indentation at the level of the UES; cricopharyngeal bar. Although rarely associated with dysphagia, its observation has been reported in 5% of patients older than 40 years who did not have symptoms.[54,59] Despite the common notion of spasm or failed relaxation, the pathogenesis of cricopharyngeal bar is not fully known. A recent study by Dantas et al.[60] has shown a normal resting pressure, as well as normal deglutitive relaxation, in individuals with cricopharyngeal bar. However, the upstream (intrabolus) pressure was found to be higher than that of normal controls. Also found was reduced dimension of UES during passage of barium, suggestive of reduced compliance of the cricopharyngeal muscle.

Ultrasonography

Ultrasound for evaluation of the oral phase of swallowing has been successfully used. Since this modality is noninvasive and does not disturb the physiology of the oral phase of swallowing, it could be used in addition to videofluoroscopy to evaluate the dysphagic patient. Using this modality, Sonies et al. have described subtle, subclinical changes of the oral phase of swallowing in the aged.[61]

MANAGEMENT

Although only a minority of the patients with oropharyngeal dysphagia are amenable to medical/surgical therapy, the majority do require retraining and use of various swallowing maneuvers and techniques in order to achieve an adequate and safe swallow.

Cricopharyngeal dilatation and myotomy has been performed for a variety of neurogenic and myogenic causes of oropharyngeal dysphagia, with variable results. However, controlled clinical trials and outcome studies are lacking. In general, myotomy yields good results in CP achalasia due to primary CP muscle involvement. The results are less predictable for primary neurogenic causes if other parts of the swallowing apparatus are also involved. The role of myotomy in secondary CP achalasia is controversial, since deglutitive relaxation and abolition resistance to flow is present in this group. The rationale for the cricopharyngeal myotomy, which

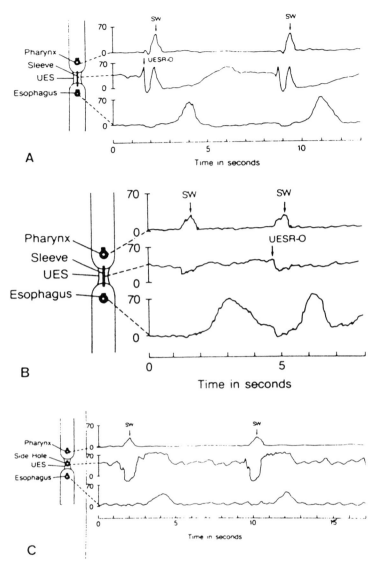

Figure 14.10. A. An example of complete manometric deglutitive UES relaxation in an elderly patient during UES manometry using a sleeve device. As seen, after the onset of UES relaxation (UESR-O), the UES pressure sharply declines to slightly below atmospheric pressure indicating complete UES relaxation. **B.** An example of UES manometry in a cricopharyngeal achalasia patient using a sleeve device. As seen with each swallow, contrary to the example in **A**, although the UES pressure reduces, it does not decline to the atmospheric pressure. The reduction in UES pressure during swallowing in this patient is felt to be due to anterocephalad displacement of cricoid cartilage as a result of suprahyoid muscle contraction. **C.** An example of UES manometry using a pneumohydraulic side hole in the patient with cricopharyngeal achalasia. During swallowing, due to orad excursion of the UES, the side hole of the manometric catheter which was within the UES during resting was displaced into the proximal esophagus and recorded esophageal pressure, thus yielding a spurious UES relaxation. (Reproduced by permission from Shaker R, Kupla JI, Kidder TM, et al. Manometric characteristics of cervical dysphagia in a patient with Kearns-Sayre syndrome. Gastroenterology 1992;103:1328–1331.)

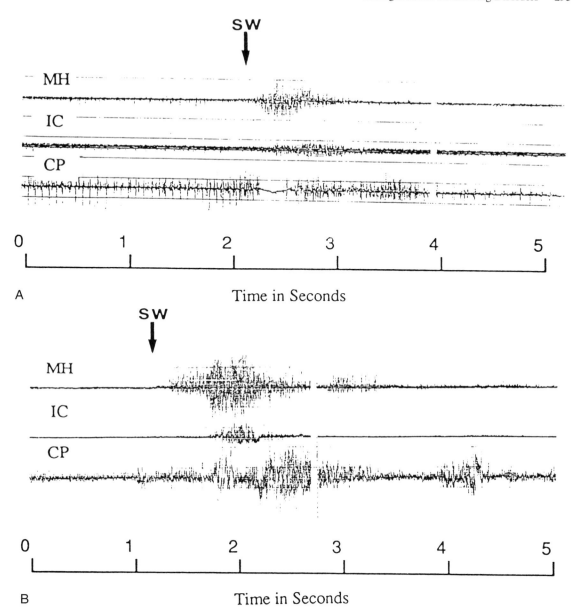

Figure 14.11. Examples of electromyographic recordings from the mylohyoid/geniohyoid muscle group (MH), inferior pharyngeal constrictor (IC) and cricopharyngeal muscle (CP) from a normal control (**A**) and a patient with CP achalasia (**B**) during dry swallow. As seen, the MH and IC do not exhibit any tone before swallow, whereas CP maintains a basal tone during resting. In the normal control subject, swallowing results in transient inhibition of CP tone, myoelectrical activity of the mylohyoid/geniohyoid group and the inferior constrictors. In the patient with CP achalasia, however, swallowing does not result in inhibition of the CP tone. (Reproduced by permission from Shaker R et al. In WJ Snape [ed], Consultations in Gastroenterology. Philadelphia: WB Saunders, 1996;177–186.)

usually is extended to the lower part of the inferior pharyngeal constrictor and upper part of the cervical esophagus, is to eliminate the resistance of the UES against the flow of the swallowed bolus. Under normal conditions, this resistance is eliminated by timely relaxation, and opening and closure of the UES. However, in a variety of conditions, because of dyscoordination of the UES and pharynx or because of ineffective pharyngeal function, the UES acts as a relative resistor to the bolus flow. It is in these conditions that cricopharyngeal myotomy may improve pharyngeal bolus transit and reduce aspiration. Recently, endoscopic transmucosal botulinum toxin injection into the CP muscle has been tried in patients with CP achalasia. However, close proximity of the injection area and the vocal cords raises special concern about possible respiratory complications. On the other hand, because of the temporary effect of the botulinum toxin, this new technique could potentially be used to select patients who will benefit from CP myotomy.

Vencovsky et al.[36] reported successful resolution of dysphagia after cricopharyngeal myotomy in a patient with acute cricopharyngeal obstruction due to dermatomyositis. Gagic[62] reported excellent results of cricopharyngeal myotomy in patients with Zenker's diverticulum and idiopathic hypertrophy of the cricopharyngeal muscle, and marked improvement in patients with vagal injuries, amyotrophic lateral sclerosis, and post CVA; however, no improvement was achieved in a patient with myotonia dystrophica. Two patients developed aspiration pneumonia and respiratory arrest. Logemann has reported[63] that the results of cricopharyngeal myotomy are superior when pathology is mainly in the UES, there are pharyngeal propulsive forces present, and patients are able to close the airway voluntarily. Since the major barrier against pharyngeal regurgitation of gastric acid, namely the UES, is ablated by myotomy, pulmonary complications of gastroesophageal reflux postoperatively remain a major concern in patients who undergo cricopharyngeal myotomy.

In patients with an inadequate deglutitive glottal closure mechanism, such as patients with Parkinson's disease or amyotrophic lateral sclerosis, the deglutitive airway closure could be augmented by injection of a nonabsorbable material such as Teflon[9,64,65] into the lateral thyroarytenoid muscle. Injection of Teflon will result in bulk formation in the injection site and displace the true cord in a fixed position toward the midline, facilitating glottal closure during swallowing, since the adduction of functioning cord will result in contact of the two cords and closure of introitus of the trachea. Teflon injection of the cords has also been successfully used to prevent aspiration in patients with various types of vocal cord paralysis, due to dysfunction of recurrent laryngeal and/or superior laryngeal nerve as a result of various central nervous system, surgical, or inflammatory disorders.[66,67]

The majority of oropharyngeal dysphagia patients, however, require specialized rehabilitation of their swallowing function. Maintaining an adequate nutrition during this period is essential.[12,68–70]

Swallow therapy is performed with the aid of videofluoroscopy[9] and more recently, with videoendoscopy.[55,56] Since swallowing studies are time consuming and must be tailored to each individual patient and the specific pathology, various techniques and maneuvers have to be tried until an efficient and safe swallow is produced.

Multiple therapeutic maneuvers (Table 14.6) are at our disposal for improvement of the oropharyngeal bolus transport and provision of airway safety. Some patients respond to a change in bolus size and/or consistency, while in others, placing the head in a specific position may assure safe passage of the bolus through the hypopharynx. For instance, flexion of the head will displace the larynx beneath the epiglot-

Table 14.6. Postural Swallowing Techniques

Utilize gravity to move the bolus
Hide away the airway from the bolus path
Possibly reduce the laryngeal entrance
Eliminate the weak side from bolus path
Direct bolus to the stronger side

tis and reduce the chance for aspiration, while rotating the head toward the weaker side will partially obstruct this weaker side and improve pharyngeal transit. Similarly, tilting the head toward the weaker side will direct the bolus laterally, and may improve pharyngeal bolus transit, and prevent aspiration.[9]

Patients with predeglutitive and deglutitive aspiration may benefit from specific therapeutic maneuvers (Table 14.7) such as supraglottic swallow.[9] In this maneuver, patients take a deep breath and hold breathing, then swallow. Swallowing is followed by a voluntary cough before resumption of respiration, which clears the larynx of aspirated material.

In patients with impaired pharyngeal transit and post deglutitive aspiration, Mendelsohn's maneuver may improve pharyngeal emptying and prevent aspiration.[2,9] In this maneuver, patients are taught to generate a sustained laryngeal and hyoid bone elevation during swallowing, in order to increase the UES traction and prolong its opening. This results in improved pharyngeal emptying. Observing the fluoroscopy monitor during this maneuver greatly enhances the patient's learning and compliance.

In the elderly, in whom the cross-sectional area of the deglutitive upper esophageal sphincter opening is reduced, isotonic and isometric head raising exercise has been shown to increase the cross sectional area of the UES.[71] This increase is accompanied by a significant decrease in hypopharyngeal intrabolus pressure, indicating a decrease in pharyngeal outflow resistance. In a preliminary study of 27 patients with pharyngeal dysphagia and documented aspiration requiring chronic tube-feeding, the use of this exercise resulted in complete resolution of aspiration in all 27. More importantly, all patients resumed modified oral diets and no longer required tube feeding.[72]

CONCLUSION

In conclusion, oropharyngeal dysphagia results from dysfunction of one or more of the highly coordinated events of the oropharyngeal phase of swallowing, leading to abnormal transport and/or airway protection. Whether due to one of a variety

Table 14.7. Swallow Maneuvers

Closes the airway before and during swallow (supraglottic-swallow)
Increases posterior tongue movement (effort-full swallow)
Prolongs UES opening and laryngeal elevation (Mendelsohn maneuver)
Increase the area of UES opening (Shaker exercise)

of muscular, peripheral, and central nervous system disorders, malignancies of oropharyngeal cavity, or surgical and radiation therapy for these malignancies, the symptoms of oropharyngeal dysphagia are highly specific and should not be dismissed as psychogenic. Physical examination should focus on detection of neurologic deficits. Although a number of useful diagnostic modalities are available, the videofluoroscopic recording of a modified barium swallow is the diagnostic modality of choice for initial investigation of the patient with oropharyngeal dysphagia. Diagnosis and optimal management of oropharyngeal dysphagia require a systematic approach by a well-trained multidisciplinary team, under the guidance of a single managing physician.

REFERENCES

1. Barclay AE. The normal mechanism of swallowing. Laryngoscope 1927;37:235–262.
2. Dodds WJ, Logemann JA, Stewart ET. Radiologic assessment of abnormal oral and pharyngeal phases of swallowing. Am J Roentgenol 1990;154:965–974.
3. Ardran GM, Kemp FH. A radiographic study of movements of the tongue in swallowing. Dent Practitioner 1955;5:252–261.
4. Shaker R, Cook IJ, Dodds WJ, Hogan WJ. Pressure-flow dynamics of the oral phase of swallowing. Dysphagia 1988;3:79–84.
5. Ardran GM, Kemp FH. The protection of the laryngeal airway during swallowing. Br J Radiol 1952;25:406–416.
6. Curtis DJ, Cruess DF, Crain M, et al. Lateral pharyngeal outpouchings: comparison of dysphagic and asymptomatic patients. Dysphagia 1988;2:156–161.
7. Shaker R, Dodds WJ, Dantas RO, et al. Coordination of deglutitive glottic closure with oropharyngeal swallowing. Gastroenterology 1990;98:1478–1484.
8. Ramsey GH, Watson JS, Gramiak R, et al. Cinefluorographic analysis of the mechanism of swallowing. Radiology 1955;64:498–518.
9. Logemann JA. Manual for the Videofluorographic Study of Swallowing. San Diego: College-Hill Press, 1986;12–14.
10. Kahrilas PJ, Dodds WJ, Dent J, et al. Upper esophageal sphincter function during deglutition. Gastroenterology 1988;92:52–62.
11. Curtis DJ, Cruess DF, Dachman AH, et al. Timing in the normal pharyngeal swallow. Invest Radiol 1984;19:523–529.
12. Logemann JA. Factors affecting ability to resume oral nutrition in the oropharyngeal dysphagic individual. Dysphagia 1990;4:202–208.
13. Donner MW, Silbiger ML. Cinefluorographic analysis of pharyngeal swallowing in neuromuscular disorders. Am J Med Sci 1966;251:600–616.
14. Duranceau A, Lafontaine ER, Taillefer R, et al. Oropharyngeal dysphagia and operations on the upper esophageal sphincter. Surg Annu 1987;19:317–362.
15. Clark G. Deglutition apnoea. J Physiol London 1920;54:59.
16. Sumi T. The activity of brain-stem respiratory neurons and spinal respiratory motoneurons during swallowing. J Neurophysiol 1963;26:466–477.
17. Kawasaki M, Ogura J. Interdependence of deglutition with respiration. Ann Otol Rhinol Laryngol 1968;77:906–913.
18. Ogura JH, Mallen RW. Partial laryngopharyngectomy for supraglottic and pharyngeal carcinoma. Trans Am Acad Opthalmol Otolaryngol 1965;69:832–845.
19. Trupe EH, Siebens H, Siebens A. Prevalence of feeding and swallowing disorders in a nursing home. Paper presented at the American Congress of Rehabilitation Medicine, Boston, 1984.
20. Groher ME. The prevalence of swallowing disorders in two teaching hospitals. Dysphagia 1986;1:3–6.
21. Doty RW. Influence of stimulus pattern on reflex deglutition. Am J Physiol 1951;166:142–158.

22. Doty R, Bosma JF. An electrophysiological analysis of reflex deglutition. J Neurophysiol 1956;19:44–60.
23. Doty R, Richmond W, Storey A. Effect of medullary lesions on coordination of deglutition. Exp Neurol 1967;17:91–106.
24. Hellemans J, Pelemans W, Vantrappen G. Pharyngoesophageal swallowing disorders and the pharyngoesophageal sphincter. Med Clin North Am 1981;65:1149–1171.
25. Ravich WJ, Wilson RS, Jones B, et al. Psychogenic dysphagia and globus: reevaluation of 23 patients. Dysphagia 1989;4:35–38.
26. Bevan K, Griffiths MV. Chronic aspiration and laryngeal competence. Laryngol Otol 1989; 103:196–199.
27. Winstein CJ. Neurogenic dysphagia. Phys Ther 1983;63:1992–1996.
28. Veis SL, Logemann JA. Swallowing disorders in persons with cerebrovascular accident. Arch Phys Med Rehabil 1985;66:372–375.
29. Horner J, Buoyer FG, Alberts MJ, et al. Dysphagia following brain-stem stroke: clinical correlates and outcome. Arch Neurol 1991;48:1170–1173.
30. Ekberg O, Nylander G. Pharyngeal dysfunction after treatment for pharyngeal cancer with radiotherapy. Gastrointest Radiol 1983;8:97–104.
31. Butcher RB II. Treatment of chronic aspiration as a complication of cerebrovascular accident. Laryngoscope 1982;92:681–685.
32. Silbiger ML, Pikielney R, Donner MW. Neuromuscular disorders affecting the pharynx. Invest Radiol 1967;2:442–448.
33. Gordon C, Hewer RL, Wade DT. Dysphagia in acute stroke. BMJ 1987;295:411–414.
34. Horner J, Massey EW, Brazer SR. Dysphagia after bilateral stroke. Neurology 1990; 40:1686–1688.
35. Lazarus C, Logemann JA. Swallowing disorders in closed head trauma patients. Arch Phys Med Rehabil 1987;68:79–84.
36. Vencovsky J, Rehak F, Pafko P, et al. Acute cricopharyngeal obstruction in dermatomyositis. J Rheumatol 1988;15:1016–1018.
37. Robbins J, Levine RL. Swallowing after unilateral stroke of the cerebral cortex: preliminary experience. Dysphagia 1988;3:11–17.
38. Stroudley J, Walsh M. Radiological assessment of dysphagia in Parkinson's disease. Br J Radiol 1991;64:890–893.
39. Jones B, Buchholz DW, Ravich WJ, et al. Swallowing dysfunction in the postpolio syndrome: a cinefluorographic study. AJR 1992;158:283–286.
40. Kagel MC, Leopold NA. Dysphagia in Hungtington's disease: a 16-year retrospective. Dysphagia 1992;7:106–114.
41. Edwards LL, Quigley EMM, Pfeiffer RF. Gastrointestinal dysfunction in Parkinson's disease: frequency and pathophysiology. Neurology 1992;42:726–732.
42. Feinberg MJ, Ekberg O, Segall L, et al. Deglutition in elderly patients with dementia: findings of videofluorographic evaluation and impact on staging and management. Radiology 1992;183:811–814.
43. Bird MR, Woodward MC, Gibson EM, et al. Asymptomatic swallowing disorders in elderly patients with Parkinson's disease: a description of findings on clinical examination and videofluoroscopy in sixteen patients. Age Ageing 1994;23:251–254.
44. Horner J, Alberts MJ, Dawson DV, et al. Swallowing in Alzheimer's disease. Alzheimer Dis Assoc Disord 1994;8:177–189.
45. Leighton SE, Burton MJ, Lund WS. Swallowing in motor neuron disease. J Royal Soc Med 1994;87:801–805.
46. Jubelt B, Drucker J. Post-polio syndrome: an update. Semin Neurol 1993;13:283–290.
47. Coelho CA, Ferranti R. The incidence and nature of dysphagia in polio survivors. Arch Phys Med Rehabil 1991;72:1071–1075.
48. Shaker R, Kupla JI, Kidder TM, et al. Manometric characteristics of cervical dysphagia in a patient with Kearns-Sayre syndrome. Gastroenterology 1992;103:1328–1331.
49. Bonavena L, Khan NA, DeMeester TR. Pharyngoesophageal dysfunctions: the role of cricopharyngeal myotomy. Arch Surg 1985;120:541–549.
50. Dodds WJ, Stewart ET, Logemann JA. Physiology and radiology of the normal oral and pharyngeal phases of swallowing. Am J Roentgenol 1990;154:953–963.

51. Montgomery WW (ed), Laryngeal Paralysis. Surgery of the Upper Respiratory System, Vol. II, 2nd Ed. Philadelphia: Lea & Febiger, 1989;607–676.

52. Logemann JA. Evaluation and Treatment of Swallowing Disorders. Boston: College-Hill Press, 1983;58–133.

53. Jones B, Donner MW. How I do it: examination of the patient with dysphagia. Dysphagia 1989;4:162–172.

54. Ekberg O. Epiglottic dysfunction during deglutition in patients with dysphagia. Arch Otolaryngol 1983;109:376–380.

55. Langmore SE, Schatz K, Olsen N. Fiberoptic endoscopic examination of swallowing safety: a new procedure. Dysphagia 1988;2:216–219.

56. Bastian RW. Videoendoscopic evaluation of patients with dysphagia: an adjunct to the modified barium swallow. Otolaryngol Head Heck Surg 1991;104:339–350.

57. Shaker R, Bowser M, Hogan WJ, et al. Videoendoscopic characterization of abnormalities in pharyngeal phase of swallowing. Gastroenterology 1991;100:A494.

58. Kahrilas PJ, Dodds WJ, Dent J, et al. A method for continuous monitoring of upper esophageal sphincter pressure. Dig Dis Sci 1987;32:121–128.

59. Seaman WB. Cineroentgenographic observations of the cricopharyngeus. Am J Roentgenol 1966;96:922–931.

60. Dantas RO, Cook IJ, Dodds WJ, et al. Biomechanics of cricopharyngeal bars. Gastroenterology 1990;99:1269–1274.

61. Shawker TH, Sonies BC, Stone M, et al. Real-time visualization of tongue movement during swallowing. J Clin Ultrasound 1983;11:485–490.

62. Gagic NM. Cricopharyngeal myotomy. Canad J Surg 1983;26:47–49.

63. Logemann JA. Swallowing physiology and pathophysiology. Otolaryngol Clin North Am 1988;21:613–623.

64. Arnold G. Vocal rehabilitation of paralytic dysphonia: IX technique of intracordal injection. Arch Otolaryngol 1962;76:358–368.

65. Sessions D, Zill R, Schwartz J. Deglutition after conservation surgery for cancer of the larynx and hypopharynx. Otolaryngol Head Neck Surg 1979;87:779–796.

66. Koufman JA, Isaacson G. Laryngoplastic phonosurgery. Otolaryngol Clin North Amer 1991; 24:1151–1177.

67. Rontal E, Rontal M. Vocal cord injection techniques. Otolaryngol Clin North Amer 1991; 24:1141–1149.

68. Ganger D, Craig RM. Swallowing disorders and nutritional support. Dysphagia 1990; 4:213–219.

69. Granieri E. Nutrition and the older adult. Dysphagia 1990;4:196–201.

70. O'Gara JA. Dietary adjustments and nutritional therapy during treatment for oral-pharyngeal dysphagia. Dysphagia 1990;4:209–212.

71. Shaker R, Kern M, Bardan E, et al. Augmentation of deglutitive UES opening in the elderly by exercise. Am J Physiol 1997;272:G1518–G1522.

72. Shaker R, Easterling C, Kern M, et al. Rehabilitation of swallowing by exercise in tube-fed patients with pharyngeal dysphagia secondary to abnormal UES opening. Gastroenterology 2002;122:1314–1321.

Chapter 15
Nutritional Support: Indications, Options, and Problems

Thomas V. Nowak

Four factors need to be considered in the decision whether to initiate parenteral or enteral nutrition in patients with neurologic disorders:

1. Whether the underlying neurologic disorder is treatable and has the potential for improvement, or whether the condition is chronic and characterized by neurologic deterioration,
2. The patient's ability to eat (orally ingest and swallow food),
3. The status of gastrointestinal function,
4. The presence of recognizable malnutrition.[1]

The nutritional status of the neurologic patient may have no direct bearing on whether either parenteral or enteral nutrition should be instituted. Rather, the presence of malnutrition will instead directly determine how soon such a decision will have to be made.

It is rather clear that patients with reversible or potentially reversible neurologic deficits should not be allowed to succumb to malnourishment. Patients with Guillain-Barré syndrome, acute cerebrovascular accidents, or acute physical brain injury are examples in which neurologic improvement can be quite substantial, particularly in younger individuals. In these conditions, the decision on whether or not to initiate nutritional support is reasonably straightforward. On the other end of the spectrum are conditions such as diffuse hypoxic brain damage, advanced Alzheimer's disease, or multiple brain metastases in which the prospect for meaningful recovery is rather guarded. In these latter circumstances, the decision to initiate nutritional support can be ethically difficult and trying.[1]

Nutritional assessment of the patient with neurologic injury or dysfunction must focus on whether or not the gastrointestinal tract is structurally and functionally intact. If the gastrointestinal tract is not compromised, then it can and should be used to maintain the patient's nutrition. If it is compromised, then total parenteral nutrition should be used on a temporary or permanent basis to address the patient's metabolic needs. If it is not clear whether nutritional needs can be adequately and safely maintained through the alimentary tract, it is prudent to institute total parenteral nutrition until the integrity of the gastrointestinal tract can be evaluated by radiologic, endoscopic, and manometric means.

Structural gastrointestinal lesions are those which constitute a mechanical impediment or blockage to the aboral movement or absorption of luminal contents. Examples of structural lesions are intraluminal malignancies, inflammatory strictures, massive small bowel resections, enteral fistulas, or obstructing duodenal ulcers. Another group of structural lesions includes mucosal diseases which effectively abolish the absorption of nutrients. Examples of such disease are Crohn's disease, small intestinal bacterial overgrowth syndromes, and celiac disease. In general, structural lesions are an unlikely cause of gastrointestinal compromise in patients with neurologic disorders unless there is a preexisting disorder. However, stress ulceration of the stomach may develop in patients with traumatic brain injury or after brain surgery, and may effectively preclude use of the stomach as an organ for maintaining the patient's nutrition. In such an instance, the small intestine remains a viable alternative for enteral alimentation.

The functional integrity of the gastrointestinal tract must be questioned if, for example, the patient shows signs and symptoms of intestinal obstruction, but no evidence of an obstructing lesion can be discerned after extensive evaluation. This situation, referred to as intestinal pseudo-obstruction, and discussed in detail in Chapter 11, can be idiopathic, or more commonly, may be secondary to a systemic disorder such as diabetes mellitus, or progressive systemic sclerosis (scleroderma). In rare cases, intestinal pseudo-obstruction may be secondary to a brain tumor, or may present as a paraneoplastic syndrome due to a visceral malignancy.[2-4] Given its muscle layers and extensive intrinsic neural network,[5] it should come as no surprise that the same diseases that affect the central or peripheral nervous systems, on the one hand, and skeletal muscle, on the other, should be associated with enteric neural and muscle dysfunction, respectively. Accordingly, pseudo-obstruction syndromes have been described in patients with multiple sclerosis[6] and myotonic muscular dystrophy,[7] and exemplify the importance of recognizing gut motor dysfunction in these patient populations and the resultant implications for nutritional support.

APPROACH TO THE NEUROLOGIC PATIENT WITH DYSPHAGIA

Nutritional support in a neurologic patient hinges on whether or not that patient can be safely fed orally. Such a question can at times be difficult to address, and the answer relies heavily on the physician's clinical assessment of the patient. Patients with swallowing dysfunction do not necessarily complain of dysphagia, even in the presence of gross aspiration during deglutition. In addition, the physical examination may offer few clues as to whether a patient with neurologic disease is likely to experience swallowing dysfunction. Hence, the physician must be vigilant and wary of signs such as drooling and dysarthria, as well as unexplained cough, episodes of wheezing and laryngospasm, and fever and pneumonia, all of which may be harbingers of subtle aspiration.[8]

It has been quite legitimately suggested that a decreased gag reflex in a patient with neurologic disease places that individual at increased risk for aspiration. Nevertheless, some healthy individuals have a diminished to near absent gag reflex, and do not aspirate. Hence, deglutition may be quite abnormal despite an intact gag reflex, while on the other hand swallowing can be quite intact with an abnormal gag reflex. Perhaps the easiest, least expensive, and clinically most useful maneuver is for the physician to observe the patient as he or she swallows several ounces of tap water. The patient swallows a sip or two at first, perhaps through a straw, and then slowly drinks the remainder. The maneuver may be performed at the bedside and while not foolproof, it will, at least, identify some patients who are likely to have difficulty clearing their own secretions, much less food, and will be at high risk for aspiration.

If the patient is able to tolerate water bolus swallows without difficulty, then the diet may be gradually advanced to clear fluids and then full liquids, and then, ultimately, to semisolid and solid food. During this dietary progression, the patient should be monitored carefully for any signs of unexplained cough, bronchospasm, or fever. If any of the latter are recorded, prudence dictates that oral feeding be withheld and that the patient's swallowing function undergo further evaluation.

VIDEOFLUOROSCOPIC SWALLOWING STUDY

The barium esophagram or "barium swallow" is designed to evaluate the pharynx and upper and lower esophagus for anatomic and structural lesions, and to record the aboral and orderly movement of a swallowed bolus of barium from the pharynx to the fundus of the stomach. However, swallowing events in the pharynx occur at a much quicker pace than those in the esophagus, and are thus not likely to be faithfully recorded by a conventional barium esophagram. Hence, in recent years, this examination has been supplemented by what in many institutions has come to be known as a formal videoflouroscopic "swallowing study." This radiologic technique utilizes fast-frame videoflouroscopy to capture the rapid motor events that propel orally ingested contrast from the mouth to, and through, the pharynx and then distally. The exam is optimally performed by a radiologist who has a dedicated interest in swallowing disorders, and with the assistance of a speech pathologist or speech therapist.

The formal videoflouroscopic swallowing study has a twofold goal:

1) A diagnostic goal; as the study may demonstrate:
   • aspiration of barium during, or immediately after, deglutition,
   • nasal regurgitation,
   • difficulty in initiating the swallow, or
   • ineffective pharyngeal clearance of barium;
2) A therapeutic goal; as the study may show that modification of bolus consistency and viscosity, as well as head position (flexion or extension) during swallowing, may reduce or eliminate the likelihood of aspiration. It is generally appreciated that flexion of the neck tends to protect the larynx from penetration of barium during deglutition, while rotation of the head toward the side of pharyngeal weakness will tend to divert the bolus to the contralateral side of the pharynx. Patients may be taught to double-swallow in order to completely clear pharyngeal residue, or to cough after swallowing, in order to prophylactically clear any anticipated laryngeal aspirate.[8]

MEDICAL TREATMENT OF NEUROGENIC DYSPHAGIA

Aside from treatment of the underlying neurologic disorder, it is unfortunate that medical treatment has no direct role in the management of a neurologic patient with dysphagia. It has been suggested that anticholinergic medications may be beneficial, as these agents decrease the volume of oropharyngeal secretions. However, whether or not these agents improve deglutition in a patient with neurologic disease and dysphagia has not been clearly demonstrated. Indeed, the resultant increase in the viscosity of pharyngeal secretions may further embarrass swallowing function, and could, in theory, impede acid clearance from the distal esophagus. These medications also carry the considerable side-effects of urinary retention and constipation, problems already not uncommon in patients with neurologic disorders.

Many neurologic patients who aspirate are almost routinely prescribed medications that inhibit gastric acid production, such as H_2 receptor antagonists and proton pump inhibitors, or promotility agents, such as metoclopramide. The inherent rationale is that at least a component of a patient's aspiration might be due to penetration of acid refluxate past the larynx. While these agents can be truly beneficial if the patient has demonstrable gastroesophageal reflux disease, in the majority of instances, such therapy is in vain. Sadly, most of these patients continue to cough and aspirate on therapy, the aspirate being oropharyngeal contents which drain into the pulmonary tree. The physician also needs to be aware that, to varying degrees, H_2 receptor antagonists can, themselves, produce mental confusion, particularly in elderly individuals, while metoclopramide can produce dystonic reactions and somnolence in an appreciable minority of patients.[9,10]

PARENTERAL VERSUS ENTERAL NUTRITION

Parenteral nutrition can be delivered via a peripheral vein or by a central venous catheter in a patient who has a disorder which precludes delivery of nutrients directly into the stomach or small intestine. In general, because of the osmolarity of the alimentation solution, a sufficient amount of nutrients cannot be delivered by the peripheral route because of the risk of phlebitis. As a consequence, peripheral venous nutrition is at best viewed as an adjunct and temporary source of nutrients in a patient with inadequate oral or enteral intake.

Central venous nutrition should be employed in a patient whose small intestine is structurally or functionally compromised and, as a result, cannot be viewed as a suitable route for maintaining the patient's nutrition. The risks (Table 15.1) of central venous hyperalimentation are significant, and warrant careful consideration before this route of nutrition is undertaken. In general, the metabolic complications of central venous hyperalimentation, such as hyperglycemia and electrolyte disturbances, can be addressed by adding insulin or adjusting glucose and electrolyte concentrations in the alimentation solution. Patients do, however, require frequent

Table 15.1. Complications of Central Venous Hyperalimentation

Metabolic	Non-Metabolic
Hyperglycemia and hyperosmolarity	Factors related to catheter placement: pneumothorax, arterial puncture, hematoma, thoracic duct puncture, air embolus
Electrolyte abnormalities	Venous thrombosis
Liver dysfunction (fatty liver)	Catheter infection
Cholelithiasis	

phlebotomies and monitoring of serum glucose and electrolyte levels, at least at the initiation of central venous hyperalimentation. Experimental evidence suggests that hepatic fat accumulation largely results from increased endogenous lipid synthesis in the liver.[11] This condition can be treated by changing the composition of the alimentation solution or the timing of its administration. Cholelithiasis results from stasis of bile in an atonic gallbladder.[11] The presence of food, particularly fat, within the duodenum stimulates the gallbladder to contract. Absence of nutrients within the intestine leads to bile sequestration in the gallbladder, gallbladder atony, the formation of sludge, and ultimately cholelithiasis.

The non-metabolic complications of central venous nutrition are those related to the physical placement of a foreign body into a vascular space. These complications may be acutely related to placement of the catheter (pneumothorax, hematoma), or due to the chronic presence of the catheter in the subclavian vein and superior vena cava, i.e., venous thrombosis. A recent study examined some of the factors associated with subclavian venous catheterization, and found that even placement of the catheter under ultrasonic guidance had no appreciable influence on improving the success rate of catheterization. The study concluded that, in patients at highest risk for complications, catheterization should be attempted by the most experienced physicians available.[12]

Catheter infection is perhaps the most frequent and serious complication of central venous nutrition. Typical organisms include Staphylococcal species, gram-negative organisms, and occasionally, fungi such as Candida species. In some instances, the catheter may be left in place, and intravenous antibiotics may be administered with the intention of sterilizing the vascular appliance. Unfortunately, in many cases, the infected catheter must be removed and the patient needs to undergo prolonged treatment with parenteral antibiotics.[13]

The daily costs of central venous hyperalimentation (Table 15.2) are considerable, and may be more than ten times those of enteral nutrition. This calculation does not consider the expense associated with the frequent phlebotomies required during central venous nutrition to monitor glucose and electrolyte levels. Likewise, the estimate does not include costs incurred to address the more frequent complications of central venous nutrition, such as prolonged parenteral antibiotic treatment for catheter-related sepsis.

ENTERAL NUTRITION

Disorders of the stomach, esophagus, or colon do not necessarily exclude use of the gastrointestinal tract from meeting the patient's nutritional needs, as the essential

Table 15.2. Daily Relative Costs of Alimentation

Total Parenteral Nutrition
2000 calories/day = $310
Net = $310.00
Enteral Nutrition
$1.33/can at 250 calories/can,
2000 calories (8 cans)
Net = $10.64

Costs are those quoted by hospital and community pharmacies in central Indiana, June 2001.

key organ is a functioning small intestine. It has been stated that the only true contraindication to enteral feeding is the absence of a gut. Other practical contraindications to enteral nutrition include perforations of the stomach, small intestine, and colon, high output enterocutaneous or entercolonic fistulas (leading to malabsorption), and frank mechanical obstruction of the gastrointestinal tract.[14] In fact, even an anatomically intact small intestine, although physiologically desirable, is not a mandatory requirement; some patients who have undergone massive small bowel resection live near normal lives with a fraction of original small intestinal length, although close medical supervision is necessary. Given an understanding of these criteria, the number of patients who should be excluded from enteral nutrition—and who conversely become candidates for central venous nutrition—falls into a minority.

Aside from considerations of cost and safety, enteral nutrition has several physiological advantages over central venous hyperalimentation. When patients are fed parenterally, rather than enterally, the small intestinal mucosa becomes atrophic. This produces an increase in mucosal permeability and a loss of gut-associated lymphoid tissue. There is evidence that this condition allows bacteria to translocate across the wall of the small intestine directly into the circulation. This situation is prevented by the presence of nutrients in the intestinal lumen.[14–16]

TUBE FEEDING IN THE NEUROLOGIC PATIENT: GENERAL CONSIDERATIONS

Some of the largest studies examining the outcome of neurologic patients who undergo placement of feeding tubes and enteral alimentation were performed over two decades ago.[17,18] In the interim, the medical management of individual neurologic disorders has improved, and newer endoscopic and surgical techniques of feeding tube placement have been developed. However, while the specific conclusions of these studies are somewhat dated and may not be strictly applicable to modern circumstances, their overall findings have stood the test of time:

1) many patients with neurologic disease who require tube feeding face a poor prognosis and appreciable mortality rate;
2) the number of truly worthwhile nutritional options for the institution and maintenance of enteral nutrition remains limited.

Aspiration is a major issue in the neurological patient. An autopsy study of 720 patients with various neurological disorders found evidence of aspiration (defined as the presence of gastric contents in the pulmonary tree) in 10%.[18] Nearly 20% of hospitalized patients had required a feeding tube to maintain their nutrition. The study found that the mere presence of a feeding tube appeared to increase the risk of aspiration almost fivefold, as nearly 24% of the patients who had feeding tubes showed evidence of pulmonary aspiration at autopsy. In contrast, only 5% of those without feeding tubes showed aspiration. These observations suggest that those patients who do require a feeding tube to maintain their nutrition exhibit more severe neurologic disease, and are particularly prone to aspirate. However, the findings also indicate that tube feeding in a neurologically impaired patient should be undertaken with deliberation and caution, and that these patients be monitored carefully as their risk for aspiration appears to be considerable.

Another retrospective study examined the clinical outcome of 83 patients with neurological disorders who underwent surgical placement of a gastrostomy or jejunostomy feeding tube.[17] Most of the patients had severe central nervous system dysfunction, and 64% were comatose at the time of surgery. Only 31 patients (37%) were still alive 30 days after tube placement. The patient's level of consciousness at the time of the surgical procedure appeared to influence mortality. Among patients who were comatose at the time of the procedure, only 22% survived 30 days, whereas 63% of those who were not comatose survived. Most (82%) of the pulmonary complications (aspiration, atelectasis, and pneumonia) occurred in comatose patients, and none of the comatose patients who developed pulmonary complications survived 30 days. Only eight patients survived six months. All of these patients had recovered from their primary disease sufficiently to have their feeding tubes removed. All but one of the fifty-four patients who were comatose at the time of surgery died within six months. The high incidence of complications and the poor survival rate described in this study suggest that surgical placement of a feeding gastrostomy or feeding jejunostomy tube offers no advantage over a nasoenteric feeding tube in a comatose individual. This same conclusion was reached by a separate investigation performed over a decade later[19]; both reinforce the concept that the presence of coma is a potent indicator of poor prognosis, and should be borne in mind when considering nutritional support.

NASOENTERIC TUBES

Nasoenteric feeding tubes constitute one mode of delivery of nutrients into the gastrointestinal tract (Table 15.3). Figure 15.1 shows the relative anatomic location of the various types of feeding tubes. The major advantage of nasoenteric feeding tubes is that their cost is relatively inexpensive and their placement is simple. Nasogastric tubes, used for either feeding or gastric suction, can be placed by a physician at the patient's bedside. However, radiologic verification of the position of the tube is mandatory prior to initiating tube feeding, in order to prevent inadvertent introduction of the tube formula diet into the pulmonary tree.[20] Figure 15.2A and B shows the intracranial position of a nasogastric tube that was blindly placed in an accident victim who had sustained head trauma and skull fractures.[21] The placement of a nasoduodenal or nasojejunal feeding tube requires fluoroscopic or endoscopic guidance to position the tip of the feeding tube distal to the pylorus. An endoscopically-placed feeding tube incurs all the risks, complications, and expenses

Table 15.3. Methods of Administrating Enteral Nutrition

Nasoenteric tube
  Nasogastric
  Nasoduodenal
  Nasojejunal
Cervical pharyngostomy
Tube enterostomy
  Percutaneous gastrostomy (endoscopic [PEG] or radiologic)
  Percutaneous gastrojejunostomy (endoscopic [PEG/J] or radiologic or direct endoscopic PEJ)
  Surgical gastrostomy
  Surgical jejunostomy

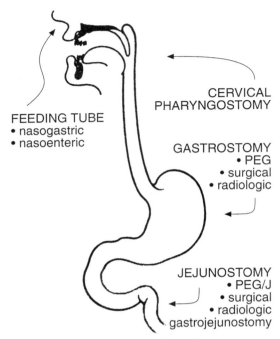

Figure 15.1. Feeding tubes and their relative anatomic position.

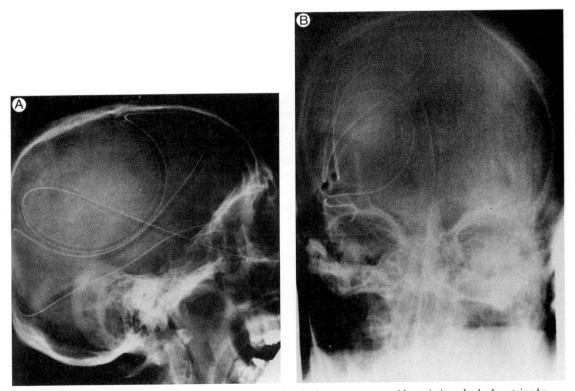

Figure 15.2. A and **B.** Intracranial placement of a nasogastric tube in a comatose accident victim who had sustained a basilar skull fracture. (Reproduced with permission from Fremstad JD, Martin SH. Lethal complication from insertion of nasogastric tube after severe basilar skull fracture. J Trauma 1978;18:820–822.)

of an upper gastrointestinal endoscopy. A fluoroscopically-placed tube incurs relatively little additional expense, and the risk related to the radiation exposure incurred is minimal.

Many of the complications of nasoenteric tubes are a mechanical consequence of the tube's physical presence in the pharynx and esophagus. Patients may experience nasopharyngeal discomfort, sinusitis, or nasal mucosal ulceration (Table 15.4).[22] Other complications are a consequence of the fact that nasoenteric tubes traverse the lower esophageal sphincter, and may act as a "wick" over which gastric acid may seep into the esophagus.[23] As a result, patients with nasoenteric tubes in place for prolonged periods of time may develop reflux esophagitis, esophageal erosions, ulcers, and strictures.[24,25] From a practical perspective, perhaps the primary source of patient dissatisfaction with nasoenteric feeding tubes is their poor cosmetic appeal. This feature prompts many patients and their families to seek other tube feeding options, such as percutaneous endoscopic gastrostomy tubes to address nutritional needs.

The concept of delivering nutrients directly into the duodenum or jejunum, and bypassing the stomach, is based upon the notion that direct delivery of a formula will reduce the risk for aspiration. Theoretically, this makes sense. In one study, a nonabsorbable marker was delivered into various portions of the duodenum and jejunum through a nasoenteric tube, and the stomach was frequently aspirated to check for enterogastric reflux.[26] Reflux into the stomach during constant perfusion of the proximal small intestine was, in fact, found to be quite variable. Three factors appeared to be associated with increased reflux into the stomach: 1) proximal location of the infusion site; 2) an infusion rate faster than 2 ml/minute; and 3) the use of anticholinergic medications. The osmolality of the test solution and its composition seemed to have no evident influence on reflux into the stomach. The study found that the optimum tube position to minimize enterogastric reflux was a location just distal to the ligament of Treitz.

Technical issues also influence success. A recent study demonstrated significant advantages, in terms of ease of positioning and risk of displacement, for a Frek Trelumina tube over a Dobhoff tube. These differences appeared to relate to the relative stiffness of the two tubes.[27] In this study, the better performing tube took, on average, 6 minutes to place and remained in position for a median of 37 days. Unfortunately, though there is some supportive evidence, feeding through a nasojejunal or nasoduodenal port has not been shown to conclusively reduce the risk of aspiration in patients fed with nasoenteric tubes.[28–31] Finally, the practicing physician needs to be aware that no method of alimentation—enteral or parenteral—will reduce the risk of aspiration of oropharyngeal contents.

Table 15.4. Complications of Nasoenteric Tubes

Aspiration pneumonia	Reflux esophagitis and ulceration
Sinusitis	Esophageal stricture
Pharyngitis	Tracheoesophageal fistula
Otitis media	Tube obstruction
Pneumothorax	Migration of tube back into stomach or esophagus
Pulmonary intubation	Poor cosmesis
Patient discomfort and intolerance	

CERVICAL PHARYNGOSTOMY

Cervical pharyngostomy was developed as a means of alimentation nearly three decades ago for patients with dysphagia secondary to maxillofacial trauma, neurologic disorders, and oropharyngeal cancer. The original technique involved an open neck dissection in order to insert the feeding catheter. Recently, a percutaneous method has been described that requires only local anesthesia and can be performed at the bedside of an awake patient.[32] Similar to the complications of enterostomy or gastrostomy feeding tubes, the complications of cervical pharyngostomy include aspiration and tube clogging by inspissated tube formula.

There are no comprehensive studies which have evaluated the relative mortality and morbidity of cervical pharyngostomy feeding tubes compared to nasoenteric feeding tubes or percutaneous endoscopic gastrostomy (PEG) tubes. However, in the case of cervical pharyngostomy alimentation, the formula is infused into the proximal esophagus in close proximity to the epiglottis and trachea. Delivery of the infused formula into the stomach is dependent on the aboral peristaltic function of the esophagus or, at the very least, gravity. If either of these factors is compromised, as in the case of the patient with gastroesophageal reflux disease and/or an atonic esophagus, or if the patient lies supine or coughs during formula infusion, then the risk of aspiration would appear to be high. In any case, cervical pharyngostomy, as a modality for tube feeding, is no longer in widespread use and has largely been supplanted by percutaneous endoscopically- or radiologically-placed gastrostomy feeding tubes.

GASTROSTOMY AND JEJUNOSTOMY FEEDING TUBES

Gastrostomy and jejunostomy feeding tubes may be placed percutaneously under local anesthesia by an endoscopist or radiologist. The procedures can be performed in the endoscopy or radiology suite, or even at the patient's bedside in the intensive care unit. A percutaneous gastrostomy involves placing a plastic feeding tube through a small incision in the anterior abdominal wall, and directly into the lumen of the stomach. Verification of tube entry into the stomach lumen is made endoscopically or by fluoroscopy. The percutaneous endoscopic gastrostomy (PEG) or radiologic gastrostomy can be used for gastrostomy tube feedings or for gastric decompression.

The percutaneous endoscopic gastrostomy-jejunostomy (PEG/J) describes a procedure in which an endoscopic gastrostomy is first formed. A second catheter is then inserted through the gastrostomy tube and delivered past the pylorus, into the small intestine. The recent introduction of specially designed double-lumen PEG/J catheters permits simultaneous gastric suction and decompression, as well as small intestinal feeding (Figure 15.3). Similarly designed double-lumen gastrostomy-jejunostomy tubes may be inserted by the radiologist under fluoroscopic guidance, and without the complications and expense of endoscopic guidance.

The theoretical advantage of jejunostomy feeding is that instillation of the tube directly into the small intestine should reduce the risk of pulmonary aspiration of the alimentation formula, a concept that has been supported by some recent studies.[33,34] As cited earlier (vide supra), physiologic investigations have shown that enterogastric reflux is reduced if the tip of the feeding tube is placed at a locus distal to the ligament of Treitz.[26] In practice, while endoscopically- or

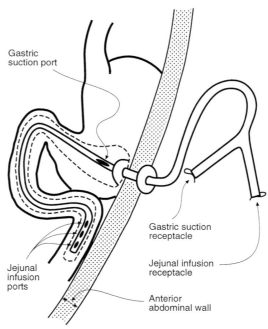

Figure 15.3. Double-lumen percutaneous gastrostomy-jejunostomy feeding tube. Such feeding tubes may be placed endoscopically or radiologically under local anesthesia. The double-lumen design allows simultaneous gastric suctioning and decompression as well as duodenal or jejunal administration of nutrients. These tubes are particularly useful in cases of gastric retention (gastroparesis).

radiologically-placed gastrojejunostomy tubes can be negotiated past the pylorus and into the small intestine, in this author's experience their successful and permanent location distal to the ligament of Treitz is infrequent. Secondly, as a consequence of the anterior-posterior configuration of the normal human stomach, gastrojejunostomy feeding tubes commonly coil in the stomach before traversing the pylorus and entering the small intestine. As a consequence, the intestinal portion of the tube may recoil into the gastric lumen, particularly when the patient is retching or vomiting.

The direct surgical approach to creation of a jejunostomy prevents proximal migration of the tube, as the tube tip can be positioned more distally in the intestine than a radiologically- or endoscopically-placed gastrojejunostomy feeding tube. The inherent disadvantage is that a surgical jejunostomy (or gastrostomy) typically requires general anesthesia, and all the attendant risks and complications.

More recently, an endoscopically-assisted technique for the direct placement of a jejunostomy feeding tube has been described (DPEG). Using either a colonoscope or an enteroscope, the tube is directed from the abdominal wall into the jejunal lumen, in a manner analogous to PEG placement. This offers significant advantages, in technical terms, over the PEG/J approach, and a direct comparison of DPEG and PEG/J has indicated a better patient outcome as well.[35] While, in this study, the success rate for placement was higher for the PEG/J (92.5% vs 72.7%), 60% of the PEG/J patients required endoscopic intervention to maintain jejunal access over the 6-month study period, in comparison to only 13.5% in the PEJ group.

EFFICACY OF PERCUTANEOUS ENDOSCOPIC GASTROSTOMY (PEG)

Percutaneous endoscopic gastrostomy was first introduced into clinical practice in 1980.[36,37] Since then, the procedure has garnered widespread application and clinical enthusiasm, particularly in patients who have neurologic disorders or resected head and neck malignancies, and who may require enteral nutrition for prolonged periods of time.

Larsen and colleagues examined the clinical course and outcome of 314 patients in whom a PEG was attempted.[37] In this particular series, as in most others, the most common indications for the PEG tube were neurologic (75%) and oropharyngeal disorders (13%). A PEG tube could be successfully placed in most, but not all, patients who underwent the procedure. The study reported a success rate of 95%. Of the 15 patients in whom a PEG tube could not be placed, 1 patient was found to have an incidental gastric cancer at the potential gastrostomy site. The procedure was not without complications: one patient aspirated, another developed laryngospasm during introduction of the endoscope, and a third developed a large hematoma at the catheter site before actual introduction of the PEG tube. In the remaining patients, it was physically impossible to appose the anterior gastric wall to the abdominal wall (i.e., unsuccessful endoscopic transillumination across the gastric and abdominal wall), or it was technically impossible to endoscopically negotiate the gastrostomy tube into the stomach (i.e., the patient had undergone a previous gastric resection or had a large diaphragmatic hernia).

In those patients in whom the PEG tube was placed, the overall procedure-related major complication rate was 3% and the mortality rate 1%. Three patients died as a direct consequence of PEG tube placement, two from aspiration and one from laryngospasm. Four patients sustained gastric perforations; all were repaired surgically with an uneventful recovery. Two patients experienced limited bleeding that eventually resolved. The overall thirty day mortality rate for the PEG tube patients was 15%. In all except three instances, the cause of death was felt to be secondary to the underlying illness and unrelated to placement of the PEG tube. Of the 46 patients who died within 30 days of PEG tube placement, 36 (78%) had neurologic disorders, the most common being cerebrovascular disease in 21 patients (46%).

The overall procedure-related minor complication rate was 13% and was, most commonly, a superficial wound infection. These typically resolved with intravenous antibiotics or incision and drainage of the wound. The PEG tube had to be removed in only one patient. Other minor procedure-related complications included transient ileus, stomal leakage, fever, aspiration, anorexia, tube migration, and hematoma formation.

Ultimately, 14% of the patients regained their ability to eat to the extent that the PEG tube could be removed without the development of a permanent gastrocutaneous fistula. The investigators concluded that PEG is a safe and effective procedure and associated with a low mortality. The study also showed that the short-term mortality rate continues to be high in those patients with neurologic disease who undergo PEG in an attempt to prevent continued aspiration. These patients die from respiratory failure, presumably from continued aspiration.

PERCUTANEOUS ENDOSCOPIC GASTROSTOMY (PEG) VS NASOENTERIC (NE) TUBES

Despite the current popularity of PEG tubes to address nutritional needs in patients who cannot tolerate oral intake, the actual superiority of PEG tubes over feeding devices such as NE tubes has not been substantiated, nor have the differences been critically examined.

One study retrospectively compared clinical outcomes in patients who received enteral nutrition via PEG (80 patients) or naso-enteric tubes (29 patients).[38] Nearly 80% of the patients in either group suffered from one or more neurologic disorders, with stroke and dementia being the most common diagnoses. There was no significant difference between the two groups with respect to their nutritional status during the study period, which was a mean of 192 days for the PEG patients and 141 days for the naso-enteric tube group. Minor short-term complications occurred at a similar frequency in both groups. Likewise, there was no significant difference in short-term mortality between the two groups. Two of the PEG patients died (one from respiratory failure, another from progression of bladder cancer), while none of the naso-enteric tube patients died. However, the frequency of aspiration pneumonia in the peri-procedure period differed significantly between the two groups in that 6% of the PEG patients and 25% of the naso-enteric tube patients developed aspiration pneumonitis within 14 days of tube placement. In no instance did the pneumonia lead to the patient's death.

Despite these differences during the peri-procedure period, there was no significant difference in the frequency of aspiration pneumonia between the two groups over the entire duration of the study. Aspiration pneumonia ultimately developed in 32% of the PEG and 46% of the naso-enteric tube patients. Other complications, such as feeding tube occlusion, occurred at a similar frequency in both groups. There was no difference between the groups with respect to the frequency of tube replacement; 31% for PEG tube patients vs 69% for naso-enteric tube patients. Per patient, this translated to a tube replacement frequency of 3.0 times for PEG and 4.3 times for the naso-enteric tube patient group.

Sixty-two or 57% of the patients died during the course of the study. There were 48 deaths in the PEG patient group and 14 in the naso-enteric tube group. Figure 15.4 shows the survival analysis and also shows that the mortality rate in both groups approaches 50% at 120 days after tube placement. There was no significant difference in mortality between the two groups in a follow-up period of up to 559 days. Altogether the most common causes of death were infections (40%) and cardiorespiratory failure (27%). Aspiration was believed to be a factor in 25% of the pneumonia and sepsis deaths in both groups.

Aspiration pneumonia has been reported to occur in 1 to 44% of patients who receive nutrition by naso-enteric feeding.[18,38–42] Among possible reasons for the large variation in frequencies are differences in study design and length, and the use of variable clinical criteria to establish the diagnosis. Published studies vary considerably in their definition of what constitutes aspiration pneumonia. Since the act of aspiration is frequently unwitnessed, the diagnosis is frequently based on circumstantial evidence. Typically—but not always—the diagnosis of aspiration is

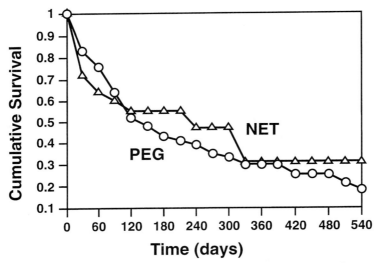

Figure 15.4. Cumulative survival of patients fed by either percutaneous endoscopic gastrostomy (PEG) or nasoenteric (NET) tube by life table calculation. (Reproduced with permission from Fay DE, Gruber M, Lance P, Poplausky M. Long-term enteral feeding: a retrospective comparison of delivery via percutaneous endoscopic gastrostomy and nasoenteric tubes. Am J Gastroenterol 1990;85:1120–1122.)

based on the finding of a new infiltrate on chest x-ray associated with tachypnea, dyspnea, fever, cough, wheezing, rales, and leukocytosis.[43] Unfortunately, not all published studies accept this definition. Rates of aspiration pneumonia after PEG tube placement likewise appear to vary quite widely, being variably reported at 5%,[44] 9%,[45] 20%,[46] and even as high as 56%.[42]

The results of these studies indicate that the mortality rates in patients who require tube feeding remain quite high, and that patients continue to aspirate and to develop pneumonia, regardless of whether the feeding appliance is a PEG or a naso-enteric tube. Contrary to popular wisdom, a PEG tube appears to offer no protective benefit over a naso-enteric tube with respect to the risk of aspiration.[31,47,48]

Patients with naso-enteric tubes do, however, appear to require more frequent replacement of their appliance than do patients with PEG tubes. Presumably, the presence of a naso-enteric tube in the nasopharynx is a source of irritation to the patient, or is more vulnerable to either deliberate or accidental removal. From a strictly practical perspective, tube replacement is quicker and less cumbersome in a patient with a mature PEG tract. Replacement of a nasoenteric tube requires fluoroscopic verification of tube position prior to resumption of tube feeding. In contrast, a PEG tube can be replaced at the bedside with either a commercially available replacement tube, or with a Foley catheter. The critical issue in PEG tube replacement is whether the gastrostomy tract, i.e., the gastrocutaneous fistula, is mature. How long it takes a fistulous tract to mature is arguable, but 30 days appears to be a reasonable, safe, and practical definition. Blind replacement of a PEG tube through an immature tract may lead to dehiscence of the gastrostomy tract, migration of the stomach away from the anterior abdominal wall, inadvertent introduction of tube formula into the peritoneal cavity, and chemical peritonitis. For these reasons, tubes that require replacement within 30 days should be repositioned under either fluoroscopic or endoscopic guidance.

ENDOSCOPIC VS RADIOLOGIC PERCUTANEOUS GASTROSTOMY/GASTROJEJUNOSTOMY

The decision as to whether to employ endoscopic or radiologic means to place a percutaneous gastrostomy or gastrojejunostomy hinges on two main considerations: 1) the clinical status of the patient; and 2) the radiologic and endoscopic expertise available at an institution. The two procedures do vary considerably in cost. However, at the present time, considerations of expense appear not to significantly affect which modality of treatment is pursued.

The clinical status of the patient determines whether there are any contraindications to percutaneous gastrostomy (Table 15.5). Massive or tense ascites or extreme obesity may make it physically impossible for either an endoscopist or radiologist to satisfactorily anesthetize and traverse the anterior abdominal wall with a needle, and place a catheter into the stomach. Either procedure requires that the patient be cooperative. In addition, an unstable cardio-respiratory status is a contraindication to endoscopy. Given this concern, the radiologic approach has a slight advantage over endoscopy, since the radiologic percutaneous gastrostomy requires little more than local anesthesia. Endoscopy generally requires parenteral sedation with benzodiazepines and narcotics, as well as close monitoring of the patient's pulse, blood pressure, and oxygenation during the period of conscious sedation. Hence, in a patient with a severely compromised cardio-respiratory status, radiologic percutaneous gastrostomy would likely present less risk than, and is preferable to, endoscopic gastrostomy.

Both radiologic and endoscopic gastrostomy should be viewed as surgical procedures, albeit minor, as both require a surgical incision under antiseptic conditions, and introduction of a plastic appliance into an intraabdominal viscus. Hemorrhage is a complication of either procedure, and coagulation disorders constitute a contraindication to either approach. Finally, technical considerations may preclude successful percutaneous endoscopic gastrostomy, and instead favor radiologic gastrostomy. Perforation of the small intestine or colon may occur during either radiologic or endoscopic approaches. To some extent, the radiologic approach is aided by fluoroscopy, and the distinctive gas patterns of the small intestine and colon may help to designate the relative positions of these organs. Endoscopic gastrostomy is, in essence, a blind procedure in that the endoscopist never knows for certain whether a loop of small intestine or colon is interposed between the stomach and the anterior abdominal wall. Some hint that the procedure can be performed safely is obtained when the abdominal wall can be transilluminated by the endoscope from within the gastric lumen, or the endoscopist is able to indent the stomach when finger pressure is placed on the

Table 15.5. Contraindications to Percutaneous Gastrostomy or Gastrojejunostomy Tube Placement

Massive ascites
Uncooperative patient
Unstable cardio-respiratory status
Severe obesity
Coagulation disorders
Altered anatomy, i.e., previous abdominal surgery (relative contraindication)

external abdominal wall ("finger press"). Many endoscopists view failure to satisfactorily perform either maneuver as a contraindication to percutaneous endoscopic gastrostomy. The presence of altered gastric anatomy, i.e., subtotal gastrectomy, constitutes a relative contraindication to endoscopic gastrostomy. Likewise, the presence of surgical scars at the potential percutaneous gastrostomy site is a harbinger that a loop of intestine may be adherent to the abdominal wall, and may constitute a relative contraindication to endoscopic feeding tube placement.

Table 15.6 compares the relative costs of radiological and endoscopic placement of feeding tubes. These costs may vary somewhat among institutions, but the table shows that radiologically-placed nasogastric or nasoenteric feeding tubes are the least expensive, while percutaneous gastrostomy or gastrojejunostomy feeding tubes are up to six times more expensive. The cost discrepancy between nasoenteric and percutaneous feeding tubes becomes clouded when one considers that disoriented and comatose patients remove or dislodge nasogastric feeding tubes far more frequently than percutaneous gastrostomy tubes. In such instances, reinsertion of a nasogastric feeding tube requires radiologic verification of tube position. If portable radiologic equipment is not available, the procedure may require an ambulance trip to the local emergency room with fluoroscopic capabilities. In contrast, a dislodged gastrostomy tube with a mature fistula tract can be reinserted by nursing personnel, on site, at the patient's bedside. In fact, in some institutions, nursing home placement is easier to obtain for patients with percutaneous gastrostomies rather than nasoenteric feeding tubes.

ADMINISTRATION OF FORMULA DIETS

There are basically four methods by which a tube formula may be administered to a given patient. These are:

1) bolus administration, in which 250 to 300 ml of formula are introduced using a syringe or bulb over 10 minutes or less;

Table 15.6. Comparative Feeding Tube Placement Costs: Radiologic or Endoscopic*

Radiology	
Nasoenteric feeding tube	
Room: $121 Radiologist $55	$ 176
Percutaneous gastrostomy	
Room: $650 Radiologist $286	$ 936
Endoscopy	
Nasoenteric feeding tube	
Room: $628 Endoscopist: $580	
Recovery room: $78	$1,286
PEG or PEG/J tube	
Room: $807 Endoscopist: $486	
Recovery room: $78	$1,371

*Costs are those in effect at several community hospitals in central Indiana, June 2001.

2) intermittent infusion, in which 250 to 300 ml of formula are infused over 30 to 60 minutes by gravity flow;

3) cyclic infusion, in which a programmable pump infuses formula over 8 to 16 hours per day;

4) continuous infusion, in which a pump delivers formula at a predetermined constant rate.

Any of the four administration methods can be used to introduce formula diet into the stomach, as this is a capacitance organ and can dilate to accept bolus or intermittent infusions of feeding. Cyclic or continuous infusions of tube formula must be used to instill tube formula directly into the small intestine. This organ does not have the reservoir capacity of the stomach, and large volume infusions may precipitate vomiting, abdominal cramping, and diarrhea. The final rate of administration is reliant upon patient tolerance, the osmolality of the formula, and whether the patient experiences abdominal cramping and diarrhea. Over time, a patient's intestinal tract becomes accustomed to the tube diet, and a continuous tube schedule may be changed to a daytime or nighttime cyclic infusion to accommodate patient and nursing schedules.

The optimum tube formula is that which addresses the patient's nutritional requirements and maintains hydration. In an otherwise healthy individual, who has simply lost the capacity to swallow and who maintains a sedentary life-style, this amounts to approximately 1500 to 1800 calories per day with a water intake of approximately 1500 ml per day. Many, but not all, tube diets are manufactured at a caloric content of one calorie per ml. Hence, a patient requiring 1600 calories per day might have the diet administered by intragastric bolus or infusions of 400 ml four times per day. If a pump is employed, the diet might be administered at a constant infusion of 67 ml per hour over 24 hours, or a cyclic infusion of 100 ml per hour over 16 hours. If the osmolality of the diet is too high, it may be diluted to ¾ or ½ strength, and the infusion rate increased accordingly to meet the caloric needs.

Decades ago, the clinician was confronted with the choice of selecting a ½, ¾, or full strength "hospital tube diet" for patients requiring enteral alimentation. This tube diet was a blenderized mixture of proteins, carbohydrate, and fat-containing foodstuffs prepared by the hospital dietary department or kitchen. Over time, this limited selection has been supplanted by an intimidating list of choices available to the practicing physician. The 2001 edition of Drug Facts and Comparisons lists nearly 78 commercially-available enteral diet formulations.[49] Some of these preparations are isosmolar to plasma while others are hyperosmolar. The formulas differ in their relative glucose, protein, and fat content. Some have added fiber. Some formulas are designed for patients who have renal, hepatic, or pulmonary failure. The clinical utility and specific application of the formulas are usually supplemented by respective clinical studies that support their focused application, although, in many instances, this author has found that the relative benefit of one formulation over another, in a patient with a functioning and anatomically intact gastrointestinal tract, is arguable.

Perhaps the main distinction among enteral tube diets is their cost (Table 15.7). The differential among the various preparations is considerable, and may vary up to fifteen-fold. Representative pharmacy charges at a tertiary care community hospital run the gamut from a low-end cost of $1.33 per carton of approximately 250 calories (Ensure), to a high range unit charge of $7.25 (Impact). Given the current economic climate and its focus on medical costs, the clinician might be best

Table 15.7. Comparative Prices of Some Enteral Formulas

Product	Unit cost to the patient
Resource	$ 3.24
Ensure	$ 1.33
Pediasure	$ 4.37
Impact	$ 7.25
Promote	$ 4.15

Prices are those quoted by several hospital and community pharmacies in central Indiana, June 2001.

advised to choose the least expensive dietary supplement available, unless the patient has some specific medical or surgical condition that requires use of a specific tube formulation.

SUMMARY AND CONCLUSIONS

Nutritional assessment in a patient with neurologic disease must consider whether the patient is able or willing to swallow. A videofluoroscopic barium contrast examination ("swallowing study") is used to determine whether a given patient can swallow properly, and to identify those individuals who are prone to aspiration. In those patients who require artificial alimentation, enteral nutrition is preferable to the parenteral route, assuming the gastrointestinal tract is structurally and functionally intact.

Enteral nutrition may be administered by radiologically- or endoscopically-placed nasogastric and nasoenteric feeding tubes, or percutaneous gastrostomy and gastrostomy/jejunostomy feeding tubes.[50] The relative merits of one tube appliance over another include patient comfort, cosmesis, cost, available local expertise, and ease of replacement if the tube becomes dislodged.

However, technical issues pale into insignificance in relation to that of patient selection. The clinician must be mindful, firstly, of the high short-term mortality in this patient population, in general,[51] and of the potential for the intervention to increase mortality further; secondly, of the failure of many of these techniques, and PEG tubes, in particular, to protect against aspiration in a population already at high risk for this complication; and, thirdly, of the absence of convincing data to indicate that these interventions significantly benefit the patient either in terms of nutrition or survival.[52] The risk of aspiration pneumonia and mortality in neurologic patients with swallowing dysfunction who require tube feeding remains high. There is, however, some evidence to suggest that tubes placed in the jejunum may substantially reduce the risk of aspiration pneumonia or death. A minority of patients may show improvement in swallowing function to the extent that percutaneous or nasoenteric feeding tubes may be removed. No study has been published which compares the benefits of tube feedings to oral feedings in dysphagic patients with advanced dementia,[53] a group who have an especially poor prognosis following PEG placement. However, three studies have demonstrated better outcome for PEGs in the patient with acute stroke.[47,48,54] It should come as no surprise, therefore, that recent reviews and guidelines suggest that the latter group are suitable candidates for PEG placement whereas the former are not.[52]

In conclusion, while clinical experience has shown that enteral nutrition can benefit the neurologically compromised patient, the decision to institute nutritional support integrates sound clinical judgment with the individual needs of each patient. In considering one of these approaches, the nature of the underlying disorder and its prognosis, as well as the risks for aspiration, must all be borne in mind if one is to avoid inflicting additional distress to a patient whose outcome is already dismal.[52,55,56]

REFERENCES

1. Twomey PL, St John JN. The Neurologic Patient. In JL Rombeau, MD Caldwell (eds), Clinical Nutrition, Vol. I. Enteral and Tube Feeding. Philadelphia: WB Saunders, 1984;292–302.
2. Wood JR, Camilleri M, Low PA, Malagelada JR. Brainstem tumor presenting as an upper gut motility disorder. Gastroenterology 1985;89:1411–1414.
3. Chinn JS, Schuffler MD. Paraneoplastic visceral neuropathy as a cause of severe gastrointestinal motor dysfunction. Gastroenterology 1988;95:1279–1286.
4. Anuras J, Anuras S. Pseudo-Obstruction Syndromes. In S Anuras (ed), Motility Disorders of the Gastrointestinal Tract. Principles and Practice. New York: Raven Press, 1992;327–344.
5. Gershon MD. The enteric nervous system: an apparatus for intrinsic control of gastrointestinal motility. Viewpoints Dig Dis 1981;13:13–16.
6. Summers RW, Anuras S, Karacic JJ. Pseudo-obstruction syndrome in multiple sclerosis. J Gastrointest Motil 1991;3:144–150.
7. Nowak TV, Anuras S, Ionasescu VV. Gastrointestinal manifestations of the muscular dystrophies. Gastroenterology 1982;82:800–810.
8. Buchholz DW. Neurogenic Dysphagia. In TM Bayless (ed), Current Therapy in Gastroenterology and Liver Disease. St Louis: Mosby, 1994;69–72.
9. Schulze-Delrieu K. Metoclopramide. Gastroenterology 1979;77:768–779.
10. Isenberg JI, Laine L, McQuaid KR, Rubin W. Acid-Peptic Disorders. In DH Alpers, C Owyang, DW Powell, et al. (eds), Textbook of Gastroenterology. Philadelphia: JB Lippincott, 1991;1241–1339.
11. Fein BI, Holt PR. Hepatobiliary complications of total parenteral nutrition. J Clin Gastroenterol 1994;18:62–66.
12. Mansfield PF, Fornage BD, Gregurich MA, et al. Complications and failures of subclavian-vein catheterization. N Engl J Med 1994;331:1735–1738.
13. Foltzer MA, Reese RE. Bacteremia and Sepsis. In RF Betts, RE Reese (eds), A Practical Approach to Infectious Disease. Boston: Little, Brown Co, 1991;19–53.
14. McClave SA, Lowen C, Snider HL. Immunonutrition and enteral hyperalimentation of critically ill patients. Dig Dis Sci 1992;37:1153–1161.
15. Alverdy JC, Aoys E, Moss GS. Total parenteral nutrition promotes bacterial translocation from the gut. Surgery 1988;104:185–190.
16. Wilmore DW, Jacobs DO, O'Dwyer ST, et al. The gut: a central organ after surgical stress. Surgery 1988;104:917–923.
17. Heimbach DM. Surgical feeding procedures in patients with neurological disorders. Ann Surg 1970;172:311–314.
18. Olivares L, Revuelta R, Segovia A. Tube feeding and lethal aspiration in neurological patients: a review of 720 autopsy cases. Stroke 1974;5:654–657.
19. Wilkinson WA, Pickleman J. Feeding gastrostomy. A reappraisal. Am Surg 1982; 48:273–275.
20. Ghahremani GG, Gould RJ. Nasoenteric feeding tubes. Radiographic detection of complications. Dig Dis Sci 1986;31:574–585.
21. Fremstad JD, Martin SH. Lethal complication from insertion of nasogastric tube after severe basilar skull fracture. J Trauma 1978;18:820–822.
22. Hafner CD, Brush BE, Wylie JH Jr. Complications of gastrointestinal intubation. Arch Surg 1961;83:163–176.
23. Nagler R, Spiro HM. Persistent gastroesophageal reflux induced during prolonged gastric intubation. N Engl J Med 1963;269:495–500.
24. McCredie JA, McDowell RF. Oesophageal stricture following intubation in a case of hiatus hernia. Br J Surg 1958;46:260–261.

25. Douglas WK. Oesophageal strictures associated with gastroduodenal intubation. Br J Surg 1956;43:404–409.

26. Gustke RF, Soergel KH, Varma RR. Gastric reflux during perfusion of the small bowel. Gastroenterology 1970;59:890–895.

27. Schwab D, Muhldorfer S, Nusko G, et al. Endoscopic placement of nasojejunal tubes: a randomized, controlled, prospective trial comparing suitability and technical success for two different tubes. Gastrointest Endosc 2002;56:858–863.

28. Strong RM, Condon SC, Solinger MR, et al. Equal aspiration rates from post-pylorus and intra-gastric placed small bore nasoenteric feeding tubes: a randomized, prospective study. J Parenter Enteral Nutr 1992;16:59–63.

29. Spain DA, Deweese RC, Reynolds MA, Richardson JD. Transpyloric passage of feeding tubes in patients with head injuries does not decrease complications. J Trauma 1995; 39:1100–1102.

30. Fox KA, Mularski RA, Sarfati MR, et al. Aspiration pneumonia following surgically placed feeding tubes. Am J Surg 1995;170:564–567.

31. Marik PE. Aspiration pneumonitis and aspiration pneumonia. N Engl J Med 2001; 344:665–671.

32. Bucklin DL, Gilsdorf RB. Percutaneous needle pharyngostomy. J Parenter Enteral Nutr 1985; 9:68–70.

33. Heyland DK, Drover JW, MacDonald G, et al. Effect of postpyloric feeding on gastroesophageal regurgitation and pulmonary microaspiration: results of a randomized, controlled trial. Crit Care Med 2001;29:1495–1501.

34. Fremstad JD, Martin SH. Lethal complication from insertion of nasogastric tube after severe basilar skull fracture. J Trauma 1978;18:820–822.

35. Fan AC, Baron TH, Rumalla A, Harewood GC. Comparison of direct percutaneous endoscopic jejunostomy and PEG with jejunal extension. Gastrointest Endosc 2002;56:890–894.

36. Gauderer MW, Izant RJ Jr, Ponsky JL. Gastrostomy without laparotomy: a percutaneous endoscopic technique. J Pediatr Surg 1980;15:872–875.

37. Larsen DE, Burton DD, DiMagno EP, Schroeder KW. Percutaneous endoscopic gastrostomy. Indications, success, complications, and mortality in 314 consecutive patients. Gastroenterology 1987;93:48–52.

38. Fay DE, Gruber M, Lance P, Poplausky M. Long-term enteral feeding: a retrospective comparison of delivery via percutaneous endoscopic gastrostomy and nasoenteric tubes. Am J Gastroenterol 1990;85:1120–1122.

39. Heymsfield SB, Ansley JD, Bethel RA, et al. Enteral hyperalimentation: an alternative to central venous hyperalimentation. Ann Int Med 1979;90:63–71.

40. Winterbauer RH, Barron E, Durning RD Jr, McFadden MC. Aspirated nasogastric feeding solution detected by glucose strips. Ann Int Med 1981;95:67–68.

41. Cataldi-Betcher EL, Jones KW, Seltzer MH, Slocum BA. Complications occurring during enteral nutrition support: a prospective study. J Parenter Enteral Nutr 1983;7:546–552.

42. Ciocon JO, Foley CJ, Graver M, Silverstone FA. Tube feedings in elderly patients. Indications, benefits and complications. Arch Intern Med 1988;148:429–433.

43. Metheny NA, Eisenberg P, Spies M. Aspiration pneumonia in patients fed through nasoenteral tubes. Heart Lung 1986;15:256–261.

44. Wolfsen HC, Ball TJ, Botoman VA, et al. Tube dysfunction following percutaneous endoscopic gastrostomy and jejunostomy. Gastrointest Endosc 1990;36:261–263.

45. Kirby DF, Craig RM, Plotnick BH, Tsang T-K. Percutaneous endoscopic gastrostomies: a prospective evaluation and review of the literature. J Parenter Enteral Nutr 1986;10:155–159.

46. Kaw M, Sekas G. Long-term follow-up of consequences of percutaneous endoscopic gastrostomy (PEG) tubes in nursing home patients. Dig Dis Sci 1994;39:738–743.

47. Park RH, Allsion MC, Lang J, et al. Randomised comparison of percutaneous endoscopic gastrostomy and nasogastric tube feeding in patients with persisting neurological dysphagia. BMJ 1992;304:1406–1409.

48. Baeten C, Hoefnagels J. Feeding via a nasogastric tube or percutaneous endoscopic gastrostomy. A comparison. Scand J Gastronterol 1992;27(Suppl 194):95–98.

49. Drug Facts and Comparisons. St Louis: Facts and Comparisons, 2001;81–88.

50. Bosco JJ, Barkun AN, Isenberg GA, et al. Endoscopic enteral nutritional access devices. Gastrointest Endosc 2002;56:796–802.

51. Grant MD, Rudberg MA, Brody JA. Gastrostomy placement and mortality among hospitalized Medicare beneficiaries. JAMA 1998;279:1973–1976.

52. Angus F, Burakoff R. The percutaneous endoscopic gastrostomy tube: medical and ethical issues in placement. Am J Gastroenterol 2003;98:272–277.

53. Finucane TE, Christmas C, Travis K. Tube feeding in patients with advanced dementia. JAMA 1999;282:1365–1370.

54. Norton B, Homer-Ward M, Donnelly MT, et al. A randomized prospective comparison of percutaneous endoscopic gastrostomy and nasogastric tube feeding after acute dysphagic stroke. BMJ 1992;27:95–98.

55. ASGE Guideline. Role of endoscopy in enteral feeding. Gastrointest Endosc 2002; 55:794–797.

56. Di Sario JA, Baskin WN, Brown RD, et al. Endoscopic approaches to enteral nutritional support. Gastrointest Endosc 2002;55:901–908.

Chapter 16

Pharmacological and Non-Pharmacological Approaches to Gastrointestinal Motor Dysfunction in Neurological Disease

Eamonn M. M. Quigley, Lorraine L. Edwards, and Waseem Ashraf

In other chapters in this volume, the various gastrointestinal problems that may occur in patients with neurological disease have been detailed and, in many cases, an approach to their management has been outlined. Most of these problems are based on motor dysfunction, be it due to dysfunction at the level of the intrinsic neuromuscular apparatus of the gut or in the brain-gut axis. In this chapter, we will focus on therapy, review the various pharmacological and non-pharmacological alternatives available, and discuss, in more detail, the management of some of the more common clinical syndromes. Given its prevalence in so many neurological disorders, particular emphasis will be given to the management of constipation.

PHARMACOLOGICAL APPROACHES TO GUT MOTOR DYSFUNCTION

While enteric neurophysiologists and pharmacologists have made tremendous progress in the study of enteric receptors and neurotransmitters in in vitro models, the translation of this information to human disease has been, given the complexity of the regulation of motility in the intact animal, far from simple.[1-4] The clinician must be mindful of the fact that many studies of motility pharmacology have concentrated on the effect of various drugs on motor patterns without attempting to assess any related changes in gut function. It tends to be forgotten in this context that improved function and not more, or fewer, pressure "waves" or different motor patterns is the goal of therapy; functional correlates of motor effects should, therefore, be sought wherever possible.

In reviewing the pharmacology of motility, a number of common themes emerge. Given the ubiquity of many types of receptors in various neuronal systems, it should come as no surprise that the usefulness of several of these agents has been limited by central nervous system and cardiovascular side effects; the former of particular relevance to their use in patients with neurological disease in general, and the latter potentially problematic for the patient with autonomic dysfunction. Metoclopramide, for example, is contraindicated in Parkinson's disease because of its potential to cause extrapyramidal side effects. For many of these agents, tolerance has also been a problem, with long-term efficacy often proving elusive. Several of these agents are somewhat site specific; we may be moving into a phase when the tailoring of drugs to specifically target organs within the gastrointestinal tract will become a reality. Another major obstacle to progress is that gastrointestinal dysmotility syndromes are, in general, poorly defined, their "definition" being based on symptom patterns rather than histopathological abnormality. Constipation, for example, may be the net result of a variety of pathophysiological processes, which may not be responsive to a single therapeutic approach. In the first part of this chapter, we will review the principal pharmacological classes of agents that may be of use in this clinical context. Table 16.1 summarizes the principal drug classes, their properties, and their applications.

Table 16.1. Pharmacological Agents that Modulate Gut Motility and/or Sensation

Category	Examples	Effects	Applications	Comments
Cholinergic agonists and antagonists	Neostigmine	Anticholinesterase inhibitor	Ogilvie's syndrome, ileus	Excellent results in decompressing acute megacolon. Little evidence for long-term efficacy
	Hyoscine, etc.	Anticholinergic	IBS	
Somatostatin analogs	Octreotide	Induces activity fronts but delays emptying and transit	Scleroderma- and neuropathy-related CIP	Anecdotal reports of efficacy in ileus; overall efficacy in CIP unclear
Prostaglandins	Misoprostol	Stimulates colonic motility and secretion	Slow transit constipation	Not evaluated in neurological patients
Serotonin agonists and antagonists	5HT$_3$ antagonists Ondansetron Alosetron	Central and peripheral antagonism of 5HT$_3$ receptors	Ondansetron etc.; effective as anti-emetics. Alosetron effective in IBS.	Alosetron restricted due to concerns reconstipation and ischemic colitis
	5HT$_4$ agonists Cisapride Tegaserod (Prucalopride)	Stimulate acetylcholine release	Cisapride and tegaserod act as pan-gut prokinetics	Cisapride withdrawn due to cardiac toxicity; tegaserod effective in IBS
Opiates	(Fedotozine)	Kappa agonist; modulates visceral afferents	Evaluated in dyspepsia; efficacy unclear	Opiates are first-line in the therapy of diarrhea; dependence is possible
	Loperamide	Agonist; precise mode of action unclear	Effective anti-diarrheal; possible effect on anal sphincter also	
Motilides	Erythromycin	Motilin agonist, prokinetic in the foregut	Effective i.v.; poor efficacy p.o.	Not suitable for long-term oral use; need alternatives
Dopamine antagonists	Metoclopramide (Domperidone)	Dopamine antagonists at the chemoreceptor trigger zone and in the periphery; anti-emetics and fore-gut prokinetics	Anti-emetics effective in gastroparesis; domperidone does not cross blood-brain barrier	Metoclopramide causes extrapyramidal side-effects; domperidone can be used in Parkinson's disease. Both cause hyperprolactinemia

IBS = irritable bowel syndrome; CIP = chronic intestinal pseudoobstruction.
Agents in parenthesis have not been approved for use in the US.

Cholinergic Agonists and Antagonists

Cholinergic agonists are the original promotility agents and relied for their effect primarily on stimulation of muscarinic M2-type receptors on the smooth muscle cell. Evidence for their effectiveness in motility disorders is, in general, inconsistent, although benefits in reflux disease and gastroparesis have been claimed.[5] Not surprisingly, given their nonspecificity, they are associated with a significant incidence of side effects and their use in the long-term management of motor disorders has diminished with the advent of newer agents. However, in the acute therapy of megacolon and other manifestations of pseudoobstruction, anticholinesterases such as neostigmine are effective and have assumed a place in the short-term management of these disorders.[6,7] Neostigmine, given in a dose of 2 mg intravenously, has been shown to reverse megacolon; in a recent report, 89% of patients had an immediate response and 61% a sustained response.[8] Females, older patients, and those not on narcotics or in the postoperative state were those most likely to respond.

Anticholinergics have been the mainstay of presumed "spastic" gut disorders, such as irritable bowel syndrome, for decades, despite a paucity of evidence for efficacy for many of these compounds.[9,10] In the past, drugs of this class have also been employed in the symptomatic therapy of nausea and vomiting[11]; their use has now been superseded by more effective agents. It is also possible that some of the efficacy attributed to antihistamines and tricyclic antidepressants in putative motor disorders and related gastrointestinal symptoms is attributable to their anticholinergic properties.

Octreotide

The somatostatin analog octreotide was introduced into gastroenterology primarily for its antisecretory affects.[12–14] Given this background of largely inhibitory effects, a prokinetic effect of octreotide was unexpected when it was shown that octreotide improved gastrointestinal symptoms, reduced bacterial overgrowth, and appeared to accelerate gastrointestinal transit among patients with scleroderma and intestinal involvement.[15,16] It was of interest that these motility effects were seen at lower doses (i.e., 10–100 µg) than employed in the treatment of diarrheal states.[15] A more detailed analysis of the effects of low-dose octreotide on motility confirmed the induction of premature, rapidly-propagating, long activity fronts and revealed a shortening of phase II of the migrating motor complex,[17] but also suggested that the net effect of octreotide on transit was to slow gastric emptying and, at doses of 25 and 50 µg, to delay small intestinal transit.[17–19] There does not appear to be any effect on colonic transit in these doses. An alternative explanation for the beneficial symptomatic response of octreotide has come from more recent studies indicating an effect of octreotide on visceral afferents. Indeed, octreotide has been shown to reverse the visceral hypersensitivity associated with irritable bowel syndrome.[20] Though one recent review[21] recommended octreotide in a dose of 50 µg at night for patients with chronic intestinal pseudoobstruction (CIP) related to either scleroderma or an enteric neuropathy, its role in CIP in general remains to be defined. It seems unlikely, on balance, and despite reports of apparent efficacy in CIP,[22] that this agent acts as a true prokinetic, given, in particular, its propensity to inhibit antral motility[23] and delay gastric emptying.[17–19] Therefore, its role in CIP remains to be defined.

Long-term treatment with octreotide may also be complicated by an inhibition of gallbladder motility and the promotion of cholelithiasis. The effects of octreotide on gallbladder function may be particularly problematic in the patient receiving high-dose octreotide therapy for acromegaly, in which gallstones have been defined in up to 20% of patients.[24–25]

Prompted by observations in animal studies of the amelioration by octreotide of postoperative ileus,[26] there have been anecdotal reports of a clinical response to octreotide among patients with ileus and Ogilvie's syndrome. These remain to be confirmed in prospective studies.

Prostaglandin Analogs

In clinical studies of the efficacy of prostaglandin analogs, such as misoprostol, in promoting gastric mucosal protection, diarrhea was noted to be a common side effect. This observation has been translated into clinical benefit through the use of misoprostol in patients with refractory slow transit constipation. In a total daily dose of 1200 μg, administered either in divided doses t.i.d. or as a single dose, misoprostol has been shown to increase stool weight and frequency and accelerate colonic transit.[27] The precise mechanism of action remains uncertain,[28] though in separate studies, a related analog, rioprostil, has been shown to accelerate gastric emptying.[29] The effects of this analog on human small intestinal activity have also been evaluated.[30] For at least this particular analog, its use is not associated with a disruption of the organization of the migrating motor complex, though contractile activity during Phase II is markedly inhibited.

Serotonin (5-HT) Agonists & Antagonists

Given the abundance of serotonergic neurons in the gastrointestinal tract, the current interest in 5-HT-receptor agonists and antagonists should come as no surprise.[31,32] The 5-HT$_3$ and 5-HT$_4$ receptors have been targeted in particular. Thus, 5-HT$_4$ agonists are, in general, prokinetics, while the primary effects of 5-HT$_3$ antagonists are to modulate visceral sensation, act as antiemetics, and delay colonic transit.

While both metoclopramide and domperidone may act as partial 5-HT$_4$ agonists, their primary effects are mediated through dopaminergic mechanisms. Cisapride, a substituted benzamide, was the prototype prokinetic agent among 5-HT$_4$ agonists. While efficacy has been demonstrated for cisapride in a number of gastrointestinal motor disorders including gastroesophageal reflux, gastroparesis of varying etiology, CIP, and constipation, a beneficial response is by no means universal in any of these disorders.[33–42] In gastroesophageal reflux, a positive response to cisapride is most likely among patients with minimal or low-grade esophagitis.[2] Among 42 patients with a neuropathic chronic intestinal motility disorder in whom there was no significant overall effect of cisapride, Camilleri and colleagues[43] identified patient subgroups that appeared to benefit in terms of symptomatic improvement from cisapride therapy. A significant response was most likely among patients who did not have extrinsic autonomic dysfunction and, in particular, among those in whom they could not detect evidence of vagal dysfunction. Rectal cisapride administered in a dose of 30 mg t.i.d. does not appear to influence the motility changes associated with surgery or to expedite the resolution of postsurgical ileus.[44] The recent association of cisapride with rare, though potentially significant and occasionally fatal, cardiac toxicity has led either to its withdrawal or to the imposition of severe restrictions on its use in many countries, including the United States. Toxicity was especially likely to occur among patients who were on other medications that affect cisapride metabolism or cardiac conduction.[4,40,45,46] This has prompted a search for an alternative; prucalopride, a full 5-HT$_4$ agonist, accelerates colonic transit[47] and benefits patients with idiopathic constipation[48] and scleroderma-related dysmotility,[49] but has not, as yet, been approved for use in the United States or Europe. Another related agent, levosulpiride, has been evaluated in gastroparesis.[50] In the meantime, and in the United States in particular, where domperidone is also unavailable, there is a distinct paucity of therapeutic alternatives for the patient who requires a prokinetic agent, a situation which has led to a variety of strategies to obtain more effective drugs from elsewhere.[41]

Tegaserod, a partial 5-HT$_4$ agonist,[51] has recently been approved in the United States for patients with constipation-predominant irritable bowel syndrome.[52,53] This agent appears to have quite generalized prokinetic properties[54–56] and to be free from cardiac side-effects.[57–59] Studies in constipation, per se, as well as in esophageal and gastric motor disorders, are underway. Tegaserod's role regarding the patient with neurological disease remains to be defined.

On the other hand, 5-HT$_3$ antagonists have been evaluated for both their central antiemetic and peripheral sensory-modulating effects. Several, such as ondansetron, granisetron, and tropisetron, are widely used in the prophylaxis and therapy of chemotherapy-related nausea and vomiting.[11] Alosetron, another 5-HT$_3$ antagonist, was introduced for therapy of irritable bowel syndrome based on its effects on visceral sensation.[60,61] These agents also inhibit motor activity,[62] an effect that led both to the recommendation that the use of alosetron in irritable bowel syndrome be restricted to those with the diarrhea-predominant variety and to the documentation of a relatively high frequency of troublesome constipation in relation to 5-HT$_3$ antagonists in general. Alosetron was temporarily withdrawn in the United States[63] because of concerns related to a reported association with ischemic colitis[64]; its recent reintroduction,[65,66] amidst some controversy,[67] has been coupled with restrictions on its use. These very same constipatory effects may, of course, be beneficial in those with carcinoid-related diarrhea.[68,69]

Opiates

Opiates and opiate-agonists and antagonists may influence gut motility through effects on central or peripheral opiate receptors. In general, mu and delta opiate agonists tend to stimulate motility, whereas kappa agonists inhibit motor activity.

Trimebutine appears to have similar affinity for mu, delta, and kappa receptor subtypes. Trimebutine has been shown to increase propagating electrical activity and accelerate colon transit among patients with idiopathic constipation who have delayed colon transit.[70] No benefit was seen among patients with constipation and normal colon transit.

Fedotozine, which acts as a peripheral kappa agonist, has been shown to abolish surgically and chemically induced ileus in a rat model. This affect does not appear to be mediated through a prokinetic action, but may be exerted through an effect on visceral afferents. The potential of kappa agonists such as fedotozine to modulate visceral afferent traffic has formed the basis for clinical studies in nonulcer dyspepsia and irritable bowel syndrome.[71] It is unclear at this time whether or not this scientific promise has been translated into clinical benefit.

The importance of opiates in motility is also emphasized by the potent constipating effects of opiate analgesics.[72,73] Indeed, the opiate antagonist naloxone can reverse opiate-induced constipation in opiate-dependent patients[74] and has even been shown to reverse chronic idiopathic constipation.[75]

Opiates, such as loperamide, remain the mainstay of symptomatic therapy for acute and short-lived diarrheal states.[76] These agents are also used in the long-term for symptomatic relief by patients with diarrheal disorders not amenable to specific therapy. There is some evidence that loperamide may not only reduce diarrhea, but may also exert beneficial effects on the anal sphincters.

Motilin Agonists

Motilin agonists, or motilides, mimic the effects of the hormone motilin on gastrointestinal motor activity. Motilin, released from the proximal duodenum, exerts potent effects on motor activity in the stomach, upper gastrointestinal tract, and gallbladder. Motilin receptors have also been identified in the distal small intestine and colon, where they appear to be present in lower density. Erythromycin, particularly when administered intravenously, is a potent motilin agonist and increases antral and duodenal contractile activity in a dose-dependent manner.[16,77–86] This is associated with an acceleration of gastric emptying and small intestinal transit. Hyperglycemia inhibits the prokinetic effect of erythromycin,[87] a factor that may limit its efficacy among this patient population. Gallbladder emptying is also accelerated.[85]

While erythromycin is an intriguing, if unexpected, addition to the prokinetic armamentarium, it has several limitations. First, it has proven far less effective when given orally in the medium- to long-term,[83,84,86] which has led some to advocate prolonged intravenous administration for highly selected cases[88] and others to explore the transdermal route.[89] Second, erythromycin is an antibiotic and is therefore prey to all of the concerns attendant on the chronic use of an antibacterial agent. Finally, erythromycin is poorly bioavailable and is possessed of far from ideal pharmacokinetic and pharmacodynamic profiles. A number of molecular modifications designed to sustain the prokinetic effect of erythromycin, while being devoid of its antibiotic activity and possessing greater bioavailability, are currently under investigation[90–93]; none are, as yet, available for clinical use.

For the moment, the most important use for erythromycin is in the therapy of acute, severe gastroparesis; here, short-term intravenous dosing may prove highly effective.[84,86,94]

Antidepressants

Antidepressants are commonly used among patients with neurological disorders. Until recently, tricyclic compounds such as amitriptyline and imipramine were the most commonly prescribed; more recently, the serotonin reuptake inhibitors have gained increasing popularity. In terms of gastrointestinal effects, the tricyclics have been shown to prolong both orocecal and whole gut transit whereas the SSRIs may actually reduce orocecal transit, but exert little effect on whole gut transit.[95]

There is accumulating evidence to suggest efficacy for these agents in a variety of functional gastrointestinal disorders, such as functional dyspepsia and irritable bowel syndrome.[96–98] These effects may also benefit the neurological patient with gastrointestinal symptoms.

Dopamine Antagonists

Metoclopramide, a central and peripheral dopamine antagonist with antiemetic and prokinetic effects, has been available for several years and has been used in the symptomatic therapy of nausea and vomiting and, more specifically, in the management of gastroesophageal reflux disease, gastroparesis of varying etiology, and other upper gastrointestinal motor disorders.[5] Though efficacy has been demonstrated in a variety of controlled trials, in these various disorders, its use has been complicated by a relatively high incidence of side effects. Most troubling among these have been neurological effects such as tremor, akathisia, myoclonus, and involuntary movements, including a parkinsonian syndrome.

Domperidone, a peripheral dopamine antagonist, does not cross the blood–brain barrier. It, therefore, maintains the prokinetic effects of metoclopramide in the periphery, as well as the antiemetic effects on the chemoreceptor trigger zone, yet, appears relatively free of central extrapyramidal side effects.[99,100] Both agents, however, may induce hyperprolactinemia and associated side effects such as gynecomastia and galactorrhea.

Domperidone has been shown to be effective in diabetic and postsurgical gastroparesis; in some instances of chemotherapy-related nausea and vomiting[11]; in the symptomatic therapy of idiopathic nausea, vomiting, and gastroparesis[101]; and in post-surgical gastroparesis.[102] The lack of penetration of the blood–brain barrier has proven attractive for those who manage gastrointestinal symptoms among patients with neurological disease. Nausea and vomiting are common among patients with Parkinson's disease and may particularly complicate therapy with a variety of dopaminergic agents. Whether a primary abnormality of gastric or duodenal motor function also contributes to these symptoms in patients with Parkinson's disease remains uncertain and has not been investigated to any extent. Gastrointestinal motor dysfunction could, however, complicate dopaminergic therapy. If these agents are not delivered in a predictable fashion to the small intestine—their site of absorption—therapeutic efficacy will be impaired and the management of patients with prominent "on/off" fluctuations will prove particularly problematic. Indeed, there is some (albeit incomplete) evidence to suggest that domperidone pretreatment may improve levodopa delivery in patients with Parkinson's disease.[103] In support of an effect on gastric emptying, a similar benefit was demonstrated in one study which used cisapride, rather than domperidone, as the prokinetic.[104] Domperidone may be particularly useful in patients with Parkinson's disease for a number of reasons. First, it is an antiemetic and prevents the gastrointestinal symptoms related to levodopa, apomorphine, bromocriptine, and other dopaminergic agents.[103,105] It may also, in theory, have a beneficial effect on any pre-existing abnormalities in gastric emptying, motility, or compliance related to the parkinsonian disease process. Second, by improving gastric motor function and accelerating gastric emptying, domperidone may increase dopamine bioavailability and thereby improve the pharmacological control of the parkinsonian process.[106,107] Finally, there is some (albeit limited) evidence to suggest that domperidone may also alleviate the cardiovascular side effects associated with levodopa and other dopaminergic agents.[108] However, it has also been suggested that in high doses (e.g., in the range of 120 mg per day), domperidone may penetrate the blood–brain barrier and lead to central blockade of the therapeutic effects of levodopa.[103]

NONPHARMACOLOGICAL APPROACHES TO THE THERAPY OF MOTOR DYSFUNCTION

Given the aforementioned frustrations and disappointments experienced in relation to pharmacological therapy, it should come as no surprise that many other approaches have been taken to the symptomatic management of the patient with gastrointestinal motor dysfunction. These are summarized in Table 16.2; most will not be discussed further here as they have been dealt with in detail elsewhere in this book. We will confine ourselves here to a few general comments regarding approaches of special relevance or interest to the neurological patient.

Neurologists will be intrigued to learn of the use of botulinum toxin (BTX) in a number of gastrointestinal motor disorders.[109] Initially, its use was explored in achalasia, but, more recently, has been employed in spastic motor disorders of the esophagus, in gastroparesis, and in "outlet" constipation. In achalasia, BTX injection into

Table 16.2. Non-Pharmacological Approaches to Motor Disorders

Approach	Techniques	Applications	Comments
Endoscopic	Dilatation	Achalasia	Pneumatic dilatation highly effective
	Insertion of tubes: Gastrostomy PEG/PEJ Jejunostomy	For decompression and/or provision of nutrition in neurological and esophageal disease, gastroparesis, CIP	PEG will not prevent aspiration; significant ethical issues in neurological patients; may provide significant decompression in CIP
	Botox injection	Achalasia, gastroparesis	Long-term efficacy unclear
	Decompression	Ogilvie's syndrome	Should be reserved for neostigmine failures; high recurrence rate
Surgical	Myotomy	Achalasia	Can now be performed by minimally-invasive approach; highly effective
	Resection	Gastroparesis, CIP, megacolon	Should be reserved for carefully selected cases
	Tube placement	Gastrostomy Jejunostomy	Indicated where endoscopic approach not feasible
	Decompressive	Venting enterostomies in CIP, cecostomy in megacolon	
	Transplantation	Severe CIP	
Electrical stimulation	Gastric	Gastroparesis	Mode of action unclear; long term efficacy to be established
	Anorectal	Incontinence	Has shown efficacy in neurological disorders
	Sacral	Constipation	Effective in spinal cord injured

PEG = percutaneous endoscopic gastrostomy; PEJ = percutaneous endoscopic jejunostomy; CIP = chronic intestinal pseudo-obstruction.

the lower esophageal sphincter improves the symptoms of chest pain and dysphagia in the short term[110–114]; long-term effects on symptoms and esophageal function are less clearly defined.[115,116] Early reports of efficacy in gastroparesis following the injection of BTX into the pyloric sphincter are encouraging[117,118]; long-term follow up studies are awaited. There are reports of good results in relation to the injection of BTX into the anal sphincters and pelvic floor muscles in patients with "outlet" type constipation.[119]

Electrical stimulation is another technique familiar to neurologists that has recently been applied to the gastrointestinal tract. Two approaches are of special interest; direct stimulation of the stomach via implanted serosal electrodes in gastroparesis and the use of stimulation of either the anal sphincter or sacral nerve roots in fecal incontinence and constipation. This approach may well be expanded to other areas.

MANAGEMENT OF ESOPHAGEAL MOTOR DYSFUNCTION, GASTROPARESIS, AND INTESTINAL AND COLONIC PSEUDOOBSTRUCTION

Each of these issues is dealt with in detail elsewhere in this book; we will confine ourselves to a few general comments.

Achalasia is perhaps the best understood motor disorder; its clinical manifestations, diagnostic criteria, pathophysiology, and management have been extensively investigated and, unlike other motor disorders, are the subject of considerable consensus. Most would agree that, in a suitable patient, the choice of optimal therapy rests between pneumatic dilatation and myotomy. Achalasia also serves as a reminder of the importance of precise diagnosis; many "motor" disorders are described among patients with dysphagia, chest pain, and other esophageal symptoms. Few withstand rigorous assessment and are best described as "non-specific." Our experience with the evaluation and management of so-called non-cardiac chest pain of presumed esophageal origin, a much more common clinical disorder, illustrates this point. Despite the description over the years of a host of manometric abnormalities among these patients, it is now evident that, for the majority, gastroesophageal reflux appears to be the major factor in initiating pain and/or esophageal spasm. For these patients, acid suppression remains the mainstay of therapy. In others, who have no evidence of reflux, a variety of "spastic" and other motor disorders of the esophagus have been documented on manometric studies and associated with episodes of pain. Therapy in this context has been far less successful, with various centers reporting less than satisfactory responses to anticholinergics, calcium-channel blockers, nitrates, bougienage, pneumatic dilatation, and even esophagomyotomy. This should not be surprising, given the often tenuous association between symptoms and motility findings. In an open label trial, Miller and colleagues have very recently reported a significant and sustained (up to 18 months) reduction in pain scores among 29 patients with noncardiac pain related to esophageal spasm who did not have achalasia or gastroesophageal reflux following injection of BTX into the lower esophageal sphincter.[120]

Patients with neurological disease commonly develop esophageal symptoms; the clinician is encouraged to exert caution in the interpretation of manometric findings and to resist the temptation to ascribe significance to motility patterns that do not fulfill criteria for well-defined entities.

The management of both gastroparesis and intestinal pseudoobstruction is complicated by the current paucity of effective therapeutic alternatives.[4,40,121,122] Cisapride has been withdrawn and potential alternatives such as prucalopride, or levosulpiride, are still at the clinical trial stage or, as in the case of tegaserod, have not as yet been shown to have efficacy beyond currently approved indications. In the United States, the clinician is left with metoclopramide—unsuitable for use in many neurological patients and of limited efficacy beyond the pylorus—and erythromycin and cholinergic agonists which, though effective in acute gastroparesis and pseudoobstruction respectively, are of little long-term use.

Gastric electrical stimulation, a procedure that requires surgical intervention and that is not without its complications, has been employed in refractory gastroparesis.[123,124] While early results appear encouraging, we await studies of long-term outcome. Stimulation is also being explored in CIP.

The patient with severe gastroparesis or advanced pseudoobstruction requires a multidisciplinary approach with attention being paid by appropriate experts to the management of such symptoms as pain and distension, as well as attending to nutrition, bacterial overgrowth, and other related illnesses. Endoscopic and surgical approaches to nutritional care and decompression may be of considerable benefit.[125–127] It needs to be stressed that optimal outcome in these situations requires a careful consideration of indications and of likely benefits and risks.[128,129] Resective surgery has a limited role in gastroparesis[130,131] and CIP.[40]

Acute colonic pseudoobstruction (Ogilvie's syndrome) is a relatively common motor disorder in the acutely ill patient and has been well described among neurological patients.[121] Untreated, there is a significant risk of perforation with an attendant mortality in the region of 40% to 50%. The clinical approach should be guided by the abdominal radiograph; a cecal diameter in excess of 9 cm should be regarded as abnormal; if this exceeds 12 cm there is a significant risk of perforation.[121] Parenteral neostigmine (2 mg intravenously) represents a significant advance in the management of this disorder and should preclude emergency decompressive colonoscopy in many instances.[6–8] If this approach fails, colonoscopy is indicated but often technically difficult, is not without risk, and is associated with a recurrence rate of up to 40%. The approach to failure at this stage must be individualized and must take into account the risk of perforation, the risks of intervention, and the patient's overall prognosis.

THE MANAGEMENT OF CONSTIPATION

Constipation and defecatory dysfunction are common in many neurological diseases including multiple sclerosis, muscular dystrophy, peripheral neuropathy, Parkinson's disease, and spinal cord injury.[132–134] Successful management of these gastrointestinal problems requires an understanding of both normal colorectal function and the pathophysiology of dysfunction.[135] In addition, careful characterization of the patient's complaint is essential. In selected patients, specialized studies of colonic and anorectal function may be indicated, a primary objective being to place patients into one of the two main categories of constipation; slow transit constipation (related to colonic hypomotility or inertia) and "outlet" constipation or defecatory dysfunction (related to pelvic floor dysfunction, rectal dyssynergia, anismus). However, in patients with central nervous system (CNS) disease the etiology of colorectal problems is often multifactorial and may include such factors as diet, inactivity, depression, mental confusion, or medications, in addition to the central and enteric effects of the underlying neurological disease. Management must be focused and individualized to each patient and, many times, relies on the combined efforts of dietitian, physical therapist, and physician.

Among patients with Parkinson's disease (PD), for example, constipation has been reported in over 50% of those attending a movement disorders clinic.[136] It has even been suggested that constipation may predate the onset of other manifestations of PD.[137] A number of factors appear to be involved in the pathophysiology of constipation in PD and include slow colon transit and defecatory dysfunction.[138] The former may, in turn, be related to the direct involvement of the colonic myenteric plexus by the Parkinson's disease process[139]—the latter appears to reflect impaired coordination of the pelvic floor and anal sphincter muscles.[140,141]

In most clinical settings, the diagnosis of constipation relies on patient history alone, although recent studies suggest that this may not be reliable in patients with idiopathic constipation.[142–144] Patients with slow transit constipation will, typically, complain of infrequent evacuation and may go for days or even weeks without a bowel movement, becoming aware of the need to evacuate only when abdominal distension and distress supervene. If central perception is blunted, as in the patient with dementia, impaction may occur. Those with defecatory dysfunction, in contrast, receive the signal to evacuate on a regular basis but defecation is ineffective, difficult, or incomplete and is often associated with prolonged straining and considerable rectal discomfort. In many situations these disorders may coexist, rendering it nigh impossible to interpret symptoms and to define the primacy of one mechanism over the other. Overlap between slow transit and outlet constipation may also go some way towards explaining the oft disappointing results of new therapies targeted at one of these pathophysiological mechanisms.

Slow-Transit Constipation

If slow transit through the colon, a disorder based primarily on propulsive failure, is considered to be the predominant factor in the pathophysiology of constipation, management involves dietary modification of fiber, fluid, and caloric intake and possibly the addition of laxatives and/or prokinetic agents.[145]

Diet

Attention should first be given to dietary changes. A dietary history can be time consuming, but also enlightening, as many patients have severely altered their diet due to the limitations of their disease. A dietitian can help to illuminate those areas which can be modified (i.e., ensuring adequate caloric, fluid, and fiber intake). Enlisting the involvement of spouses and families in these discussions can be most helpful, and working toward a balanced, healthy diet for both partners will generally be more successful.

A major problem complicating the assessment of bowel habit or any other gastrointestinal function in relation to neurological disease in the older patient is the relatively poor state of our knowledge of age-related changes in motor function in the normal population.[146–149] Is constipation a normal accompaniment of aging, or is it, as some have suggested, simply a consequence of an age-related decrease in caloric intake?[150] Furthermore, many debilitated patients, those with dysphagia in particular, have difficulty in consuming the recommended daily allowance of 18 to 20 gm of fiber.[151] Thus, we found that our patients with Parkinson's disease (and their spouses) had a mean daily dietary fiber intake of only 11 grams. Their caloric intake, however, was similar to that of their spouses.[136] Achieving appropriate fiber supplementation may, therefore, be a considerable challenge despite the evidence for its benefits in preventing constipation.[152] Astarloa and colleagues also reported that a diet rich in insoluble fiber produced a significant improvement in constipation in PD, as indicated by an increase in stool frequency and an improvement in stool consistency.[153] A most fascinating observation in this study was that of a parallel improvement in extrapyramidal function, which, in turn, appeared to be related to an increase in the bioavailability of orally administered L-dopa. They suggested that this increase in L-dopa absorption and the resultant improvement in clinical status were related to an augmentation in gastrointestinal motility and, thereby, drug delivery by the high fiber diet. Given the description that constipation, rectal distention, and suppression of defecation can result, perhaps through a cologastric reflex, in a delay in gastric emptying,[154–156] one could also speculate that the beneficial effects of the high fiber diet could have resulted from the improvement in constipation and mediated this same reflex.

Fiber Supplementation

If dietary modification alone is unsuccessful or unacceptable to the patient, fiber supplements or bulking agents such as psyllium may be added. Though there is evidence for efficacy for these compounds in simple, apparently slow-transit, constipation,[157] there have been few studies in the patient with neurological disease. We have demonstrated a beneficial effect for psyllium in constipation related to Parkinson's disease.[158] Both stool frequency and stool weight increased significantly after 8 weeks of psyllium treatment,[158] in a manner similar to that reported in idiopathic constipation[157] (Figure 16-1).

On psyllium, patients experienced an average of three additional bowel movements per week. No significant improvement was observed, however, in symptoms that reflected difficulty with the process of defecation itself, such as straining and incomplete evacuation. As these latter symptoms may dominate in many patients with Parkinson's disease and constipation, this may represent a limitation of psyllium therapy. There is no information on the effects of psyllium on L-dopa bioavailability and motor function.

An association between improved bowel function and a beneficial effect on neurological status may not be unique to Parkinson's disease. Among children with autism and other neuro-developmental disorders in which bowel dysfunction is also common, relief of constipation—whether slow transit or "outlet" in type— is often accompanied by striking improvements in behavior and performance. Various interpretations have been applied to this clinical observation; some contend that it supports the existence of a specific gastrointestinal disorder[159] or that it provides evidence for a role for the gut in perpetuating neurological dysfunction,[160] while many would contend that these improvements reflect the removal of the considerable stress and discomfort attendant on constipation and ineffective defecation.

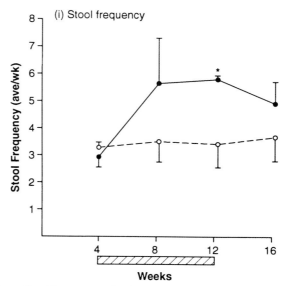

Figure 16-1. Effects of psyllium on constipation in Parkinson's disease. Note significant increase in stool frequency during treatment period *(indicated by hatched bar)* in those PD patients who receive psyllium *(continuous line)* but not in those who received placebo *(broken line)*. *p*<.05 psyllium vs placebo. (From Ashraf W, Pfeiffer RF, Park F, et al. Constipation in Parkinson's disease. Objective assessment and response to psyllium. Mov Dis 1997;12:946-951, with permission.)

Laxatives

When additional fiber is still insufficient, osmotic agents such as lactulose have been the traditional next step. During the first few days of lactulose therapy, gaseous distention, belching, flatulence, borborygmi, and abdominal pain and cramping may be avoided by starting with a lower dosage and advancing as tolerated.[161] Diarrhea indicates overdose and usually responds to dose reduction. Dosage ranges from 7.5 to 30 ml (5–20 gm) are initially given every morning, but may be given twice a day if necessary. If given per nasogastric tube, lactulose should be well diluted to prevent induction of vomiting.

A recent innovation has been the development of laxative doses and preparations of the same polyethylene glycol-based balanced electrolyte solutions that are used in large volume for bowel preparation prior to colonoscopy.[162,163] Therapy is usually commenced with 1 to 2 sachets mixed in an appropriate volume of water and increased as tolerated until an effect is achieved.

Chronic use of other laxatives (such as mineral oil or phenolphthalein) is not routinely recommended, in constipation in general, due to potential side effects. Mineral oil has been associated with lipid pneumonia following aspiration and may lead to systemic lipid granulomatosis. Phenolphthalein has been withdrawn from use in the United States. The chronic abuse of stimulant laxatives, such as senna and the anthraquinone derivatives, leads to pigment deposition in the colon (melanosis coli) and has been associated with fluid/electrolyte abnormalities, malabsorption, and the so-called "cathartic colon." With regard to the latter, whether these agents actually cause the enteric neural or muscle injury thought to cause this radiological appearance, indicative of colonic inertia, remains unresolved. These morphological changes may, indeed, be reflective of a primary disorder of enteric muscle or nerve that has in turn caused constipation, rather than of an iatrogenic injury. The balance of evidence is currently against a neurotoxic effect of laxatives. A risk/benefit ratio assessment may, therefore, support their use in some patients with neurological disease when the risks of impaction outweigh potential side-effects, especially in those with a considerably reduced life expectancy. In these patients, the regular administration of suppositories or enemas may be essential to prevent impaction.[164]

Prokinetic Agents

While many pharmacological therapies have been advocated for the treatment of constipation in Parkinson's disease and other neurological conditions, few have been subjected to clinical trial. Jost reported both symptomatic improvement and an acceleration of colon transit in PD patients with constipation treated with the prokinetic agent cisapride.[165] Other studies—in spinal cord injured patients, for example—have also been encouraging, though data is scanty and far from conclusive. Prucalopride, a new alternative to cisapride, shows promise in treating constipation.[48]

While most prokinetic agents have little direct effect on colonic motility, misoprostol, a prostaglandin E_1 analog, holds more promise. Misoprostol accelerates orocecal transit time[27] and is effective in patients with slow transit constipation; dosage should begin at 200 μg given 30 minutes prior to meals and increased up to 800 μg, or it may be given in one dose. Two recent and unexpected additions to this category have been colchicine[166] and the neurotrophic factor, neurotrophin-3 (NT-3).[167,168] The interest in these compounds as prokinetic agents again stemmed from serendipitous observations in clinical trials for other conditions.

Attention to Psychological Factors

One must always be mindful of the possible role of psychological factors in patients with constipation. An association between psychological distress and slowed colonic transit has been identified; it is unclear, however, whether constipation contributed to the psychological distress or whether the psychological distress adversely affected bowel motility.[150] In general, chronically constipated patients with normal colonic transit manifest a higher degree of psychological distress compared to constipated patients with slow transit.[144,169] Depression, anxiety, and somatization have been associated with chronic constipation[170,171] and are certainly common in patients with neurological disease. Recognition of these processes is important, since therapy directed at them may result in improvement of constipation. The clinician should, in particular, be aware of elderly patients who present with apparently intractable constipation, appear obsessed by the need to evacuate, and are severely frustrated by their failed efforts. This is frequently a manifestation of depression and may respond dramatically to antidepressant therapy.

Invasive Approaches

Among patients with chronic, resistant, slow-transit constipation, surgery in the form of subtotal colectomy has been performed in a minority of patients. Patient selection is crucial to success; the ideal surgical candidate exhibits no evidence of pelvic floor or anal sphincter dysfunction, is free of motor dysfunction elsewhere in the gastrointestinal tract, and is well adjusted in psychological terms.[135,145,161,172,173] Apart from anecdotal reports of colectomy in extreme cases, such as in association with chronic megacolon, there is little data on the use of this surgical strategy in the patient with underlying neurological disease. It is apparent that many in the latter group of patients would be poor candidates for surgery because of their underlying disease process.

An alternative, non-pharmacological approach that has been evaluated to some extent in the spinal cord-injured patient, in particular, is that of spinal stimulation.[174–177] Patients with spinal cord injuries often have bowel and bladder dysfunction. Establishing a bowel regimen is important in these patients to avoid complications and improve their quality of life. While the mainstay of therapy has been suppositories, routine enemas, and digital extraction, sacral anterior root stimulation can be effective in improving defecation in patients with spinal cord injury.[174] An intradural sacral anterior root stimulator is implanted and the patient activates the device by holding a transmitter over the implanted receiver. Although study groups have been small, all patients showed improvement, with 50% achieving complete rectal evacuation.[174] This procedure should be reserved for those patients with spinal cord injuries who do not respond to conventional therapy and in centers that are familiar with their use and the implantation procedure.

Defecatory Dysfunction—"Outlet"-type Constipation

When transit time is normal and the primary abnormality is defecatory dysfunction or "outlet" obstruction, the approach to management is different.[135,178,179] Commonly, affected individuals complain of difficulty in evacuation with multiple prolonged attempts at straining, or in more severe cases, digital extraction. Recognition of this particular form of constipation is extremely important, as the use of the therapeutic modalities employed in slow-transit constipation may, in some instances, compound the problem. While stool softeners will aid defecation by modifying stool consistency, the use of agents that act to increase stool bulk may well prove counterproductive for a patient who is unable to effectively defecate.

These reservations notwithstanding, it is important to remember that among debilitated patients with neurological disease, severe constipation and defecatory dysfunction in particular may significantly affect quality of life and may actually exacerbate their neurological condition. Therefore, with respect to slow-transit constipation, avoiding obstipation and impaction by whatever means available must be a part of their routine medical regimen.

Biofeedback

As pelvic floor dysfunction may be a learned abnormal response, biofeedback has been shown in several small, uncontrolled studies to be an effective means of improving constipation associated with anismus.[180–184] Several techniques have been employed.

In one of the most widely used biofeedback techniques, an electromyographic recording device is attached to an anal plug, which the patient inserts. The device provides both audio output and a visual tracing on a monitor. The patient then attempts to reduce sphincteric EMG activity visually on the monitor and by altering the auditory output in order to achieve normal pelvic floor relaxation. The patient is instructed on the use of the device at home with close follow up and support. A physical therapist can be of great assistance in training the patient to use the device and providing encouragement and positive verbal feedback, which enhances the therapeutic benefit.

Alternatively, oatmeal enemas may be used to train patients in achieving effective defecation. The patient is instructed to instill a 300 cc oatmeal porridge enema, and 15 minutes later to attempt to evacuate the porridge. Initially, the patient practices six times per day in conjunction with EMG feedback and then graduates to the porridge alone.[180] It is important to remember that an intact mental status and motivation are prerequisites for successful biofeedback, and therefore, these techniques may not be applicable to many patients with neurological disease.

Bowel Regimen

For many patients with neurological disease and "outlet" obstruction, a bowel regimen utilizing a fiber-restricted diet and regularly scheduled enemas works quite well.[132] Some may do well with rectal suppositories every other day to establish a satisfactory elimination pattern. One must again remember, however, that each patient's bowel regimen may need to be tailored to his or her special needs.

Dopaminergic Agents

In Parkinson's disease (PD), it has been shown that constipation and defecatory dysfunction are directly related to PD severity, suggesting that optimum treatment of the underlying disease could have a beneficial effect on constipation.[136,185] The use of apomorphine, a dopamine agonist used in the treatment of on/off fluctuations in PD, has been shown to normalize puborectalis function and improve defecation in some patients.[186,187] For anorectal dysfunction, apomorphine is usually administered subcutaneously in the morning at a dose of 1 mg to 6 mg. Initially, nausea may be a significant side effect; however, this usually subsides with continued use. Orthostatic hypotension is a side effect of which the clinician should be aware, and PD patients should be monitored closely when initiating therapy. Patient education is an important aspect of this therapy and may limit its use. The advent of an intranasal form has simplified the use of this drug and may be more useful in PD patients with constipation. The dosage varies from one to four puffs, and has a mean latency of onset from 5 to 15 minutes, with a duration of 26 to 90 minutes.[188,189] This medication should be reserved for those patients with severe fluctuating PD and documented anorectal dysfunction.

Botulinum Toxin (BTX)

In neurological disease associated with spasticity involving the anal sphincter, injection of BTX may be useful when more conservative measures fail. Some patients with refractory constipation due mainly to anismus (inappropriate contraction of the puborectalis, i.e., pelvic floor dystonia), have experienced good success with this treatment.[119,190] The dosage must be individualized beginning with 1.5 mg injected to each side of the puborectalis muscle. The effects usually last 6 to 12 weeks and must, therefore, be repeated. The main difficulty with this therapy is the development of fecal incontinence; however, it is important to reassure patients that this is a temporary problem that will improve as the drug effect wears off. The prevalence and severity of incontinence may be minimized by ensuring the delivery of the appropriate dose to each individual patient. This approach has been successfully employed in a small number of PD patients with obstructed defecation.[191]

Surgery

Surgery for constipation or anorectal dysfunction should not be taken lightly. Each candidate needs a complete evaluation and trial of all other modalities.[172,173,192,193] By using quantitative tests of colonic, rectal, and anal canal function, patients with constipation can be divided into those with slow transit, pelvic floor dysfunction, a combination of both, or irritable bowel syndrome. Those with pure slow transit may respond well to colectomy with or without ileorectostomy; however, objective evidence of diffuse colonic slowing must be present in the absence of generalized intestinal pseudoobstruction before subtotal colectomy is considered since there is a 50% complication rate.[192–194]

For patients with combined slow transit and pelvic floor dysfunction, successful pelvic floor retraining done preoperatively improves the outcome of ileorectostomy and colectomy.[193] Pelvic floor dysfunction alone, unless associated with anatomic abnormalities (rectal prolapse, rectocele, Hirschsprung), does not respond well to surgery. Likewise, surgery should be avoided in irritable bowel syndrome.

FECAL INCONTINENCE

Fecal continence requires intact rectal and anal sensation, an adequate reservoir, competent anal sphincters, and appropriate coordination of the pelvic floor musculature.[194–197] In neurological disease, colorectal abnormalities may be present that alter one or a combination of these factors and result in fecal incontinence.[198] The most common cause is fecal impaction with overflow incontinence. Unfortunately, all too commonly, this condition is overlooked by the clinician. Initial treatment is aimed at cleansing of the entire colon, first with enemas, followed by colonic irrigation with a balanced electrolyte solution, if necessary. Once the colon has been cleansed, treatment will depend on the nature of the underlying problem, the functional level of the patient, and the motivation of the patient. In those patients who are totally immobilized or functionally impaired, a regimen of biweekly enemas and a fiber-restricted diet should prevent recurrent soiling.

Among incontinent patients with motivation, ability to comprehend directions, and at least some level of rectal sensation, biofeedback has been widely employed.[199–205] Despite widespread enthusiasm for this approach, there have been few randomized trials and results have not always demonstrated added benefits for biofeedback over conservative approaches.[204,205] While there have been reports of success with biofeedback in multiple sclerosis,[133,134,182] this approach may not be feasible for many patients with neurological disease or may require adaptation to the specific needs and capabilities of the patient.[183,206]

In some patients, fecal incontinence is associated with, and exacerbated by, chronic diarrhea. This may be due to impaired rectal reservoir capacity or be related to neurogenic abnormalities affecting colorectal function. In these patients, bowel training and fiber restriction should decrease fecal soiling; however, if soiling persists, loperamide can be taken to decrease stool frequency. One must be vigilant to prevent fecal impaction in patients taking loperamide, and enemas may need to be administered once or twice weekly.[199,200] One must also be mindful of other complications associated with fecal incontinence, especially in the paralyzed patient, such as skin breakdown and infection.

Sacral nerve stimulation has also been employed, with reported success, in the management of fecal incontinence.[207–214] In one study among five patients with scleroderma and incontinence, continence was achieved following permanent placement of an electrode in relation to the S2–3 roots.[215] As for the situation for this technique in constipation, data must be reviewed with caution, as there have been few large prospective trials, a situation which led the authors of one recent systematic review to conclude that there was "insufficient data to allow reliable conclusions to be drawn."[216]

Surgery for patients with fecal incontinence should be considered carefully, because there are few controlled studies that compare long-term outcome with conservative treatment.[217] Each patient should be fully evaluated and surgery considered only after identification of a specific abnormality that does not respond to conservative therapy.[199,200] If rectal prolapse is present, resuspension or rectopexy can be performed, either alone or in combination with rectosigmoidectomy to restore continence.[173] In the absence of rectal prolapse, a variety of surgical procedures may be considered, such as postanal repair, external sphincter repair, creation of a neosphincter with a gracilis flap, and subsequent activation of the muscle using an implanted stimulator,[173,217,218] or, in a less invasive approach, by injecting a silicone-based biomaterial into the area of the sphincters.[219] There is insufficient experience with any of these techniques in the patient with neurological disease to allow one to make general recommendations; it stands to reason that any procedure contemplated must be mindful of the primary disease process and of the physiological deficit.

REFERENCES

1. Dent J (ed). Pharmacotherapy of gastrointestinal motor disorders. Sydney: Reed Healthcare Communications 1991.
2. Ramirez B, Richter JE. Review article: Promotility drugs in the treatment of gastroesophageal reflux disease. Aliment Pharmacol Ther 1993;7:5–20.
3. Quigley EMM. The clinical pharmacology of motility disorders: the perils (and pearls) of prokinesia. Gastroenterology 1994;106:1112–1114.
4. Quigley EMM. Pharmacotherapy of gastroparesis. Expert Opin Pharmacother 2000; 1:881–887.
5. Malagelada JR, Rees WDW, Mazzotta LJ, Go VLW. Gastric motor abnormalities in diabetic and post vagotomy gastroparesis: effect of metoclopramide and bethanechol. Gastroenterology 1980;78:286–293.
6. Ponec RJ, Saunders MD, Kimmey MB. Neostigmine for the treatment of acute colonic pseudo-obstruction. N Engl J Med 1999;341:137–141.
7. Daboul B, Eaker EY. Successful decompression of colonic pseudo-obstruction with neostigmine. Am J Gastroenterol 1999;94:3371–3372.
8. Loftus CG, Harewood GC, Baron TH. Assessment of predictors of response to neostigmine for acute colonic pseudo-obstruction. Am J Gastroenterol 2002;97:3118–3122.
9. Brandt LJ, Bjorkman D, Fennerty MB, et al. Systematic review on the management of irritable bowel syndrome in North America. Am J Gastroenterol 2002;97(Suppl 2):S7–S26.
10. Jaiwala J, Imperiale TF, Kroenke K. Pharmacologic treatment of the irritable bowel syndrome: a systematic review of randomized, controlled trials. Ann Intern Med 2000; 133:136–147.

11. Quigley EMM, Hasler WL, Parkman HP. AGA technical review on nausea and vomiting. Gastroenterology 2001;120:263–286.
12. Buchler MW, Binder M, Freiss H. Role of somatostatin and its analogues in the treatment of acute and chronic pancreatitis. Gut 1994;Suppl 3:S15–S19.
13. Farthing MJG. Octreotide in the treatment of refractory diarrhea and intestinal fistulae. Gut 1994;Suppl 3:S5–S10.
14. Harris AG. Somatostatin and somatostatin analogues: pharmacokinetic and pharmacodynamic effects. Gut 1994;Suppl 3:S1–S4.
15. Soudah HC, Hasler WL, Owyang C. Effect of octreotide on intestinal motility and bacterial overgrowth in scleroderma. N Engl J Med 1991;325:1461–1467.
16. Verne GN, Eaker EY, Hardy E, Sninsky CA. Effect of octreotide and erythromycin on idiopathic and scleroderma-associated intestinal pseudoobstruction. Dig Dis Sci 1995; 40:1892–1901.
17. Haruma AK, Wiste JA, Camilleri M. Effect of octreotide on gastrointestinal pressure profiles in health and in functional and organic gastrointestinal disorders. Gut 1994;35:1064–1069.
18. O'Donnell LJD, Watson AJM, Cameron D, Farthing MJG. Effect of octreotide on mouth-to-cecum transit time in healthy subjects and in the irritable bowel syndrome. Aliment Pharmacol Ther 1990;4:177–182.
19. Chen JDZ, Lin ZY, Edmunds MC, McCallum RW. Effects of octreotide and erythromycin on gastric myoelectrical and motor activities in patients with gastroparesis. Dig Dis Sci 1998;43:80–89.
20. Hasler WL, Soudah HC, Owyang C. A somatostatin analogue inhibits afferent pathways mediating perception of rectal distension. Gastroenterology 1993;104:1390–1397.
21. Malagelada J-R. Chronic intestinal psudoobstruction. Curr Treat Options Gastroenterol 2000;3:335–340.
22. Perlemuter G, Cacoub P, Chaussade S, et al. Octreotide treatment of chronic intestinal pseudoobstruction secondary to connective tissue disorders. Arthritis Rheum 1999; 42:1545–1549.
23. Di Lorenzo C, Lucanto C, Flores AF, et al. Effect of octreotide on gastrointestinal motility in children with functional gastrointestinal symptoms. J Pediatr Gastroenterol Nutr 1998; 27:508–512.
24. Ewins DL, Javaid A, Coskeran PB, et al. Assessment of gall bladder dynamics, cholecystokinin release and the development of gallstones during octreotide treatment for acromegaly. QJM 1992;83:295–306.
25. Catnach SM, Anderson JV, Fairclough PD, et al. Effect of octreotide on gall stone prevalence and gall bladder motility in acromegaly. Gut 1993;34:270–273.
26. Cullen JJ, Eagon JC, Dozois EJ, Kelly KA. Treatment of acute postoperative ileus with octreotide. Am J Surg 1993;165:113–119.
27. Soffer EE, Launspach J. Effect of misoprostol on postprandial intestinal motility and orocecal transit time in humans. Dig Dis Sci 1993;38:851–855.
28. Rutgeerts P, Vantrappen G, Hiele M, et al. Effects on bowel motility of misoprostol administered before and after meals. Aliment Pharmacol Therap 1991;5:533–542.
29. Penston JG, Wormsley KG. The effects of prostaglandins on gastric emptying. Scand J Gastroenterol 1989;24:127–132.
30. Vantrappen G, Janssens J. Effect of rioprostil 600 μg on the interdigestive myoelectrival activity of the human small intestine. Scand J Gastroenterol 1989;24:133–139.
31. Talley NJ. Review article: 5-hydroxytryptamine agonists and antagonists in the modulation of gastrointestinal motility and sensation-clinical implications. Aliment Pharmacol Therap 1992;6:273–290.
32. Talley NJ. Serotonergic neuroenteric modulators. Lancet 2001;358:2061–2068.
33. Camilleri M, Malagelada J-R, Abell TL, et al. Effect of six weeks of treatment with cisapride in gastroparesis and intestinal pseudo-obstruction. Gastroenterology 1989;96:705–712.
34. Abell TL, Camilleri M, DiMagno EP, et al. Long-term efficacy of oral cisapride in symptomatic upper gut dysmotility. Dig Dis Sci 1991;36:621–626.
35. Wehrmann T, Lembcke B, Caspary WF. Influence of cisapride on antroduodenal motor function in healthy subjects and diabetics with autonomic neuropathy. Aliment Pharmacol Therap 1991;5:599–608.

36. McHugh S, Lico S, Diamant NE. Cisapride versus metoclopramide: an acute study in diabetic gastroparesis. Dig Dis Sci 1992;37:997–1001.
37. Heading RC, Wood JD. Gastrointestinal dysmotility. Focus on cisapride. Raven Health Care Communications 1992.
38. Richards RD, Valenzuela JA, Davenport KS, et al. Objective and subjective results of a randomized, double-blind, placebo-controlled trial using cisapride to treat gastroparesis. Dig Dis Sci 1993;38:811–816.
39. Dworkin BM, Rosenthal WS, Casellas AR, et al. Open label study of long-term effectiveness of cisapride in patients with idiopathic gastroparesis. Dig Dis Sci 1994;39:1395–1398.
40. Quigley EMM. Chronic intestinal pseudo-obstruction. Curr Treat Options Gastroenterol 1999;2:239–250.
41. Jones MP. Access options for withdrawn motility-modifying drugs. Am J Gastroenterol 2002;97:2184–2188.
42. Braden B, Enghofer M, Schaub M, et al. Long-term cisapride treatment improves diabetic gastroparesis but not glycaemic control. Aliment Pharmacol Ther 2002;6:1341–1346.
43. Camilleri M, Balm RK, Zinsmeister AR. Determinants of response to a prokinetic agent in neuropathic chronic intestinal motility disorder. Gastroenterology 1996;106:916–923.
44. Benson MJ, Roberts JP, Wingate DL, et al. Small bowel motility following major intra-abdominal surgery: the effects of opiates and rectal cisapride. Gastroenterology 1996;106:924–936.
45. Tonini M, De Ponti F, Di Nuci A, Crema F. Review article: cardiac adverse effects of gastrointestinal prokinetics. Aliment Pharmacol Ther 1999;13:1585–1591.
46. Wang SH, Lin CY, Huang TY, et al. QT interval effects of cisapride in the clinical; setting. Int J Cardiol 2001;80:179–183.
47. Bouras EP, Camilleri M, Burton DD, McKinzie G. Selective stimulation of colonic transit by the benzofuran 5-HT$_4$ agonist, prucalopride, in healthy humans. Gut 1999;44:682–686.
48. Emmanuel AV, Roy AJ, Nicholls TJ, Kamm MA. Prucalopride, a systemic enterokinetic, for the treatment of constipation. Aliment Pharmacol Ther 2002;16:1347–1356.
49. Boeckxstaens GE, Bartelsman JFWM, Lauwers L, Tytgat GNJ. Treatment of GI dysmotility in scleroderma with a new enterokinetic agent prucalopride. Am J Gastroenterol 2002;97:194–197.
50. Mansi C, Borro P, Giacomini M, et al. Comparative effects of levosulpiride and cisapride on gastric emptying and symptoms in patients with functional dyspepsia and gastroparesis. Aliment Pharmacol Ther 2000;14:561–569.
51. Camilleri M. Review article: tegaserod. Aliment Pharmacol Ther 2001;15:277–289.
52. Muller-Lissner SA, Fumagalli I, Bardhan KD, et al. Tegaserod, a 5-HT(4) receptor partial agonist, relieves symptoms in irritable bowel syndrome patients with abdominal pain, bloating and constipation. Aliment Pharmacol Ther 2001;15:1655–1666.
53. Novick J, Miner P, Krause R, et al. Randomized, double-blind, placebo-controlled trial of tegaserod in female patients suffering from irritable bowel syndrome with constipation. Aliment Pharmacol Ther 2002;16:1877–1888.
54. Prather CM, Camilleri M, Zinsmeister AR, et al. Tegaserod accelerates orocecal transit in patients with constipation-predominant irritable bowel syndrome. Gastroenterology 2000;118:463–468.
55. Kahrilas PJ, Quigley EM, Castell DO, Spechler SJ. The effects of tegaserod (HTF 919) on oesophageal acid exposure in gastro-oesophageal reflux disease. Aliment Pharmacol Ther 2000;14:1503–1509.
56. Degen L, Matzinger D, Merz M, et al. Tegaserod, a 5-HT4 receptor partial agonist, accelerates gastric emptying and gastrointestinal transit in healthy male subjects. Aliment Pharmacol Ther 2001;15:1745–1751.
57. Fidelholtz J, Smith W, Rawls J, et al. Safety and tolerability of tegaserod in patients with irritable bowel syndrome and diarrhea symptoms. Am J Gastroenterol 2002;97:1176–1181.
58. Tougas G, Snape WJ Jr, Otten MH, et al. Long-term safety of tegaserod in patients with constipation-predominant irritable bowel syndrome. Aliment Pharmacol Ther 2002;16:1701–1708.

59. Morganroth J, Ruegg PC, Dunger-Baldauf C, et al. Tegaserod, a 5-hydroxytryptamine type 4 receptor partial agonist, is devoid of electrocardiographic effects. Am J Gastroenterol 2002; 97:2321–2327

60. Camilleri M, Northcutt AR, Kong S, et al. Efficacy and safety of alosetron in women with irritable bowel syndrome: randomized, placebo-controlled trial. Lancet 2000;355: 1035–1040.

61. Camilleri M, Chey WY, Mayer EA, et al. A randomized controlled trial of the serotonin type 3 receptor antagonist alosetron in women with diarrhea-predominant irritable bowel syndrome. Arch Intern Med 2001;161:1733–1740.

62. Viramontes BE, Camilleri M, McKinzie S, et al. Gender-related differences in slowing colonic transit by a 5-HT3 antagonist in subjects with diarrhea-predominant irritable bowel syndrome. Am J Gastroenterol 2001;96:2671–2676.

63. Lisi DM. Lotronex withdrawal. Arch Intern Med 2002;162:101.

64. Friedel D, Thomas R, Fisher RS. Ischemic colitis during treatment with alosetron. Gastroenterology 2001;120:557–560.

65. McCarthy M. FDA allows controversial bowel drug back on to market. Lancet 2002; 359:2095.

66. Crawford LM Jr. From the Food and Drug Administration. JAMA 2002;288:688.

67. Moynihan R. Alosetron: a case study in regulatory capture, or a victory for patients rights? BMJ 2002;325:592–595.

68. Steadman CJ, Talley N, Phillips SF, Zinsmeister AR. Selective 5-hydroxytrytamine type 3 receptor antagonism with ondansetron as treatment for diarrhea-predominant irritable bowel syndrome. A pilot study. Mayo Clin Proc 1992;67:732–738.

69. Saslow SB, Scolapio JS, Camilleri M, et al. Medium-term effects of a new 5HT3 antagonist, alosetron, in patients with carcinoid diarrhea. Gut 1998;42:628–634.

70. Schang JC, Devroede G, Pilote M. Effects of trimebutine on colonic function in patients with chronic idiopathic constipation: evidence for the need of a physiologic rather than clinical selection. Dis Colon Rectum 1993;36:330–336.

71. Fraitag B, Homerin M, Hecketsweiler P. Double-blind dose-response multicenter comparison of fedotozine and placebo in treatment of non-ulcer dyspepsia. Dig Dis Sci 1994;39: 1072–1077.

72. Sandgren JE, McPhee MS, Greenberger NJ. Narcotic bowel syndrome treated with clonidine. Ann Intern Med 1984;101:331–334.

73. Pappagallo M. Incidence, prevalence, and management of opioid bowel dysfunction. Am J Surg 2001;182(Suppl 5A):11S–18S.

74. Culpepper-Morgan JA, Inturrisi CE, Portenoy RK, et al. Treatment of opioid-induced constipation with oral naloxone: a pilot study. Clin Pharmacol Ther 1992;52:90–95.

75. Kreek M-J, Schaefer RA, Hahn EF, Fishman J. Naloxone, a specific opioid antagonist, reverses chronic idiopathic constipation. Lancet 1983;1:261–262.

76. Wingate D, Phillips SF, Lewis SJ, et al. Guidelines for adults on self-medication for the treatment of acute diarrhea. Aliment Pharmacol Ther 2001;15:773–782.

77. Janssens J, Peeters TL, Vantrappen G, et al. Improvement of gastric emptying in diabetic gastroparesis by erythromycin. N Engl J Med 1990;322:1028–1031.

78. Tack J, Janssens J, Vantrappen G, et al. Effect of erythromycin on gastric motility in controls and in diabetic gastroparesis. Gastroenterology 1992;103:72–79.

79. Fraser R, Shearer T, Fuller J, et al. Intravenous erythromycin overcomes small intestinal feedback on antral, pyloric and duodenal motility. Gastroenterology 1992;103:116–119.

80. Weber FH, Richards RD, McCallum RW. Erythromycin: a motilin agonist and gastrointestinal prokinetic agent. Am J Gastroenterol 1993;88:485–490.

81. Keshavarzian A, Isaac RM. Erythromycin accelerates gastric emptying of indigestible solids and transpyloric migration of the tip of an enteral feeding tube in fasting and fed states. Am J Gastroenterol 1993;88:193–197.

82. Mantides A, Xynos E, Chrysos E, et al. The effect of erythromycin in gastric emptying of solids and hypertonic liquids in healthy subjects. Am J Gastroenterol 1993;88:198–202.

83. Richards RD, Davenport K, McCallum RW. The treatment of idiopathic and diabetic gastroparesis with acute intravenous and chronic oral erythromycin. Am J Gastroenterol 1993; 88:203–207.

84. Camilleri M. The current role of erythromycin in the clinical management of gastric empty-ing disorders. Am J Gastroenterol 1993;88:169–171.

85. Fiorucci S, Distrutti E, Gerli R, Morelli A. Effect of erythromycin on gastric and gall blad-der emptying and gastrointestinal symptoms in scleroderma patients is maintained medium term. Am J Gastroenterol 1994;89:550–555.

86. Maganti K, Onyemere K, Jones MP. Oral erythromycin and symptomatic relief of gastro-pareis: a systematic review. Am J Gastroenterol 2003;98:259–263.

87. Rayner CK, Su YC, Doran SM, et al. The stimulation of antral motility by erythromycin is attenuated by hyperglycemia. Am J Gastroenterol 2000;95:2233–2241.

88. DiBiase JK, Quigley EMM. Efficacy of prolonged administration of intravenous erythromy-cin in an ambulatory setting as treatment of severe gastroparesis: one center's experience. J Clin Gastroenterol 1999;28:131–134.

89. Brand RM, Lof J, Quigley EMM. Transdermal delivery of erythromycin lactobionate – impli-cations for the therapy of gastroparesis. Aliment Pharmacol Therap 1997;11:589–592.

90. Verhagen MAMT, Samsom M, Maes B, et al. Effects of a new motilide, ABT-229, on gastric emptying and postprandial antroduodenal motility in healthy volunteers. Aliment Pharmacol Ther 1997;11:1077–1086.

91. Van Herwaarden MA, Samsom M, Van Nispen CH, et al. The effect of motilin agonist ABT-229 on gastroesophageal reflux, oesophageal motility and lower oesophageal sphincter char-acteristics in GERD patients. Aliment Pharmacol Ther 2000;14:453–462.

92. Talley NJ, Verlinden M, Geenen DJ, et al. Effects of a motilin receptor agonist (ABT-229) on upper gastrointestinal symptoms in type I diabetes mellitus: a randomized double blind, placebo controlled trial. Gut 2001;49:395–401.

93. Tack J, Peeters T. What comes after macrolides and other motilin stimulants? Gut 2001; 49:317–318.

94. Clanton LJ Jr, Bender J. Refractory spinal cord injury induced gastroparesis: resolution with erythromycin lactobionate, a case report. J Spinal Cord Med 1999;22:236–238.

95. Gorard DA, Libby GW, Farthing MJG. Influence of antidepressants on whole gut and oroce-cal transit times in health and irritable bowel syndrome. Aliment Pharmacol Ther 19948:159–166.

96. Clouse RE. Antidepressants for functional gastrointestinal syndromes. Dig Dis Sci 1994; 39:2352–2363.

97. Drossman DA, Camilleri M, Mayer EA, Whitehead WE. AGA technical review on irritable bowel syndrome. Gastroenterology 2002;123:2108–2131.

98. Clouse RE. Antidepressants for irritable bowel syndrome. Gut 2003;52:598–599.

99. Brogden RM, Carmine AA, Heel RC, et al. Domperidone. Drugs 1982;24:360–400.

100. Champion MC, Hartnett M, Yen M. Domperidone: a new dopamine antagonist. CMAJ 1986;135:457–461.

101. Davis RH, Clench MH, Mathias JR. Effects of domperidone in patients with chronic unex-plained upper gastrointestinal symptoms: a double-blind, placebo-controlled study. Dig Dis Sci 1988;33:1505–1511.

102. Molino D, Mosca S, Angrisani G, Magliacano V. Symptomatic effects of domperidone in post-vagotomy gastric stasis. Curr Ther Res 1987;41:313–316.

103. Parkes JD. Domperidone and Parkinson's disease. Clin Neuropharmacol 1986;9:517–532.

104. Neira WD, Sanchez V, Mena MM, de Yebenes JG. The effects of cisapride on plasma L-dopa levels and clinical response in Parkinson's disease. Mov Disord 1995;10:66–70.

105. Hughes AH, Bishop S, Kleedorfer B, et al. Subcutaneous apomorphine in Parkinson's disease: response to chronic administration for up to five years. Mov Disord 1993; 8:165–170.

106. Delev D, Ebinger G, Michotte Y. Clinical and pharmacokinetic comparison of oral and duo-denal delivery of levodopa/caribdopa in patients with Parkinson's disease with a fluctuating response to levodopa. Eur J Clin Pharmacol 1991;41:453–458.

107. Robertson DR, Higginson I, Macklin BS, et al. The influence of protein containing meals on the pharmacokinetics of levodopa in healthy volunteers. Br J Clin Pharmacol 1991; 31:413–417.

108. Merello M, Pirtosek Z, Bishop S, Lees AJ. Cardiovascular reflexes in Parkinson's disease: effect of domperidone and apomorphine. Clin Auton Res 1992;2:215–219.

109. Bhutani MS. Gastrointestinal uses of botulinum toxin. Am J Gastroenterol 1997;92:929–933.
110. Pasricha PJ, Ravich WH, Hendrix TR, et al. Intrasphincteric botulinum toxin for treatment of achalasia. N Engl J Med 1995;32:774–778.
111. Gordon JM, Eaker EY. Prospective study of esophageal botulinum toxin injection in high-risk achalasia patients. Am J Gastroenterol 1997;92:1812–1817.
112. Katzka DA, Castell DO. Use of botulinum toxin as a diagnostic/therapeutic trial to help clarify an indication for definitive therapy in patients with achalasia. Am J Gastroenterol 1999;94:637–642.
113. Annese V, Basciani M, Perri F, et al. Controlled trial of botulinum toxin injection versus placebo and pneumatic dilatation in achalasia. Gastroenterology 1996;111:1418–1424.
114. Cuillier C, Ducrotte P, Zerbib F, et al. Achalasia: outcome of patients treated with intrasphincteric injection of botulinum toxin. Gut 1997;41:87–92.
115. Annese V, Bassotti G, Coccia G, et al. A multicentric randomized study of intrasphincteric botulinum toxin in patients with oesophageal achalasia. Gut 2000;46:597–600.
116. Vaezi MF, Richter JE, Wilcox CM, et al. Botulinum toxin versus pneumatic dilatation in the treatment of achalasia: a randomized trial. Gut 1999;44:231–239.
117. Ezzeddine D, Jit R, Katz N, et al. Pyloric injection of botulinum toxin for treatment of diabetic gastroparesis. Gastrointest Endosc 2002;55:920–923.
118. Miller LS, Szych GA, Kantor SB, et al. Treatment of idiopathic gastroparesis with injection of botulinum toxin into the pyloric sphincter muscle. Am J Gastroenterol 2002; 97:1653–1660.
119. Ron Y, Avni Y, Lukovetski A, et al. Botulinum toxin type-A in therapy of patients with anismus. Dis Colon Rectum 2001;44:1821–1826.
120. Miller LS, Pullela SV, Parkman HP, et al. Treatment of noncardiac, nonreflux, nonachalasia spastic esophageal motor disorders using botulinum toxin injection into the gastroesophageal junction. Am J Gastroenterol 2002;97:1640–1646.
121. Quigley EMM. Acute intestinal pseudo-obstruction. Curr Treat Options Gastroenterol 2000; 3:273–285.
122. Talley NJ. Diabetic gastropathy and prokinetics. Am J Gastroenterol 2003;98:264–271.
123. Bortolotti M. The "electrical way" to cure gastroparesis. Am J Gastroenterol 2002; 97:1874–1883.
124. McCallum RW, Chen JDZ, Lin Z, et al. Gastric pacing improves emptying and symptoms in patients with gastroparesis. Gastroenterology 1998;114:456–461.
125. Michaud L, Guimber D, Carpentier B, et al. Gastrostomy as a decompression technique in children with chronic gastrointestinal obstruction. J Pediatr Gastroenterol Nutr 2001;32:82–85.
126. Devendra D, Millward BA, Travis SP. Diabetic gastroparesis improved by percutaneous endoscopic jejunostomy. Diabetes Care 2000;23:426–427.
127. Allen JW, Ali A, Wo J, et al. Totally laparoscopic feeding jejunostomy. Surg Endosc 2002;16:1802–1805.
128. Sanders DS, Carter MJ, D'Silva J, et al. Percutaneous endoscopic gastrostomy: a prospective audit of the impact of guidelines in two district general hospitals in the United Kingdom. Am J Gastoenterol 2002;97:2239–2246.
129. Angus F, Burakoff R. The percutaneous endoscopic gastrostomy tube: medical and ethical issues in placement. Am J Gastroenterol 2003;98:272–277.
130. Schnedl WJ, Wenzl HH, Obermayer-Pietsch B, et al. Is gastroparesis in diabetes cured by gastrectomy? Diabetes Care 1999;22:1920–1921.
131. Forstner-Barthell AW, Murr MM, Nitecki S, et al. Near-total completion gastrectomy for severe postvagotomy gastric stasis: analysis of early and long-term results in 62 patients. J Gastrointest Surg 1999;3:15–21.
132. Spinal Cord Medicine Consortium. Clinical Practice Guidelines: Neurogenic bowel management in adults with spinal cord injury. J Spinal Cord Med 1998;21:248–293.
133. Wiesel PH, Norton C, Glickman S, Kamm MA. Pathophysiology and management of bowel dysfunction in multiple sclerosis. Eur J Gastroenterol Hepatol 2001;13:441–448.
134. Wiesel PH, Norton C, Brazzelli M. Management of faecal incontinence and constipation in adults with central neurological diseases. Cochrane Database Syst Rev 2001;(4):CD002115.
135. Locke GR III, Pemberton JH, Phillips SF. AGA technical review on constipation. American Gastroenterological Association. Gastroenterology 2000;119:1766–1778.

136. Edwards LL, Pfeiffer RF, Quigley EMM, et al. Gastrointestinal symptoms in Parkinson's disease. Mov Disord 1991;6:151–156.

137. Abbott RD, Petrovitch H, White LR, et al. Frequency of bowel movements and the future risk of Parkinson's disease. Neurology 2001;57:456–462.

138. Edwards LL, Quigley EMM, Harned RK, et al. Characterization of swallowing and defecation in Parkinson's disease. Am J Gastroenterol 1994;89:15–25.

139. Singaram C, Ashraf W, Gaumnitz EA, et al. Dopaminergic defect of enteric nervous system in Parkinson's disease patients with chronic constipation. Lancet 1995;346:861–864.

140. Ashraf W, Pfeiffer RF, Quigley EMM. Anorectal manometry in the assessment of anorectal function in Parkinson's disease: a comparison with chronic idiopathic constipation. Mov Disord 1994;9:655–663.

141. Ashraf W, Wszolek ZK, Pfeiffer RF, et al. Anorectal function in fluctuating (on-off) Parkinson's disease: evaluation by combined anorectal manometry and electromyography. Mov Disord 1995;10:650–657.

142. Manning AP, Wyman JB, Heaton KW. How trustworthy are bowel histories? Comparison of recalled and recorded information. Br Med J 1970;2:213–214.

143. Probert CSJ, Emmett PM, Cripps HA, Heaton KW. Evidence for the ambiguity of the term constipation: the role of irritable bowel syndrome. Gut 1994;35:1455–1458.

144. Ashraf W, Park F, Lof J, Quigley EMM. An examination of the reliability of reported stool frequency in the diagnosis of idiopathic constipation. Am J Gastroenterol 1996;91:26–32.

145. Bharucha AE, Phillips SF. Slow transit constipation. Gastroenterol Clin North Am 2001; 30:77–95.

146. Wade PR. Aging and neural control of the GI tract: I. Age-related changes in the enteric nervous system. Am J Physiol 2002;283:G489–G495.

147. Hall KE. Aging and neural control of the GI tract: II. Neural control of the aging gut; can an old dog learn new tricks? Am J Physiol 2002;283:G827–G832.

148. Orr WC, Chen CL. Aging and neural control of the GI tract: IV. Clinical and physiological aspects of gastrointestinal motility and aging. Am J Physiol 2002;283:G1226–G1331.

149. O'Mahony D, O'Leary P, Quigley EMM. Aging and intestinal motility. Drugs Aging 2002; 19:515–527.

150. Towers AL, Burgio KL, Locher JL, et al. Constipation in the elderly: influence of dietary, psychological and physiological factors. J Am Geriatr Soc 1994;42:701–706.

151. Block G, Hartman AM, Dresser CM, et al. A data-based approach to diet questionnaire design and testing. Am J Epidemiol 1986;124:453–469.

152. Dukas L, Willett W, Giovannucci EL. Association between physical activity, fiber intake and other lifestyle variables and constipation in a study of women. Am J Gastroenterol 2003.

153. Astarloa R, Mena MA, Sanchez V, et al. Clinical and pharmacologic effects of a diet rich in insoluble fiber on Parkinson's disease. Clin Neuropharmacol 1992;15:375–380.

154. Kellow JE, Gill RC, Wingate DL. Modulation of human upper gastrointestinal motility by rectal distention. Gut 1987;28:864–868.

155. Tjeerdsma HC, Smout AJPM, Akkermans LMA. Voluntary suppression of defecation delays gastric emptying. Dig Dis Sci 1993;38:832–836.

156. Zighelboim J, Talley NJ, Phillips SF. Response of gastric fundus to rectal distension in healthy persons. Dig Dis Sci 1994;39:1441–1445.

157. Ashraf W, Park F, Lof J, Quigley EMM. Effects of psyllium therapy on stool characteristics, colon transit and anorectal function in chronic idiopathic constipation. Aliment Pharmacol Therap 1995;9:639–647.

158. Ashraf W, Pfeiffer RF, Park F, et al. Constipation in Parkinson's disease. Objective assessment and response to psyllium. Mov Disord 1997;12:946–951.

159. Wakefield AJ, Anthony A, Murch SH, et al. Enterocolitis in children with developmental disorders. Am J Gastroenterol 2000;95:2285–2295.

160. Wakefield AJ, Puleston JM, Montgomery SM, et al. Review article: the concept of enterocolonic encephalopathy, autism and opioid receptor ligands. Aliment Pharmacol Ther 2002; 16:663–674.

161. Schiller LR. Review article: the therapy of constipation. Aliment Pharmacol Ther 2001; 15:749–763.

162. Corazziari E, Badiali D, Habib FI, et al. Small volume isosmotic polyethylene glycol electrolyte balanced solution (PMF-100) in treatment of chronic non-organic constipation. Dig Dis Sci 1996;41:1636–1642.

163. DiPalma JA, Smith JR, Cleveland MVB. Overnight efficacy of polyethylene glycol laxative. Am J Gastroenterol 2002;97:1776–1779.

164. Price KJ, Elliott TM. What is the role of stimulant laxatives in the management of childhood constipation and soiling? Cochrane Database Syst Rev 2001;(3):CD002040.

165. Jost WH. The effects of cisapride on colonic transit time in PD patients. Wien Klin Wochenschr 1994;106:673–676.

166. Verne GN, Davis RH, Robinson ME, et al. Treatment of chronic constipation with colchicine: randomized double blind, placebo-controlled, crossover trial. Am J Gastroenterol 2003; 98:1112–1116.

167. Coulie B, Szarka LA, Camilleri M, et al. Recombinant human neurotrophic factors accelerate colonic transit and relieve constipation in humans. Gastroenterology 2000; 119:41–50.

168. Parkman HP, Rao S, Reynolds JC, et al. Neurotrophin-3 (NT-3) improves functional constipation. Am J Gastroenterol 2003;98:1338–1347.

169. Wald A, Burgio K, Holeva K, Locher J. Psychological evaluation of patients with severe idiopathic constipation: which instrument to use? Am J Gastroenterol 1992;87: 977–980.

170. Rose JDR, Troughton AH, Harvey JS, Smith PM. Depression and functional bowel disorders in gastrointestinal outpatients. Gut 1986;27:1025–1028.

171. Merkel IS, Locher J, Burgio K, et al. Physiologic and psychologic characteristics of an elderly population with chronic constipation. Am J Gastroenterol 1993;88:1854–1859.

172. Pemberton JH, Rath DM, Ilstrup DM. Evaluation and surgical treatment of severe chronic constipation. Ann Surg 1991;214:403–413.

173. Rotholtz NA, Wexner SD. Surgical treatment for constipation and fecal incontinence. Gastroenterol Clin North Am 2001;30:131–166.

174. MacDonagh RP, Sun WM, Smallwood R, et al. Control of defecation in patients with spinal injuries by stimulation of sacral anterior nerve roots. Br Med J 1990;300:1494–1497.

175. Chan CL, Saunders J, Williams NS. Permanent sacral nerve stimulation for treatment of idiopathic constipation. Br J Surg 2002;89:1482.

176. Kenefick NJ, Nicholls RJ, Cohen RG, Kamm MA. Permanent sacral nerve stimulation for treatment of idiopathic constipation. Br J Surg 2002;89:882–888.

177. Kenefick NJ, Vaizey CJ, Cohen CR, et al. Double-blind placebo-controlled crossover study of sacral nerve stimulation for idiopathic constipation. Br J Surg 2002;89:1570–1571.

178. Wald A. Outlet dysfunction constipation. Curr Treat Options Gastroenterol 2001;4:293–297.

179. Rao SS. Dyssynergic defecation. Gastroenterol Clin North Am 2001;30:97–114.

180. Bleijenberg G, Kuijpers HC. Treatment of the spastic pelvic floor syndrome with biofeedback. Dis Colon Rectum 1987;30:108–111.

181. Kawimbe BM, Papachrysostomou M, Binnie NR, et al. Outlet obstruction constipation (anismus) managed by biofeedback. Gut 1991;32:1175–1179.

182. Wiesel PH, Norton C, Roy AJ, et al. Gut focused behavioural treatment (biofeedback) for constipation and faecal incontinence in multiple sclerosis. J Neurol Neurosurg Psychiatry 2000;69:240–243.

183. Brazzelli M, Griffiths P. Behavioural and cognitive interventions with or without other treatments for defaecation disorders in children. Cochrane Database Syst Rev 2001;(4):CD002240.

184. Mason HJ, Serrano-Ikkos E, Kamm MA. Psychological state and quality of life in patients having behavioural treatment (biofeedback) for intractable constipation. Am J Gastroenterol 2002;97:3154–3159.

185. Jost WH, Schimrigk K. Constipation in Parkinson's disease. Klin Wochenschr 1991; 69:906–909.

186. Mathers SE, Kempster PA, Swash M, Lees AJ. Constipation and paradoxical puborectalis contraction in anismus and Parkinson's disease: a dystonic phenomenon? J Neurol Neurosurg Psychiatry 1988;51:1503–1507.

187. Edwards LL, Quigley EMM, Harned RK, et al. Defecatory function in Parkinson's disease: response to apomorphine. Ann Neurol 1993;33:490–493.

188. Kleedorfer B, Turjanski N, Ryan R, et al. Intranasal apomorphine in Parkinson's disease. Neurology 1991;41:761–762.

189. Van Laar T, Jansen ENH, Essink AWG, Neef C. Intranasal apomorphine in Parkinsonian on-off fluctuations. Arch Neurol 1992;49:482–484.

190. Hallan RI, Melling J, Womack NR, et al. Treatment of anismus in intractable constipation with botulinum A toxin. Lancet 1988;2:714–717.

191. Albanese A, Maria G, Bentivoglio AR, et al. Severe constipation in Parkinson's disease relieved by botulinum toxin. Mov Disord 1997;12:764–766.

192. Yoshioka K, Keighley MRB. Clinical results of colectomy for severe constipation. Br J Surg 1989;76:600–604.

193. Wald A. Surgical treatment for refractory constipation - more hard data about hard stools? Am J Gastroenterol 1990;85:759–760.

194. Wald A, Caruana BJ, Freimanis MG, et al. Contributions of evacuation proctography and anorectal manometry to evaluation of adults with constipation and defecatory difficulty. Dig Dis Sci 1990;35:481–487.

195. Fogel R. Fecal incontinence. Curr Treat Options Gastroenterol 2001;4:261–266.

196. Rudolph W, Galandiuk S. A practical guide to the diagnosis and management of fecal incontinence. Mayo Clin Proc 2002;77:271–275.

197. Fernandez-Fraga X, Azpiroz F, Malagelada J-R. Significance of the pelvic floor muscles in anal incontinence. Gastroenterology 2002;123:1441–1450.

198. Wald A. Constipation and fecal incontinence in the elderly. Gastroent Clin N Amer 1990; 19:405–418.

199. Soffer EE, Hull T. Fecal incontinence: a practical approach to evaluation and treatment. Am J Gastroenterol 2000;95:1873–1880.

200. Whitehead WE, Wald A, Norton NJ. Treatment options for fecal incontinence. Dis Colon Rectum 2001;44:131–142.

201. Chiaroni G, Bassotti G, Stegagnini S, et al. Sensory retraining is key to biofeedback therapy for formed stool fecal incontinence. Am J Gastroenterol 2002;97:109–117.

202. Norton C, Kamm MA. Anal sphincter biofeedback and pelvic floor exercises for faecal incontinence in adults – a systematic review. Aliment Pharmacol Ther 2001;15:1147–1154.

203. Norton C, Kamm MA. Outcome of biofeedback for faecal incontinence. Br J Surg 1999; 86:1159–1163.

204. Norton C, Hosker G, Brazzelli M. Biofeedback and/or sphincter exercises for the treatment of faecal incontinence in adults. Cochrane Database Syst Rev 2000;(2):CD002111.

205. Norton C, Chelvanayagam S, Kamm MA. Randomised controlled trial of biofeedback for fecal incontinence. Gastroenterology 2002;122:A–70.

206. Smith LJ, Franchetti B, McCoull K, et al. A behavioural approach to retraining bowel function after long-standing constipation and faecal impaction in people with learning disabilities. Dev Med Child Neurol 1994;36:41–49.

207. Matzel KE, Stadelmaier U, Hohenfellner M, Gall FP. Electrical simulation of sacral spinal nerves for treatment of faecal incontinence. Lancet 1995;346:1124–1127.

208. Mander BJ, Williams NS. Electrical stimulation of sacral nerves for treatment of incontinence. Lancet 1996;347:63–64.

209. Ganio E, Luc AR, Clerico G, Trompetto M. Sacral nerve stimulation for treatment of fecal incontinence: a novel approach for intractable fecal incontinence. Dis Colon Rectum 2001;44:619–629.

210. Vaizey CJ, Kamm MA, Turner IC, et al. Effects of short-term sacral nerve stimulation on anal and rectal function in patients with anal incontinence. Gut 1999;44:407–412.

211. Vaizey CJ, Kamm MA, Roy AJ, Nicholls RJ. Double-blind crossover study of sacral nerve stimulation for fecal incontinence. Dis Colon Rectum 2000;43:298–302.

212. Malouf AJ, Vaizey CJ, Nicholls RJ, Kamm MA. Permanent sacral nerve stimulation for fecal incontinence. Ann Surg 2000;232:143–148.

213. Leroi AM, Michot F, Grise P, Denis P. Effect of sacral nerve stimulation on anal and rectal function in patients with fecal and urinary incontinence. Dis Colon Rectum 2001; 44:779–789.

214. Kenefick NJ, Vaizey CJ, Cohen RC, et al. Medium-term results of permanent sacral nerve stimulation for faecal incontinence. Br J Surg 2002;89:896–901.

215. Kenefick NJ, Vaizey CJ, Nichols RJ, et al. Sacral nerve stimulation for faecal incontinence due to systemic sclerosis. Gut 2002;51:881–883.
216. Hosker G, Norton C, Brazzelli M. Electrical stimulation for faecal incontinence in adults. Cochrane Database Syst Rev 2000;2:CD001310.
217. Bachoo P, Brazzelli M, Grant A. Surgery for faecal incontinence in adults. Cochrane Database Syst Rev 2000;(2):CD001757.
218. Mander BJ, Williams NS. The electrically stimulated gracilis neo-anal sphincter. Eur J Gastroenterol Hepatol 1997;9:435–441.
219. Kenefick NJ, Vaizey CJ, Malouf AJ, et al. Injectable silicone material for faecal incontinence due to internal anal sphincter dysfunction. Gut 2002;51:225–228.

Index

Note: Page numbers followed by f refer to figures; page numbers followed by t refer to tables.

Aspiration (*Continued*)
in Parkinson's disease, 65
in progressive supranuclear palsy, 73
Ataxia, with pyridoxine excess, 234
Autism, gluten and, 241
Autonomic dysreflexia, in spinal cord injury,
103
Autonomic nervous system, 11–12, 35–38,
36f, 37f
evaluation of, 50–53, 51f, 52f, 53t
Autonomic neuropathy, 83–96. *See also*
specific disorders.
acute, 83–89
cholinergic, 86
clinical features of, 84
criteria for, 85
differential diagnosis of, 85–86
drug-induced, 88–89
evaluation of, 84–85, 95–96
in botulism, 87–88
in Guillain-Barré syndrome, 86–87
in porphyria, 88
paraneoplastic, 86
toxin-induced, 89
amyloid, 92–93
chronic, 89–92
differential diagnosis of, 85
evaluation of, 95–96
in Adie's syndrome, 90–91
in Chagas' disease, 91
in chronic idiopathic anhidrosis, 90
in dopamine β-hydroxylase deficiency, 92
in idiopathic distal small fiber
neuropathy, 89–90
combined sympathetic and parasympathetic,
86, 92–94
in Riley-Day syndrome, 94
in Sjögren's syndrome, 93–94
intermittent, 94–95
management of, 95–96
paroxysmal, 94–95
Autonomic neuropathy with neuronal
intranuclear inclusions, gastroparesis
in, 170

B

Bassen-Kornzweig disease, 230–231
Becker muscular dystrophy, 118
Belch reflex, in achalasia, 155
Belching, in Parkinson's disease, 67
Beta-carotene, 222
Bezoar, 186
Bile duct obstruction, malabsorption in, 207t
Biofeedback
in defecatory dysfunction, 337–338
in diabetes-related fecal incontinence, 261

Biopsy
in celiac disease, 240f, 241
in intestinal pseudo-obstruction, 193
in Sjögren's syndrome, 94
in Whipple's disease, 243f, 244–245
Blind loop syndrome, malabsorption in,
207t
Blindness, in vitamin A deficiency, 222
Botulinum toxin, 330–331
in cricopharyngeal achalasia, 296
in defecatory dysfunction, 338–339
in parkinsonian drooling, 64
Botulism, 87–88, 123
Bowel movements, frequency of. *See also*
Constipation; Fecal incontinence.
in Parkinson's disease, 70
in spinal cord injury, 105
Bowel regimen, in defecatory dysfunction,
338
Brain injury
dysphagia after, 62–63
gastric emptying after, 46, 63
Brain tumor, 62
Brainstem disease
gastric dysfunction in, 172
intestinal pseudo-obstruction with, 182–183
vomiting with, 46, 62

C

C fibers, in nociception, 38, 95
Cajal, interstitial cells of, 9–10
Cancer
brain, 46, 62
head and neck, 151
lung, 190
neuropathy with, 49, 169
pseudoachalasia with, 155
Cardio-intestinal syndrome, in Duchenne
muscular dystrophy, 118
Catheter infection, with parenteral nutrition,
305
Celiac disease, 205t, 235–242
atypical presentation of, 238, 238t
clinical features of, 237–238, 238t
diagnosis of, 241–242
environmental factors in, 237
epidemiology of, 237
epilepsy in, 239–240
genetics of, 236–237
gluten in, 237
neurologic associations of, 238–241, 239t,
240f
pathogenesis of, 235–237, 235f–236f
psychiatric disorders in, 240–241
treatment of, 242
vitamin deficiencies in, 239, 239t